D1252018

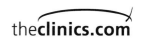

CLINICS IN
PERINATOLOGY

Late Preterm Pregnancy and the Newborn

GUEST EDITORS
Lucky Jain, MD, MBA
Tonse N.K. Raju, MD, DCH

December 2006 • Volume 33 • Number 4

SAUNDERS

An Imprint of Elsevier, Inc.
PHILADELPHIA   LONDON   TORONTO   MONTREAL   SYDNEY   TOKYO

W.B. SAUNDERS COMPANY
A Division of Elsevier Inc.

Elsevier, Inc., 1600 John F. Kennedy Blvd., Suite 1800, Philadelphia, PA 19103-2899

http://www.theclinics.com

CLINICS IN PERINATOLOGY	**Volume 33, Number 4**
December 2006	**ISSN 0095-5108**
Editor: Carla Holloway	**ISBN-10: 1-4160-3899-X**
	ISBN-13: 978-1-4160-3899-3

Copyright © 2006 by Elsevier Inc. All rights reserved. No part of this publication may be reproduced or transmitted in any form or by any means, electronic or mechanical, including photocopy, recording, or any information retrieval system, without written permission from the publisher.

Single photocopies of single articles may be made for personal use as allowed by national copyright laws. Permission of the publisher and payment of a fee is required for all other photocopying, including multiple or systematic copying, copying for advertising or promotional purposes, resale, and all forms of document delivery. Special rates are available for educational institutions that wish to make photocopies for non-profit educational classroom use. Permissions may be sought directly from Elsevier's Rights Department in Philadelphia, PA, USA: phone: (+1) 215 239 3804, fax: (+1) 215 239 3805, e-mail: healthpermissions@elsevier.com. Requests may also be completed on-line via the Elsevier homepage (http://www.elsevier.com/locate/permissions). In the USA, users may clear permissions and make payments through the Copyright Clearance Center, Inc, 222 Rosewood Drive, Danvers, MA 01923, USA; phone: (978) 750-8400; fax: (978) 750-4744, and in the UK through the Copyright Licensing Agency Rapid Clearance Service (CLARCS), 90 Tottenham Court Road, London W1P 0LP, UK; phone: (+44) 171 436 5931; fax: (+44) 171 436 3986. Others countries may have a local reprographic rights agency for payments.

Reprints. For copies of 100 or more of articles in this publication, please contact the commercial Reprints Department, Elsevier Inc., 360 Park Avenue South, New York, New York 10010-1710. Tel: (212) 633-3813 Fax: (212) 462-1935, e-mail: reprints@elsevier.com.

The ideas and opinions expressed in *Clinics in Perinatology* do not necessarily reflect those of the Publisher. The Publisher does not assume any responsibility for any injury and/or damage to persons or property arising out of or related to any use of the material contained in this periodical. The reader is advised to check the appropriate medical literature and the product information currently provided by the manufacturer of each drug to be administered, to verify the dosage, the method and duration of administration or contraindications. It is the responsibility of the treating physician or other health care professional, relying on independent experience and knowledge of the patient, to determine drug dosages and the best treatment for the patient. Mention of any product in this issue should not be construed as endorsement by the contributors, editors, or the Publisher of the product or manufacturers' claims.

Clinics in Perinatology (ISSN 0095-5108) is published in quarterly by Elsevier Inc., 360 Park Avenue South, New York, NY 10010-1710. Months of issue are March, June, September, and December. Business and Editorial offices: 1600 John F. Kennedy Blvd., Suite 1800, Philadelphia, PA 19103-2899. Customer Service Office: 6277 Sea Harbor Drive, Orlando, FL 32887-4800. Periodicals postage paid at New York, NY and additional mailing offices. Subscription prices are $182.00 per year for (US individuals), $270.00 per year for (US institutions), $215.00 per year (Canadian individuals), $335.00 per year (Canadian institutions), $248.00 per year (foreign individuals), $335.00 per year (foreign institutions) $88.00 per year (US students), and $121.00 per year (foreign students). Foreign air speed delivery is included in all Clinics subscription prices. All prices are subject to change without notice. **POSTMASTER:** Send address changes to *Clinics in Perinatology*; Elsevier Periodicals Customer Service, 6277 Sea Harbor Drive, Orlando, FL 32887-4800. **Customer Service: 1-800-654-2452 (US). From outside of the US, call 1-407-345-1000.** E-mail: elspcs@elsevier.com

Clinics in Perinatology is also pubilshed in Spanish by McGraw-Hill Interamericana Editores S.A., P.O. Box 5-237, 06500 Mexico D.F., Mexico.

Clinics in Perinatology is covered in *Index Medicus, Current Contents, Excepta Medica, BIOSIS* and *ISI/BIOMED.*

Printed in the United States of America.

GUEST EDITORS

LUCKY JAIN, MD, MBA, Professor of Pediatrics and Physiology, Executive Vice Chairman, Division of Neonatology, Emory University School of Medicine, Atlanta, Georgia

TONSE N.K. RAJU, MD, DCH, Medical Officer/Program Scientist, Pregnancy and Perinatology Branch, CDBPM/NICHD, National Institutes of Health, Bethesda, Maryland

CONTRIBUTORS

DAVID H. ADAMKIN, MD, Professor of Pediatrics, Director of Neonatal Medicine, Director of Neonatal Nutrition Program, University of Louisville School of Medicine, Louisville, Kentucky

IRA ADAMS-CHAPMAN, MD, Director, Developmental Progress Clinic, Assistant Professor of Pediatrics, and Department of Pediatrics, Division of Neonatology, Emory University School of Medicine, Atlanta, Georgia

RONALD L. ARIAGNO, MD, Professor of Pediatrics, Department of Pediatrics, Stanford University School of Medicine, Stanford, California

DANIEL K. BENJAMIN, JR, MD, PhD, MPH, Associate Professor, Department of Pediatrics, Duke Clinical Research Institute, Duke University, Durham, North Carolina

SARAID S. BILLIARDS, PhD, Department of Pathology, Children's Hospital Boston, Boston, Massachusetts; Harvard Medical School, Boston, Massachusetts

JOHN CHENG, MD, Assistant Professor of Pediatrics, Division of Pediatric Emergency Medicine, Emory University; Attending Physician, Children's Healthcare of Atlanta at Egleston, Atlanta, Georgia

JANE CLEARY-GOLDMAN, MD, Assistant Clinical Professor, Department of Obstetrics and Gynecology, Division of Maternal-Fetal Medicine, Columbia University Medical Center, New York, New York

MARY E. D'ALTON, MD, Chair, Department of Obstetrics and Gynecology, Willard C. Rappleye Professor of Obstetrics and Gynecology, Columbia University Medical Center, New York, New York

ROBERT A. DARNALL, MD, Professor of Pediatrics and of Physiology, Departments of Pediatrics and Physiology, Dartmouth Medical School, Lebanon, New Hampshire

SHERIN U. DEVASKAR, MD, Division of Neonatology and Developmental Biology, Department of Pediatrics, David Geffin School of Medicine at University of California Los Angeles and Mattel Children's Hospital at University of California Los Angeles, Los Angeles, California

WILLIAM J. DOBAK, DO, Maternal-fetal Medicine Fellow, Department of Gynecology and Obstetrics, Emory University School of Medicine, Atlanta, Georgia

GOLDE G. DUDELL, MD, Associate Professor of Pediatrics, Emory University School of Medicine, Atlanta, Georgia

REBECCA D. FOLKERTH, MD, Department of Pathology, Children's Hospital Boston; Department of Pathology, Brigham and Women's Hospital; Department of Neurology, Children's Hospital, Boston, Massachusetts

KARIN FUCHS, MD, Division of Maternal-fetal Medicine, Department of Obstetrics and Gynecology, Columbia University Medical Center, Presbyterian Hospital, New York, New York

MICHAEL O. GARDNER, MD, MPH, Professor, Department of Gynecology and Obstetrics, Emory University School of Medicine, Atlanta, Georgia

MEENA GARG, MD, Division of Neonatology and Developmental Biology, Department of Pediatrics, David Geffen School of Medicine at University of California Los Angeles and Mattel Children's Hospital at University of California Los Angeles, Los Angeles, California

ROBIN L. HAYNES, PhD, Department of Pathology, Children's Hospital Boston; Harvard Medical School; Department of Neurology, Children's Hospital, Boston, Massachusetts

LUCKY JAIN, MD, MBA, Professor of Pediatrics and Physiology, Executive Vice Chairman, Division of Neonatology, Emory University School of Medicine, Atlanta, Georgia

SHABNAM JAIN, MD, Assistant Professor of Pediatrics, Division of Pediatric Emergency Medicine, Emory University; Attending Physician, Children's Healthcare of Atlanta at Egleston, Atlanta, Georgia

HANNAH C. KINNEY, MD, Department of Pathology, Children's Hospital Boston; Harvard Medical School, Boston, Massachusetts

YOUNG MI LEE, MD, Maternal-Fetal Medicine Fellow, Department of Obstetrics and Gynecology, Columbia University Medical Center, New York, New York

CHRISTOPHER R. PIERSON, MD, PhD, Department of Pathology, Children's Hospital Boston; Harvard Medical School; Department of Pathology, Brigham and Women's Hospital, Boston, Massachusetts

TONSE N.K. RAJU, MD, DCH, Medical Officer/Program Scientist, Pregnancy and Perinatology Branch, CDBPM/NICHD, National Institutes of Health, Bethesda, Maryland

BARBARA J. STOLL, MD, George Brumley, Jr Chair, and Professor, Department of Pediatrics, Emory University; Medical Director, Children's Healthcare of Atlanta, Atlanta, Georgia

RONALD WAPNER, MD, Professor, Division of Maternal-Fetal Medicine, Department of Obstetrics and Gynecology, Columbia University Medical Center, Presbyterian Hospital, New York, New York

JON F. WATCHKO, MD, Division of Newborn Medicine, Department of Pediatrics, University of Pittsburgh School of Medicine; Magee-Womens Research Institute, Magee-Womens Hospital, Pittsburgh, Pennsylvania

CONTENTS

The preterm birth rate (births before 37 completed weeks of gestation) has been increasing in the United States, largely driven by an
increase in infants delivered between 34 and 36 weeks, often called
near-term, but referred to as late preterm in this article. In 2004, the
preterm birth rate was 12.5%, the highest rate since the National
Center for Health Statistics began tracking such data. This article
reviews the epidemiology of late preterm births and proposes a research agenda.

The late preterm infant represents a significant portion of preterm
deliveries. Historically, this cohort has been referred to as near
term, which may not address adequately the increased perinatal
morbidity these neonates experience. The changing demographics
of pregnant women also are increasing the number of inductions
in this gestational age group. More women with chronic hypertension, diabetes, and other chronic medical problems are getting
pregnant, and often these pregnancies may require induction during this gestational age. The increasing numbers of multi-fetal gestations also have an average gestational age at delivery in this
range of 34 to 36.6 weeks. Preeclampsia is another factor that can
lead to delivery and induction during this gestational age. This article discusses some of the physiologic causes behind late preterm
deliveries.

This article focuses on the less-explored problem of severe hypoxic respiratory failure in the late preterm infant and discusses potential strategies for management.

the extremely low birth weight infants and the intrauterine growth-restricted infants, adequately powered studies restricted to only the late preterm infants are required and need future consideration.

Late preterm neonates have unique susceptibilities to infection. The closed setting of the neonatal ICU (NICU) and the immunologic immaturity of premature infants set the stage for the development of nosocomial infections. This article discusses infections that might be seen in this population and gives options for diagnosis and treatment.

The brainstem development of infants born between 33 and 38 weeks' gestation is less mature than that of a full-term infant. During late gestation, there are dramatic and nonlinear developmental changes in the brainstem. This translates into immaturity of upper airway and lung volume control, laryngeal reflexes, chemical control of breathing, and sleep mechanisms. Ten percent of late preterm infants have significant apnea of prematurity and they frequently have delays in establishing coordination of feeding and breathing. Unfortunately, there is a paucity of clinical, physiologic, neuroanatomic, and neurochemical data in this specific group of infants. Research focused on this group of infants will not only further our understanding of brainstem maturation during this high risk period, but will help develop focused plans for their management.

This article addresses the issue of whether the late preterm infant is more susceptible to gray matter injury induced by hypoxia-ischemia than the term infant. Although different gray matter regions display varying patterns of neuronal injury in the face of hypoxia-ischemia during advancing gestational development, little is known about the specific patterns of injury faced by the late preterm infant. This changing pattern of neuronal vulnerability with age likely reflects developmental changes of susceptibility and protective factors essential for responding to energy deprivation at the molecular, cellular, biochemical, and vascular levels. Future research involving closer examination of the late preterm period is essential to provide a greater understanding of the neuronal vulnerability in the face of hypoxic-ischemic injury.

GOAL STATEMENT

The goal of *Clinics in Perinatology* is to keep practicing neonatologists and maternal-fetal medicine specialists up to date with current clinical practice in perinatology by providing timely articles reviewing the state of the art in patient care.

ACCREDITATION

The *Clinics in Perinatology* is planned and implemented in accordance with the Essential Areas and Policies of the Accreditation Council for Continuing Medical Education (ACCME) through the joint sponsorship of the University of Virginia School of Medicine and Elsevier. The University of Virginia School of Medicine is accredited by the ACCME to provide continuing medical education for physicians.

The University of Virginia School of Medicine designates this educational activity for a maximum of 60 *AMA PRA Category 1 Credits*™. Physicians should only claim credit commensurate with the extent of their participation in the activity.

The American Medical Association has determined that physicians not licensed in the US who participate in this CME activity are eligible for *AMA PRA Category 1 Credits*™.

Credit can be earned by reading the text material, taking the CME examination online at http://www.theclinics.com/home/cme, and completing the evaluation. After taking the test, you will be required to review any and all incorrect answers. Following completion of the test and evaluation, your credit will be awarded and you may print your certificate.

FACULTY DISCLOSURE/CONFLICT OF INTEREST

The University of Virginia School of Medicine, as an ACCME accredited provider, endorses and strives to comply with the Accreditation Council for Continuing Medical Education (ACCME) Standards of Commercial Support, Commonwealth of Virginia statutes, University of Virginia policies and procedures, and associated federal and private regulations and guidelines on the need for disclosure and monitoring of proprietary and financial interests that may affect the scientific integrity and balance of content delivered in continuing medical education activities under our auspices.

The University of Virginia School of Medicine requires that all CME activities accredited through this institution be developed independently and be scientifically rigorous, balanced and objective in the presentation/discussion of its content, theories and practices.

All authors/editors participating in an accredited CME activity are expected to disclose to the readers relevant financial relationships with commercial entities occurring within the past 12 months (such as grants or research support, employee, consultant, stock holder, member of speakers bureau, etc.). The University of Virginia School of Medicine will employ appropriate mechanisms to resolve potential conflicts of interest to maintain the standards of fair and balanced education to the reader. Questions about specific strategies can be directed to the Office of Continuing Medical Education, University of Virginia School of Medicine, Charlottesville, Virginia.

The authors/editors listed below have identified no professional or financial affiliations for themselves or their spouse/partner:
Ira Adams-Chapman, MD; Ronald L. Ariagno, MD; Saraid S. Billards, PhD; John Cheng, MD; Jane Cleary-Goldman, MD; Mary D'Alton, MD; Robert A. Darnall, MD; Michael J. Davidoff; William J. Dobak, DO; Rebecca D. Folkerth, MD; Karin Fuchs, MD; Michael Gardner, MD, MPH; Meena Garg, MD; Robin L. Haynes, PhD; Carla Holloway (Acquisitions Editor); Shabnam Jain, MD; Hannah C. Kinney, MD; Young Mi Lee, MD; Christopher R. Pierson, MD, MPH; Tonse N. K. Raju, MD, DCH (Guest Editor); Barbara Stoll, MD; Ronald Wapner, MD; and, Jon F. Watchko, MD.

The authors/editors listed below identified the following professional or financial affiliations for themselves or their spouse/partner:
David H. Adamkin, MD is a consultant for Mead Johnson and for Ross Labs.
Daniel K. Benjamin, Jr., MD, PhD, MPH received research support from Cape Cod Associates, Astellas, MedImmune, NIAID, NICHD, Pediatrix, and Rockeby; and, has received research fellowships from Thrasher Research, Astra Zeneca, and Johnson and Johnson.
Sherin U. Devaskar, MD serves as faculty for research presentations by fellows for Mead-Johnson.
Golde Dudell, MD is on the speaker's bureau for INO Therapeutics.
Lucky Jain, MD, MBA (Guest Editor) is a research consultant for Schering Corporation and is on the speaker's bureau for INO Therapeutics.

Disclosure of Discussion of non-FDA approved uses for pharmaceutical products and/or medical devices:
The University of Virginia School of Medicine, as an ACCME provider, requires that all faculty presenters identify and disclose any "off label" uses for pharmaceutical and medical device products. The University of Virginia School of Medicine recommends that each physician fully review all the available data on new products or procedures prior to instituting them with patients.

TO ENROLL

To enroll in the Clinics in Perinatology Continuing Medical Education program, call customer service at 1-800-654-2452 or visit us online at www.theclinics.com/home/cme. The CME program is available to subscribers for an additional fee of $195.00

FORTHCOMING ISSUES

RECENT ISSUES

The Clinics are now available online!

Access your subscription at
www.theclinics.com

CLINICS IN
PERINATOLOGY

Clin Perinatol 33 (2006) xv–xvi

Preface

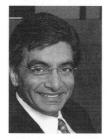 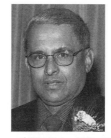

Lucky Jain, MD, MBA   Tonse N.K. Raju, MD, DCH
Guest Editors

In North America, births at 34 to 36.9 weeks gestation, often referred to as *late preterm* or *near-term* births, account for up to 75% of all preterm births. In spite of concerted efforts to decrease prematurity, the total and late preterm birth rates have been increasing during the past decade, raising concerns about the reasons for such trends. Higher rates of induced deliveries and cesarean births have also caused concern about their collective impact on morbidity and health care cost.

Although late preterm infants are the largest subgroup of preterm infants, there has been little research on this group until recently. This is mainly because having been labeled "near-term," such infants were being looked upon as "almost mature," and hence there was no need to be concerned. However, recent research has revealed a contrary trend. While serious morbidities are rare, the late preterm group has 2 to 3 fold increased rates for mild to moderate morbidities, such as hypothermia, hypoglycemia, delayed lung fluid clearance and respiratory distress, poor feeding, jaundice, infection, and readmission rates after initial hospital discharge. Because the late preterm subgroup accounts for 9% of all births, even a modest increase in any morbidity will have a huge impact on the overall health care resources. Thus, it is not surprising that the absolute number of late preterm infants being admitted to NICUs has been increasing worldwide.

The issue gets even more complex: because more than 80% of all deliveries occur in community hospitals, the health care teams may not always be equipped to assess and manage sick, late preterm infants. Moreover, since such infants may initially appear mature and healthy, they may be admitted

0095-5108/06/$ - see front matter © 2006 Elsevier Inc. All rights reserved.
doi:10.1016/j.clp.2006.10.002   *perinatology.theclinics.com*

to term nurseries, or allowed to "room in" with their mothers until the clinical status deteriorates.

Recent work in developmental and neurobiology has revealed startling facts about the growth and maturation of the brain during the final few weeks of gestation. These processes include maturation of oligodendroglia, increasing neuronal arborization and connectivity, maturation of neurotransmitter systems especially in the brainstem, and about 30% increase in brain size. Thus, at least with regard to the brain, the late preterm infant is not "almost term and mature," but in fact, a very vulnerable and immature infant who needs close monitoring and diligent follow-up.

We are delighted that an entire issue of the *Clinics in Perinatology* has been devoted to bring some of the above issues to focus. The articles cover a large array of topics that will interest clinicians as well as stimulate researchers. The overarching theme is to provide a state-of-the-art review of the topics and to present an outline for multidisciplinary research agenda. The authors stress the need for prospective data collection to accurately define the scope and public health impact of late preterm births. They also point out the need for designing clinical trials management to formulate evidence-based strategies in the care of the late preterm pregnancies and the newborn infants.

Finally, we would like to thank all the authors for their valuable contributions on this difficult topic, and Carla Holloway at Elsevier for her untiring efforts in getting them published.

Lucky Jain, MD, MBA
Department of Pediatrics and Physiology
Division of Neonatology
Emory University School of Medicine
2015 Uppergate Drive NE
Atlanta, GA 30322, USA

E-mail address: ljain@emory.edu

Tonse N.K. Raju, MD, DCH
Pregnancy and Perinatology Branch
CDBPM/NICHD, National Institutes of Health
6100 Executive Boulevard, Room 4B03
Bethesda, MD 20892

E-mail address: rajut@mail.nih.gov

ELSEVIER
SAUNDERS

CLINICS IN
PERINATOLOGY

Clin Perinatol 33 (2006) 751–763

Epidemiology of Late Preterm (Near-Term) Births

Tonse N.K. Raju, MD, DCH

National Institute of Child Health and Human Development, National Institutes of Health,
6100 Executive Boulevard, 4B03, Bethesda, MD 20892, USA

"Of the time of birth and which is called natural or unnatural: The due season is most commonly after the ninth month or about forty weeks after the conception, although some be delivered sometimes, in the seventh month, and the child proves very well. But such as are borne in the eight month, either they be dead before the birth, or else live not long after." The Byrthe of Mankynde, Book II, Chap. 1 Circa 1540 by Thomas Raynalde [1].

Since antiquity, it has been taught that borderline preterm infants born at 8 months of gestation (near-term or late preterm in today's terminology) may not survive, whereas those born at 7 months can survive [1,2]. A plausible physiological explanation for this paradox may be the overlapping timelines between the changing alveolar shape during development [3] relative to surfactant surge. Infants born around 28 weeks of gestation have more saccular (less circular) alveoli with longer radii of curvature. This may be physiologically advantageous, because such alveoli require less surfactant for stability. By contrast, infants at 32 to 33 weeks of gestation with more circular alveoli, born especially before the well known, surfactant surge (around 34 to 35 weeks), may suffer from relative surfactant deficiency and respiratory distress.

A more pragmatic explanation for the paradox may be one of recollection bias. Being small and frail, infants born at 7 months gestation would require special care for survival. Should such infants survive, they were more likely to be remembered. By contrast, infants born at 8 months appear healthy and were expected to survive; thus, only their death, unexpected as it would be, was more likely to be remembered.

Whatever the explanation, preterm birth remains one of the leading causes of infant mortality and morbidity globally, and experts contend that there is no such thing as a healthy premature infant. Even borderline

---

E-mail address: rajut@mail.nih.gov

0095-5108/06/$ - see front matter © 2006 Elsevier Inc. All rights reserved.
doi:10.1016/j.clp.2006.09.009

preterm birth has been shown to increase morbidity and mortality risk [4–15] compared with term. Furthermore, increasing preterm birth rates over the past two decades in the United States and internationally [15–18] have added new measures of concern [19,20].

Definitions

In 1948, the First World Health Assembly recommended that infants who weighed 5.5 lbs (2500 g) or less at birth, and those born less than 37 weeks gestation be considered immature infants. In 1950, the World Health Organization (WHO) revised this definition after recognizing that many preterm infants weighed more than 2500 g, and many term infants weighed less than 2500 g at birth. The new version defined preterm births as those occurring less than 37 completed weeks of gestation, counting from the first day of the last menstrual period (LMP) [21]. The American Academy of Pediatrics (AAP) and the American College of Obstetricians and Gynecologists (ACOG) have endorsed this definition [22].

Despite unanimity in defining preterm, there is less uniformity in defining its subgroups. The common subgroup terminologies used are: very preterm (less than 32 weeks), extremely preterm (less than 28 weeks), and moderately preterm (32 to 26 weeks). In addition, many permutations and combinations of gestational age ranges between 32 and 36 weeks have been used to describe the near-term births [23]. An expert panel at a workshop convened by the National Institute of Child Health and Human Development (NICHD) of the National Institutes of Health (NIH) in July 2005 [24] recommended that births between 34 completed weeks (34 $^{0/7}$ weeks or day 239) and less than 37 completed weeks (36 $^{6/7}$ weeks or day 259) of gestation be referred to as late preterm. This suggestion was based on the recognition that the 34th week marks an obstetrical milestone after which antenatal steroids typically are not administered [25], and on the fact that late preterm infants have higher risks for mortality and morbidity compared with term infants [4–15]. The phrase late preterm also conveys the concept that these infants are indeed premature, not almost term, as the near-term phrase might convey [24].

Trends in late preterm birth

Unless otherwise noted, the US data presented in this article were calculated by the March of Dimes Perinatal Data Center using birth certificate data from US natality files of the National Center for Health Statistics (NCHS), or modified (with permission) from those reported by Davidoff and colleagues [26].

Of the more than 4 million annual live births in the United States, approximately 360,000 occur at late preterm gestations. Fig. 1 shows the

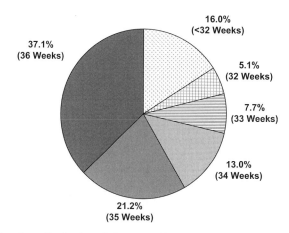

Fig. 1. Gestational age distribution of all preterm births, United States, 2003, based on 499,008 preterm singleton births. (*Adapted from* Davidoff MJ, Dias T, Damus K, et al. Changes in the gestational age distribution among US singleton births: impact on rates of late preterm birth, 1992 to 2002. Semin Perinatol 2006;30:9; with permission.)

distribution of all US preterm births in 2003. More than 71% of preterm births occurred in late preterm gestations. When analyzed by plurality, 61% of preterm multiple births and 73% of preterm singleton births were late preterm gestations. This difference reflects the higher likelihood for multiple than singleton pregnancies to deliver before 34 weeks.

In the United States the rate of late preterm birth has increased at a faster pace than the overall rate of preterm birth [16]. Between 1981 and 2003, the overall preterm birth rate increased by 31% (from 9.4% to 12.3%), whereas the rate of late preterm birth increased by 40% (from 6.3% to 8.8%). During this period, the rate of very preterm birth also increased, but at a slower pace, by about 11%.

The increasing proportion of births at late preterm gestations in the United States is part of a larger trend. Fig. 2 shows the distribution of singleton births by week of gestation at delivery for the years 1992, 1997, and 2003. There has been a clear shift from higher to lower gestational ages, causing the most frequent length of singleton gestation in the United States to shift from 40 to 39 weeks. A detailed study of singleton births over the same period also reported similar shifts to earlier gestations for births with the birth certificate-identified diagnosis of: premature rupture of membranes (PROM), medical interventions (cesarean deliveries or inductions without PROM), and spontaneous births [26].

A closer evaluation of gestational age categories reveals a drop in the proportions of infants delivered post-term (Table 1). After controlling for maternal age and race/ethnicity, there was a 18.6% decrease in the proportion of births at 40 and 41 weeks of gestation and a 36.6% decrease in the proportion of births at or beyond 42 weeks. This trend was associated with an

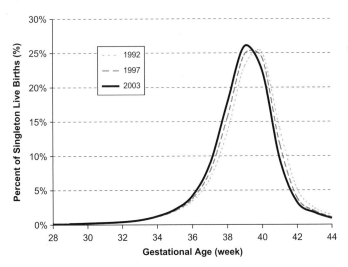

Fig. 2. Shifting distribution of gestational age among all live births, United States, 1992, 1997 and 2003. (*Adapted from* Davidoff MJ, Dias T, Damus K, et al. Changes in the gestational age distribution among US singleton births: impact on rates of late preterm birth, 1992 to 2002. Semin Perinatol 2006;30:11; with permission.)

increase in the proportion of births between 37 and 39 weeks of gestation. Among preterm gestations, late preterm births had the largest proportional increase of nearly 15%. Changes in the distribution of maternal age and race/ethnicity between 1992 and 2003 accounted for little to none of the observed change in each category.

Table 1
Changes in gestational age distribution among singleton live births, United States 1992 and 2003

Weeks	Distribution proportion (%)		Percent change	
	1992	2003	Unadjusted[a]	Adjusted[b]
<32	1.5	1.4	−6.7	−6.7
32–33	1.3	1.3	0.0[c]	0.0
34–36	6.9	7.9	14.5	14.5
37–39	43.1	53.0	23.0	21.7
40–41	37.8	30.6	−19.0	−18.6
42–44	9.4	5.8	−38.3	−36.6

[a] All rates between 1992 and 2002 significantly different ($P < .01$) except when indicated.
[b] Adjusted for maternal race/ethnicity and maternal age.
[c] Rates not significantly different between 1992 and 2002.

Adapted from Davidoff MJ, Dias T. Damus K. et al. Changes in the gestational age distribution among US singleton births: impact on rates of late preterm birth 1992 to 2002. Semin Perinatol 2006;30(1):8–15.

Racial/ethnic trends

Preterm birth rates have been 1.5 times higher for non-Hispanic black infants than for Hispanic and non-Hispanic white infants [16]. This differential persists among late preterm births, albeit at narrower margins. Between 1992 and 2003, the late preterm birth rate was 10.7% for singleton non-Hispanic black infants, 8.1% for Hispanic infants, and 7.2%, for non-Hispanic white infants (Fig. 3).

Despite having the lowest rate of late preterm births, non-Hispanic white infants had the largest increase (approximately 25%) in late preterm births between 1992 and 2003. Because they account for most US births, the overall increase in preterm birth rate in the United States can be explained largely by an increase in late preterm births among non-Hispanic white infants.

International trends

It is difficult to directly compare preterm birth rates between the United States and other countries because of variations in the definition of live births and fetal deaths, differences in measurement of gestational age, and a lack of published data [19]. One study using the Medical Birth Registry of Norway found a 25% increase in preterm births between 1980 and 1998 (4.12% to 5.16%) [17]. Multivariate analyses showed that the increase was mainly caused by an increase in obstetric interventions, especially cesarean deliveries. Trends in gestational age subgroups, however, were not provided in this study.

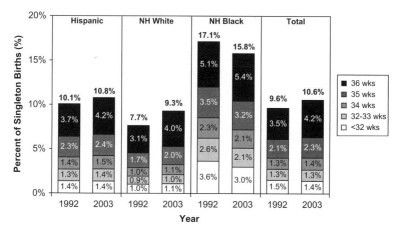

Fig. 3. Comparison of singleton preterm birth rates by gestational age and race/ethnicity, 1992 and 2003. (*Adapted from* Davidoff MJ, Dias T, Damus K, et al. Changes in the gestational age distribution among US singleton births: impact on rates of late preterm birth, 1992 to 2002. Semin Perinatol 2006;30:12; with permission.)

Joseph and colleagues reported that in Canada, between 1981 and 1983 (average) and 1997, the preterm birth rate increased by 15% (from 6.25% to 7.19% of live births) [27]. Among singleton births, they found that the late preterm births increased by 6% between the aggregated years 1985 to 1989 and 1990 to 1996. Similar to the Norwegian study, they also attributed an increase in preterm birth rate to an increase in obstetric interventions.

A study from Denmark [18] reported that there was a 22% increase in spontaneous singleton preterm births between 1995 and 2004 for white European women who were 20 to 24 years of age (from 5.2% to 6.3% of live births). The gestational age breakdown showed that there was a 40.9% increase in extremely preterm (22 to 27 weeks) births, a 21.8% increase in very preterm (28 to 31 weeks) births, and a 21.8% increase in moderately preterm (32 to 36 weeks) births. It is worth noting that the largest increase in the preterm subcategory in United States occurred in the late preterm births, not in the extremely preterm births, as was in Denmark. More studies are needed to understand the reasons for differences in the trends in preterm birth among various countries.

Trends associated with late preterm births

Cesarean deliveries and labor inductions

The rates of cesarean deliveries and inductions of labor have been increasing in the United States [16,28]. Although the cesarean delivery rates declined between 1989 and 1996, the rate increased to 29% of all births in 2004—the highest ever reported [29]. Between 1990 and 2003, the rate of induction increased from 9.5% of live births to 20.6%, and this change probably contributed to the increasing rate of preterm birth in the United States [16]. Fig. 4 shows gestational age-specific cesarean and induction rates for singleton live births between 1992 and 2003. Although both rates increased among late preterm births (31% and 78% respectively), cesarean rates increased more at earlier gestations, and induction rates increased more at later gestations.

Traditional causes of preterm births

Preeclampsia and premature rupture of the membranes are among the well-known causes of preterm birth [30,31]. Because national data on their trend and prevalence are not available, however, their contribution to the recent increase in the preterm birth rate remains to be quantified.

Reductions in stillbirth rates

Several investigators have proposed that the declining US stillbirth rates and increasing US preterm births are causally related [28,32–37]. Some have

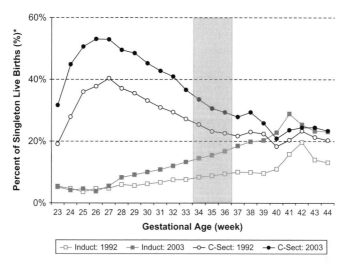

Fig. 4. Proportion of births with cesarean section and labor induction among singleton live births by gestational age, United States, 1992 and 2003. Shaded area: late preterm gestations. *Adapted from* Davidoff MJ, Dias T, Damus K, et al. Changes in the gestational age distribution among US singleton births: impact on rates of late preterm birth, 1992 to 2002. Semin Perinatol 2006;30:13; with permission.)

shown that an increase in cesarean deliveries and labor inductions have contributed to reductions in stillbirth among singletons [33] and twins [34], but not among triplets [35]. These studies imply that to prevent stillbirths, timed obstetrical interventions for at-risk groups are needed, and an increase in preterm birth rates may be the price. More work is needed, however, to ascertain the causal association between increasing obstetric interventions and decreasing stillbirths, and their combined role in increasing the overall and late preterm birth rates. Prospective studies exploring the gestational age-specific reasons for preterm births are needed to address these issues.

Practice guidelines

Because of higher perinatal mortality among post-term births [38,39], practice guidelines have changed considerably over the past two decades. In 1989, the ACOG recommend that labor be induced in low-risk pregnancies in the 43rd week of gestation, and in 1997, it recommended close fetal surveillance beginning at 42 weeks [40]. The Society of Obstetricians and Gynecologists of Canada recommended routine induction of labor at 41 weeks [41]. It is possible that the welcome trend of preventing post-term births might have shifted the distribution of all births to earlier gestations.

Measurement of gestational age

Assessment of gestational age is an imperfect science [42–45]. It typically is estimated using the mother's LMP, or based on fetal ultrasound measures [19]. When performed before 20 weeks, fetal ultrasound is considered to be more accurate than the LMP method. Early ultrasound for accurate estimations of gestational age have been shown to prevent post-term births and increase preterm birth [44]. One study demonstrated that this explained a significant proportion of a temporal increase in preterm births in Canada [46]. More studies are needed to assess the impact of temporal trends in the methods of estimating fetal gestational age on increasing overall and late preterm births in the United States.

Delayed childbearing, increasing use of assisted reproductive technology and multiple births

Three inter-related factors during the past decade might have contributed, in part, to increasing overall and late preterm births in the United States. These include:

- Increasing proportion of women choosing to have babies later in life [47]
- Increasing demand for assisted reproductive technology (ART)
- Increasing rates of twins, triplets, and higher-order multiples [19,48,49]

The individual contributions of each of these factors to increasing preterm rates are difficult to discern. Some epidemiological observations, however, can be summarized.

The relationship between maternal age and the frequency of preterm birth assumes a u-shaped curve, with higher preterm births occurring among younger and older women. A recent analysis using a pooled dataset from 1998 to 2000 showed that women younger than 16 and older 35 years of age had 2% to 4% higher rates of preterm births compared with those 21 to 24 years of age [19]. Considerable differences, however, existed in the trends for different racial/ethnic groups. Among non-Hispanic African American women, preterm birth rates began to rise at younger ages (27 to 29 years) than for non-Hispanic white women (33 to 35 years). More work is needed to address the interaction effects of race and ethnicity and maternal age [19].

The ART use rate has been increasing in the United States within a 6-year span. In 2002, 33,000 American women delivered following successful infertility treatment—an approximately twofold increase compared with 1996. Because an unintended consequence of ART is an increase in the incidence of multiple pregnancies, a well-recognized risk factor for preterm births [19,48,49], increasing rates of ART use can be causally linked to increasing overall and late preterm birth rates. It is also known that ART increases the risk of preterm births even among singleton pregnancies [19].

Obesity and fetal macrosomia

Numerous studies have shown that there is an epidemic of overweight and obesity in all US population subgroups [50]. Because high body mass index is a risk factor for preterm delivery [51], the epidemic of overweight and obesity among women of reproductive age may be contributing, in part, to an overall increase in US preterm births. Fetal imaging with ultra-sound to estimate gestational age is more difficult in overweight and obese women, compounding the difficulty in choosing an optimal time for obstetric intervention. Fetal macrosomia in such pregnancies may lead an overestimation of gestational age, and the obstetrician may end up choosing an earlier date for cesarean section or induction of labor to prevent complications associated with macrosomia. More research is needed to discern the individual and collective roles of these variables on increasing overall and late preterm birth rates in the United States.

Morbidity, mortality, and late preterm births

Although the survival rates for infants born at 34 to 36 weeks are higher compared with infants born at earlier gestations, Kramer and colleagues [15] showed that at the population level, the etiologic fraction (defined as the proportion of infant deaths in a population attributable to being born at 34 to 36 weeks) can be considerable. In the US and Canadian populations, between 6.8% and 8.0% of all infant deaths were attributable to being born at 34 to 36 weeks of gestation, compared with an almost identical range, between 7.1% and 7.3% of all infant deaths attributable to being born at 28 to 32 weeks of gestation [15].

Using a population-based cohort study of healthy, singleton late preterm infants delivered vaginally, Tomashek and colleagues showed that late preterm infants discharged within 48 hours of age were 1.8 times more likely to be readmitted than term infants [5]. Using the same dataset, Shapiro-Mendoza and colleagues [6] identified some specific risk factors for increased postdischarge morbidity, including (among others), being firstborn, breast fed at discharge, and a history of labor and delivery complications. These and other studies [4–14] clearly show that late preterm birth increases the risk for neonatal and postneonatal morbidity and mortality. Other articles in this issue address specific conditions leading to excess morbidity and mortality among late preterm infants.

Societal and economic costs

According to estimates by the Institute of Medicine (IOM), the economic burden caused by preterm births in the United States in 2005 was, at a minimum, $26.2 billion, or $51,600 per preterm infant [19]. Thus, even a modest reduction in preterm birth rate at any gestation will reduce the burden of disease and lead to substantial cost savings. Using a population-based dataset for 1996, Gilbert and colleagues concluded that preventing nonmedically indicated births between 34 and 37 weeks of gestation could have saved

49.9 million dollars in California [7]. Some experts contend that in regional perinatal centers, preterm births for nonmedical indications are very rare [52]. State and national data, however, are lacking to estimate the proportion of nonindicated (and hence potentially preventable) preterm births. Thus, the findings of Gilbert and colleagues [7] need to be validated at the regional and national levels to assess the prevalence of potentially preventable preterm births, their causes, and their economic and societal burden.

Summary

One of the objectives of the US Healthy People 2010 is to achieve a preterm birth rate of no more than 7.6%. The NCHS data presented in this article indicate that unless the present trend is reversed, the 2010 target cannot be achieved, especially considering the pace of increase in late preterm births. The 2006 IOM report recommended that more research to address the health care burden from increasing preterm births [19] as did the expert panel at the NICHD workshop [24].

Research topics and opportunities in epidemiology of late preterm births include:

- Changing trends in the contribution of gestational age-specific preterm birth rate to the neonatal and infant mortality, and morbidity rates
- The distribution of gestational age at birth for different ethnic and socio–demographic subgroups and changing trends at the national level.
- Causes of late preterm birth stratified by place of delivery, payer status, and level of hospital care
- Gestational age-specific prevalence trends of known causes for preterm births, with an intent to identify potentially preventable and nonpreventable causes
- The effect of efforts to prevent extreme preterm births on late preterm birth rates
- The effect of efforts to prevent post-term births on the late preterm birth rates
- The impact of routine early ultrasound for assessing fetal gestational age on the temporal trends in US preterm birth rates
- The cost versus benefit analyses of prolonging pregnancies at late preterm gestations
- Long-term neuro–developmental outcomes at school age for late preterm births and the economic and societal impact of such outcomes

It is gratifying that despite an increase in the preterm birth rate, perinatal mortality rates have been dropping in the United States. Larger studies that evaluate gestational week-specific short- and long-term morbidity and mortality by cause of death would help solidify current knowledge of late preterm outcomes, however. It remains to be seen whether increasing late preterm births have any relation to the place of birth and level of hospital care. Regional and national trends are needed to assess the potential contribution of nonmedically indicated late preterm births to the overall preterm birth rate.

One of the major concerns of public health importance is the need to study the long-term neurological and school-age outcomes of late preterm infants. Because one out of 11 births in this country is a late preterm birth (nearly 9% of all births), and since the brain of the late preterm infant is less mature than that of the term infant [53], even a minor increase in the rate of neurological disability and scholastic failure in this group can have a huge impact on the health care and educational systems.

Research is needed to understand the etiology of all preterm births. Toward this end, the US Senate unanimously passed a Preemie Act recommending various measures to help address the problem of preterm births [20]. There is also an urgent need for educating health care providers and parents about the vulnerability of late preterm infants, who need diligent monitoring and care during the initial hospital stay, and a comprehensive follow-up plan for postneonatal and long-term evaluations.

Acknowledgments

The author sincerely thanks Michael Davidoff, MPH, March of Dimes, White Plains, NY for analyzing and updating all of the NCHD data presented in the article and for help during the preparation of this manuscript. The author also thanks the following scientists from the March of Dimes for their critical appraisal of the manuscript: Todd Davis, MS; Rebecca Russell, MSPH; Tomoko Kushnir, PH; Nancy Green, MD; and Joann Petrini, PhD, MPH.

References

[1] Clendening L. Source book of medical history. New York: Dover Publications Incorporated; 1942. p. 170–3.
[2] Tempkin O. Soranus' gynecology. Baltimore (MD): Johns Hopkins University Press; 1956. p. 32–4.
[3] Snyder JM. Regulation of alveolarization. In: Polin RA, Fox WW, Abman SH, editors. Fetal and neonatal physiology. 3rd edition. New York: Elsevier; 2004. p. 795–801.
[4] Wang ML, Dorer DJ, Fleming MP, et al. Clinical outcomes of near-term infants. Pediatrics 2004;114:372–6.
[5] Tomashek KM, Shapiro-Mendoza CK, Weiss J, et al. Early discharge among late preterm and term newborns and risk of neonatal morbidity. Semin Perinatol 2002;30:61–8.
[6] Shapiro-Mendoza CK, Tomashek KM, Kotelchuck M, et al. Risk factors for neonatal morbidity and mortality among healthy, late preterm newborns. Semin Perinatol 2006;30:54–60.
[7] Gilbert WM, Nesbitt TS, Danielsen B. The cost of prematurity: quantification by gestational age and birth weight. Obstet Gynecol 2003;102:488–92.
[8] Sarici SU, Serdar MA, Korkmaz A, et al. Incidence, course, and prediction of hyperbilirubinemia in near-term and term newborns. Pediatrics 2004;113:775–80.

[9] Klassen AF, Lee SK, Raina P, et al. Health status and health-related quality of life in a population-based sample of neonatal intensive care unit graduates. Pediatrics 2004;113:594–600.

[10] Jones JS, Istwan NB, Jacques D, et al. Is 34 weeks an acceptable goal for a complicated
singleton pregnancy? Manag Care 2002;11:42–7.

[11] Huddy CL, Johnson A, Hope PL. Educational and behavioral problems in babies of 32–35
weeks gestation. Arch Dis Child Fetal Neonatal Ed 2001;85:F23–8.

[12] Arnon S, Dolfin T, Litmanovitz I, et al. Preterm labour at 34–36 weeks of gestation: should
it be arrested? Paediatr Perinat Epidemiol 2001;15:252–6.

[13] Seubert DE, Stetzer BP, Wolfe HM, et al. Delivery of the marginally preterm infant: what are
the minor morbidities? Am J Obstet Gynecol 1999;81:1087–91.

[14] Alexander GR, Kogan M, Bader D, et al. US birth weight/gestational age-specific neonatal
mortality: 1995–1997 rates for whites, Hispanics, and blacks. Pediatrics 2003;111:e61–6.

[15] Kramer MS, Demissie K, Yang H, et al. The contribution of mild and moderate preterm
birth to infant mortality. Fetal and Infant Health Study Group of the Canadian Perinatal
Surveillance System. JAMA 2000;284:843–9.

[16] Martin JA, Hamilton BE, Sutton PD, et al. Births: final data for 2003. Natl Vital Stat Rep
2005;54(2):1–116.

[17] Thompson JMD, Irgens LM, Rasmussen S, et al. Secular trends in socioeconomic status and
the implications for preterm birth. Paediatr Perinat Epidemiol 2006;20:182–7.

[18] Langhoff-Roos J, Kesmodel U, Jacobsson B, et al. Spontaneous preterm delivery in primiparous women at low risk in Denmark: population-based study. BMJ 2006;332:937–9.

[19] Berhman RE, Butler AS, editors. Preterm birth: causes, consequences and prevention.
Washington (DC): Institute of Medicine of the National Academies; 2006.

[20] Prematurity Research Expansion and Education for Mothers who deliver Infants Early Act
or the 'PREEMIE Act'. [S.707.ES]. Available at: http://thomas.loc.gov/cgi-bin/query/
D?c109:2:./temp/~c109Wjiyqx. Accessed August 17, 2006.

[21] World Health Organization Expert Group on Prematurity. Final report on a meeting held in
Geneva, 12–21, April 1950. Geneva (Switzerland): WHO; 1950. p. 1–12.

[22] American Academy of Pediatrics and the American College of Obstetricians and Gynecologists. Guidelines for Perinatal Care. 5th edition. Elk Grove Village (IL); 2005.

[23] Engle WA. A recommendation for the definition of late preterm (near-term) and the birth
weight–gestational age classification system. Semin Perinatol 2006;30:2–7.

[24] Raju TNK, Higgins RD, Stark AR, et al. Optimizing care and outcome for late-preterm
(near-term) infants: a summary of the workshop sponsored by the NICHD. Pediatrics
2006;118:1207–14.

[25] Cunningham FG, Leveno KJ, Bloom SL, et al. Williams obstetrics. 22nd edition. New York:
McGraw-Hill; 2005.

[26] Davidoff MJ, Dias T, Damus K, et al. Changes in the gestational age distribution among US
singleton births: impact on rates of late preterm birth, 1992 to 2002. Semin Perinatol 2006;30:
8–15.

[27] Joseph KS, Demissie K, Kramer MS. Obstetric intervention, stillbirth, and preterm birth.
Semin Perinatol 2002;26:250–9.

[28] MacDorman MF, Mathews TJ, Martin JA, et al. Trends and characteristics of induced
labour in the United States, 1989–98. Paediatr Perinat Epidemiol 2002;16:263–73.

[29] National Center for Health Statistics. 2004 Preliminary birth data: maternal and infant
health. Available at: http://www.cdc.gov/nchs/products/pubs/pubd/hestat/highlights/2004/
prebirth.htm. Accessed August 19, 2006.

[30] Sibai BM. Preeclampsia as a cause of preterm and late preterm (near-term) births. Semin
Perinatol 2006;30:16–9.

[31] Hauth JC. Preterm labor and premature rupture of membranes: to deliver or not to deliver.
Semin Perinatol 2006;30:98–102.

[32] Hankins GDV, Longo M. The role of stillbirth prevention and late preterm (near-term)
births. Semin Perinatol 2006;30:20–3.

[33] Ananth CV, Joseph KS, Oyelese Y, et al. Trends in preterm birth and perinatal mortality among singletons: United States, 1989 through 2000. Obstet Gynecol 2005;105:1084–91.

[34] Ananth CV, Joseph KS, Kinzler WL. The influence of obstetric intervention on trends in twin stillbirths: United States, 1989–9. J Matern Fetal Neonatal Med 2004;15:380–7.

[35] Getahun D, Amre DK, Ananth CV, et al. Temporal changes in rates of stillbirth, neonatal and infant mortality among triplet gestations in the United States. Am J Obstet Gynecol 2006;2, in press.

[36] Ananth CV, Liu S, Kinzler WL, et al. Stillbirths in the United States, 1981–2000: an age, period, and cohort analysis. Am J Public Health 2005;95:2213–7.

[37] Feldman GB. Prospective risk of stillbirth. Obstet Gynecol 1992;79(4):547–53.

[38] Hannah ME, Hannah WJ, Hellmann J, et al. Induction of labor as compared with serial antenatal monitoring in post-term pregnancy. A randomized controlled trial. The Canadian multi-center Post-term Pregnancy Trial Group. N Engl J Med 1992;326:1587–92.

[39] Smith GC. Life table analysis of the risk of perinatal death at term and post-term in singleton pregnancies. Am J Obstet Gynecol 2001;184:489–96.

[40] ACOG Committee on Practice Bulletins-Obstetrics. Clinical management guidelines for obstetricians-gynecologists. Number 55, September 2004 (replaces practice pattern number 6, October 1997). Management of Post-term pregnancy. Obstet Gynecol 2004;104(3):639–46.

[41] Crane J. Induction of labour at term. Maternal–Fetal Medicine Committee, SOGC Practice Guidelines. Number 107. August 2001. Available at: http://www.sogc.org/guidelines/index_e.asp. Accessed September 3, 2006.

[42] Savitz DA, Terry JW Jr, Dole N, et al. Comparison of pregnancy dating by last menstrual period, ultrasound scanning, and their combination. Am J Obstet Gynecol 2002;187(6):1660–6.

[43] Taipale P, Hilesmaa V. Predicting deliver date by ultrasound and last menstrual period in early gestation. Obstet Gynecol 2001;97:189–94.

[44] Yang H, Kramer MS, Platt RW, et al. How does early ultrasound scan estimation of gestational age lead to higher rates of preterm birth? Am J Obstet Gynecol 2002;186(3):433–7.

[45] Kramer MS, McLean FH, Boyd ME, et al. The validity of gestational age estimation by menstrual dating in term, preterm and post-term gestation. JAMA 1988;26:3306–9.

[46] Joseph KS, Kramer MS, Marcoux S, et al. Determinants of preterm birth rates in Canada from 1981 through 1983 and from 1992 through 1994. N Engl J Med 1998;339(20):1434–9.

[47] Mathews TJ, Hamilton BE. Mean age of mother, 1970–2000. Natl Vital Stat Rep 2002;(51):1–13.

[48] Russell RB, Petrini JR, Damus K, et al. The changing epidemiology of multiple births in the United States. Obstet Gynecol 2003;101(1):129–35.

[49] Lee YM, Cleary-Goldman J, D'Alton ME. Multiple gestations and late preterm (near-term) deliveries. Semin Perinatol 2006;30:103–12.

[50] Hedley AA, Ogden CL, Johnson CL, et al. Prevalence of overweight and obesity among US children, adolescents, and adults, 1999–2002. JAMA 2004;291(23):2847–50.

[51] Rosenberg TJ, Garber S, Lipkind H, et al. Maternal obesity and diabetes as risk factors for adverse pregnancy outcomes: differences among 4 racial/ethnic groups. Am J Public Health 2005;95:1545–51.

[52] Leveno KJ. Optimizing care and long-term outcome of near-term pregnancy and near-term newborn infant. Available at: http://www.nichd.nih.gov/cdbpm/pp/PastMeetings/workshop_optimizing_agenda.htm. Accessed September 3, 2006.

[53] Kinney HC. The near-term (late preterm) human brain and risk for periventricular leukomalacia: a review. Semin Perinatol 2006;30:81–8.

CLINICS IN
PERINATOLOGY

Clin Perinatol 33 (2006) 765–776

Late Preterm Gestation: Physiology of Labor and Implications for Delivery

William J. Dobak, DO*,
Michael O. Gardner, MD, MPH

*Department of Gynecology and Obstetrics, Emory University School of Medicine,
Room 412, 66 Jesse Hill Junior Drive, Atlanta, GA 30303, USA*

The gestational ages known as near-term or late preterm represent about 75% of preterm births [1]. These infants range in gestational age from 34.0 to 36.6 weeks and are at greater risk of morbidity than term infants. The increasing rate of preterm deliveries in the United States is a growing concern. The rate has increased from 9.4% of live births in 2005 to nearly 13% today, and much of this increase is because of deliveries of 32- to 36-week fetuses. This group of neonates has an increased risk of respiratory distress syndrome, hypoglycemia, hypothermia, and hyperbilirubinemia. In addition, they have greater lengths of stays in neonatal intensive care units than term infants [2–5].

An increase from 5.8% to 7.0% in non-Hispanic white infants between 34 and 36 weeks from 1992 to 2002 helps explain the increase in preterm deliveries seen in that time frame, since most deliveries in the United States occur in non-Hispanic whites. During this same period, there was a decrease in the overall delivery rate of late preterm deliveries in non-Hispanic black women from 10.9% to 10.5% [6].

Historically, prematurity was defined based on a birth weight of 2500 g or less. This definition was chosen by the inaugural World Health Assembly in 1948. Later, it was noted by investigators that many preterm infants were being labeled as term simply because their weight was greater than 2500 g. Observations like those helped in developing a relationship between gestational age and birth weight. Lubchenco and Battaglia were among the first to develop a classification system for newborns based on gestational age

---

* Corresponding author.
E-mail address: wjdobak@aol.com (W.J. Dobak).

0095-5108/06/$ - see front matter © 2006 Elsevier Inc. All rights reserved.
doi:10.1016/j.clp.2006.09.001
perinatology.theclinics.com

and birth weight [7]. They defined nine distinct categories and assessed risk for perinatal mortality within each group [8].

The American College of Obstetricians and Gynecologists and the World Health Organization define prematurity as birth on or before the last day of the 37th week (259th day) following the onset of the last menstrual period. Term is delivery between the 260th day and the 294th day (first day of the 38th week to the last day of the 42nd week). Post-term is birth of an infant from the beginning of the first day of the 43rd week (295th day) after the start of the last menstrual period [9–11].

There has not been a consistent definition for late preterm delivery; however, many consider 34 completed weeks as when late preterm begins. Many obstetricians use 34 weeks as a milestone to discontinue steroids and tocolytics. In addition, patients with stable preterm premature rupture of membranes often are induced at this gestational age. This is also the period where neonatal ICU (NICU) admissions begin to fall. Almost all neonates born at 33 weeks are admitted to the NICU. This falls to 44% to 84% of infants born at 34 weeks [12–14]. Because of the high admission rate to the NICUs for late preterm infants, many advocate trying to avoid the phrase near term, because this gives the false impression of being mature.

Common causes of late preterm birth include:

- Preeclampsia
- Intrauterine growth restriction
- Preterm labor
- Multiple gestation

Causes of late preterm delivery

Preterm premature rupture of membranes

Preterm premature rupture of membranes (PPROM) is responsible for one third of all preterm deliveries. The pathophysiology of PPROM is multi-factorial and represents more than one pathophysiologic process occurring simultaneously. One major factor may be choriodecidual infection. Although this plays a larger role in PPROM at an earlier gestation, it also can be a factor in the late preterm pregnancy. Lower socioeconomic status, cigarette smoking, sexually transmitted infections, prior cervical surgery (conization or cerclage), uterine distension from multiple gestation or polyhydramnios, amniocentesis, and a history of vaginal bleeding also are implicated in PPROM [15].

The diagnosis of rupture of membranes is a clinical one based on a suspicious history and documentation by positive Nitrazine/positive ferning fluid passing from the cervix. Documentation of low fluid by ultrasound is also a helpful feature. Semen and blood may create a false-positive nitrazine test. Cervical mucus may make the fern test falsely positive, so the sample should be obtained from the posterior vaginal fornix or lateral vaginal sidewalls. A false-negative test may occur if there is prolonged leaking with only a small residual of fluid within the vagina. There are situations in which the testing may be equivocal, but the history and ultrasound findings are strongly suggestive of rupture of membranes. For these situations, the injection of indigo carmine by ultrasound-guided amnioinfusion is appropriate to make a definitive diagnosis.

Studies have shown an increased risk of infectious morbidity and a decreased latency with digital cervical examinations [16,17]. Therefore, it is suggested to avoid digital cervical examinations with the diagnosis of PPROM. Visual examination with the aid of a speculum can help estimate the cervical dilation. During the speculum examination, cultures should be obtained for *Chlamydia* and gonorrhea. An anovaginal culture for group B *Streptococcus* also should be obtained with the initial examination.

When PPROM occurs between 34 and 37 weeks, corticosteroids are not administered for fetal lung maturation. The National Institutes of Health Consensus Development Panel does not recommend the use of corticosteroids after 34 weeks. Mercer and colleagues [15] looked at 93 women with PPROM at 32 to 36 weeks gestation. All 93 women had confirmed fetal lung maturity and were randomized to either immediate delivery or expectant management. The authors found a significant increase in chorioamnionitis with the expectant management group (28% versus 11%, $P < .05$). A trend toward increased prevalence of sepsis also was noted. Naef and colleagues looked at conservative versus aggressive management of rupture of membranes during this gestation [18]. They found an increased risk of amnionitis with conservative management (16% versus 2%, $P = .001$). In addition, there was prolonged maternal hospitalization (5.2 versus 2.6 days, $P = .006$), and a lower mean umbilical cord pH at delivery (7.25 versus 7.35, $P = .009$). They did not find the benefit of a significant reduction of perinatal complications related to prematurity with the conservative management [18]. Therefore, expeditious delivery is recommended with preterm premature rupture of membranes after 34 weeks.

Multiple gestation

Multiple gestation is another important cause of late preterm delivery. The National Vital Statistics Report for 2003 showed a 67% increase in the rate of twins since 1980. There has been an increase of more than 500% in the same time period for triplets and higher order multiples [19,20]. Multiple gestations deliver in the late preterm gestational age range on average and have higher incidents of maternal and neonatal complications than their singleton counterparts.

In 2002, the mean age for delivery of twins was 35.3 weeks. The mean age was 32.2 weeks for triplets and 29.9 weeks for quadruplets [21]. The prevention of preterm delivery in multiples has been as challenging as the prevention of preterm delivery in singletons. The only therapies that have proven to work to decrease the adverse outcomes caused by prematurity are surfactant and corticosteroids. Newman and colleagues looked at prophylactic cerclage in a randomized trial with 128 patients with twins [22]. Those randomized to cerclage at 18 to 26 weeks did not have a lower preterm delivery rate [22]. This could mean that there are more factors than just cervical insufficiency when it comes to preterm delivery in multiples, or that cerclages in general do not work.

A Cochrane database review of six randomized trials, which included over 600 multiples, did not show any benefit from routine bed rest or early hospitalization for multiples [23]. In fact, there was a paradoxical increased risk of delivery at less than 34 weeks with bed rest. There also may be an increased risk of deep venous thrombosis and thromboembolic disease caused by the uterus obstructing venous return and sedentary activity [23].

Many late preterm deliveries occur for fetal/maternal indications with multiples. All major obstetric complications are seen with increased rates in multiples. Gestational diabetes, intrauterine growth retardation (IUGR), preeclampsia, abruption, hemorrhage, and low birth weight (LBW) can be seen in as many as 80% of multiples, while they may be seen in only 25% of singletons [24,25].

Monoamniotic twins make up less than 1% of monozygotic twins, and they may have a high perinatal mortality rate. Fetal mortality rates have been reported as high as 50%, but studies by Rodis and Allen put the mortality rate between 10% and 21%. Cord entanglement and cord accidents are common, and management of these pregnancies to prevent those complications is somewhat controversial. Some have argued for early hospitalization, at the point of viability, and delivery at 34 weeks if the pregnancy remains uncomplicated, with earlier delivery as indicated [26–29].

Twin–twin transfusion syndrome (TTTS) is another potential complication in monozygotic twins. TTTS is the uneven distribution of blood flow across the placenta shared by the two fetuses. Up to 15% to 20% of monochorionic twin pregnancies may develop this syndrome despite the fact that all monochorionic twins share some portion of their vasculature [25,27,28].

The diagnosis of TTTS is made by visualization of a single placenta, fetuses of the same gender, weight discordance, and differences in amniotic fluid surrounding the two fetuses. The twin receiving the extra blood will demonstrate signs of heart failure and hydrops consistent with fluid overload. The twin donating the blood would demonstrate signs consistent with a lack of blood, IUGR, and a stuck appearance. There are three treatment methods for TTTS. It should be stated that if found early enough, termination of the recipient twin or both twins may be offered. One treatment option that has been used the most is serial amnioreduction. Septostomy is another option, where a hole is created between the two amniotic sacs so that fluid may flow evenly between the two. The option one that shows the most promise is the selective fetoscopic coagulation of the communicating vessels. Three studies (two nonrandomized and one randomized) have shown a 71% to 83% survival of at least one twin with use of the fetoscopic surgery. In addition, lower rates of neurologic complications were shown when compared with serial amnioreduction. Without clear therapies, delivery late preterm remains an option [25,27–34].

There has been a lot of discussion of the utility of late preterm delivery for multiples. The logic behind the debate is that the risk of fetal death increases at an earlier gestational age for multiples than for singletons. Studies have shown that the prospective risk of fetal death for twins at 36 to 37 weeks is equivalent to that of post-term singletons. Another way to consider this debate is to analyze where the risks of neonatal death and fetal death intersect. For twins, this is at 39 weeks, but for triplets it is at 36 weeks. Using these data, some have advocated for late preterm delivery of multiples. Of course, the risks of prematurity need to be considered, and studies are not consistent in showing benefit of late preterm delivery [25,35–37].

Barigye and colleagues [36] evaluated the risk of fetal death in uncomplicated monochorionic twin pregnancies. There were 10 unexpected fetal deaths seen in the study, and these occurred during the late preterm period, with a median gestational age of 34 weeks and 1 day. Unfortunately, there were no antenatal markers such as IUGR or TTTS in these pregnancies with the intrauterine fetal demises (IUFDs) [36]. These authors suggested late preterm delivery of uncomplicated monochorionic twins might eliminate the increased risk of fetal death. Other authors have added that late preterm delivery at 34 to 35 weeks after the administration of corticosteroids and thorough counseling may be appropriate [25].

Preeclampsia

Preeclampsia affects 5% to 8% of singleton pregnancies. The rates for twins is 2 to 2.6 times higher. Although preeclampsia is generally a disease of later pregnancy, it occurs earlier in multiple gestations. Because no interventions have been shown to reduce or prevent the incidence of preeclampsia, delivery remains the only cure. The incidence of preterm delivery and placental abruption are also higher in multiple gestation pregnancies complicated by preeclampsia [25,38]. Davidson and colleagues also showed that women with multiple gestation are at increased risk of developing acute fatty liver of pregnancy [25].

There is an increased rate of intrauterine growth restriction with multiples, and there is also the risk of discordant growth with multiples. Discordant growth is defined as at least 20% difference in weight between fetuses as compared with the larger fetus. Fetal growth discordance may be seen in 15% of twins [39]. Risk factors for discordant growth include monochorionicity, velamentous cord insertion, antenatal bleeding, uteroplacental insufficiency, and gestational hypertension. Studies have not been consistent on the adverse outcomes of discordant growth [25,39,40]. Blickstein and colleagues reviewed more than 10,000 discordant twins and found neonatal mortality rates were 29 versus 11 per 1000 live births when the smaller twin was less than the 10th percentile compared with those above it [41]. A study from Amaru and colleagues suggests that 20% growth discordance may increase some adverse outcomes, but not for serious sequelae [42].

Another area of interest is the development of gestational hypertension–preeclampsia in the late preterm gestation. Because gestational hypertension–preeclampsia is seen in 6% to 10% of pregnancies, it is probably the most common medical complication of pregnancy. Additionally, its incidence is increasing with the changing demographics of women who are getting pregnant [43]. Women at greatest risk of developing maternal and perinatal complications are those with a history of prior pregnancy complicated by preeclampsia, those women with severe preeclampsia, women with pre-existing medical disorders, multi-fetal gestation, and those who develop gestational hypertension–preeclampsia before 35 weeks [44,45].

Delivery remains the only treatment for preeclampsia [46]. Delivery is recommended for all women who develop gestational hypertension–preeclampsia after 37 weeks. Delivery is recommended for all women who develop severe preeclampsia at or after 34 weeks [45]. Delivery is recommended at 35 to 37 weeks if gestational hypertension–preeclampsia is complicated by severe hypertension–preeclampsia, preterm labor or premature rupture of membranes, suspected intrauterine growth restriction with oligohydramnios, vaginal bleeding, or abnormal fetal testing that includes variable or late decelerations, absent or reverse umbilical artery diastolic flow, or a biophysical profile of no more than 6 [43]. These recommendations were made by considering the potential complications that could develop at this gestational age with expectant management [44,47].

Recommendations for late preterm delivery include:

- Delivery at 34 weeks for PPROM
- Corticosteroids before 34 weeks
- Avoid vacuum delivery before 35 weeks
- Need for accurate dating before elective cesarean delivery
- Notify pediatricians prior to delivery

Knuist, Hauth, and Sibai have evaluated the rates of preterm delivery in women who developed mild gestational hypertension [48,49]. The rates of preterm delivery did not exceed 7.0% in any of the studies. The rate of preterm delivery approaches 22% in women who develop recurrent preeclampsia. The difficulty with any of these studies is knowing whether the preterm delivery was spontaneous, caused by preterm rupture of membranes, or iatrogenic. The numbers from these studies were obtained from academic centers. Barton and colleagues found that 15% of women with mild gestational hypertension are delivered between 34 and 36 weeks when community hospitals are included [47]. The average length of hospitalization for these neonates was 5 days [46,48–50].

Sibai and colleagues reviewed the admissions to the NICU in the studies that looked at mild preeclampsia and found that there was a significantly higher percentage of admission to the NICU of term infants than there were inductions for preterm/late preterm preeclampsia. In the study by Hauth and colleagues, there was a 7.0% preterm delivery rate in those with mild hypertension, yet 18.2% admission rate to the NICU. Similar numbers were seen in the study by Sibai. This indicates that most admissions to the NICU were of term newborns. This could be in part because of the high induction rate resulting in high use of cervical ripening agents, prolonged labor with resultant development of chorioamnionitis, oxytocin use, nonreassuring fetal heart tracings, and increases cesarean delivery rates [46,48].

If the obstetrician is forced to deliver a late preterm infant, what is preferred method of delivery: spontaneous vaginal delivery, operative vaginal delivery, or cesarean delivery? US national statistics report 1 million fetal deaths per year, with 90% occurring in the first 20 weeks. Only 2% of fetal deaths occur beyond 28 weeks. Copper and colleagues have found a consistent rate of stillbirths between 23 and 40 weeks with a rate of 5% per week of gestation [51]. Froen and colleagues found a significant increase in both explained and unexplained IUFD starting around 36 to 37 weeks [52].

There are many causes of intrauterine fetal demise, and these can be broken into the large categories of congenital anomalies, infection, maternal injury, cord accidents and hemorrhage, and maternal medical conditions. Maternal medical conditions that increase the risk of stillbirth include hypertensive disorders, diabetes mellitus, obesity, lupus, chronic renal disease, thyroid disorders, and cholestasis of pregnancy [53].

Romero and colleagues found maternal age, maternal smoking, placental abruption, umbilical cord accidents, and multi-parity to be risk factors for stillbirth in their study population in Mexico [54]. They also found a significant reduction in stillbirth with antenatal care (odds ratio 0.1, confidence interval [CI] 0.08–0.4). It unfortunately is the case that 50% of stillbirths had a benign antenatal course and no identifiable risk factors. Petersson and colleagues found that 11.5% of intrauterine fetal demises, which most likely would not have been explained, were explained by infection with parvovirus, cytomegalovirus, or enterovirus with the use of polymerase chain reaction (PCR) [55].

Methods of delivery

Another area of interest in late preterm delivery is the use of vacuum extractors. Since vacuum extractors and forceps are used in about 10% of all deliveries, and vacuum extractors are used twice as often as forceps, it is important to know the risks [56,57].

The subgaleal hemorrhage is the major concern when using vacuum extractors. Subgaleal hemorrhage occurs when veins that bridge the subgaleal space are damaged, and blood accumulates in this subaponeurotic space.

There are no boundaries in this space, which allows blood to gather from the orbital ridges to the nape of the neck. This is an area with a potential space of several hundred milliliters [56–58].

Other complications associated with the use of vacuum extraction include retinal hemorrhage, cephalohematoma, intracranial hemorrhage (subdural, subarachnoid, intraventricular, and cerebral), subconjunctival hemorrhage, skull fracture, and large caput succedaneum. Because of the potential complications, the American College of Obstetricians and Gynecologists has published guidelines for the use of vacuum extractors. One of the relative contraindications is prematurity with a gestational age less than 37 weeks. An absolute contraindication is gestational age less than 34 weeks. Other contraindications include prior fetal scalp sampling and midpelvic delivery [56–58].

Some predisposing risk factors for complications associated with vacuum extractors include failed forceps application, use of vacuum greater than three times or duration more than 20 minutes, excessively applied suction pressure (500 to 600 mm Hg), fetal hemorrhagic diathesis, vacuum application over anterior fontanel, and fetal malpresentation [56–58].

Historically, some practitioners used a sequential approach with forceps and vacuums. Williams and colleagues did not find any significantly increased morbidity with use of forceps after vacuum or vacuum after forceps. Ezengau and colleagues also found that the sequential use of vacuum and forceps did not have higher rates of maternal or neonatal morbidity [59]. Studies by Castro and colleagues, Al-Kadri and colleagues, Towner and colleagues, and others, however, have shown increased fetal/neonatal complications when there is sequential use of forceps and vacuum extractors [60–62].

The question of mode of delivery for small neonates has been examined, but there is no clear consensus. Some studies seem to suggest that cesarean delivery may be beneficial for infants with birth weights less than 1000 g [63]. To date, there are no known studies that show a benefit to cesarean delivery over vaginal delivery for the late preterm infant [64–70]. Therefore, it remains the recommendation to perform cesarean delivery for standard indications in the late preterm group.

Summary

The late preterm gestation is an area that has seen an increase in deliveries for multiple reasons. Although the mortality rate for these deliveries is quite low, there is still an increase in cost because of extended nursery stay and supportive care. Nevertheless, when indicated, delivery in this gestational age range may be preferable in cases of PPROM or severe preeclampsia. Because of the substantial perinatal morbidity associated with this gestation, further randomized studies need to be done.

References

[1] Martin JA, Hamilton BE, Sutton PD, et al. Births: final data for 2003. Natl Vital Stat Rep 2005;54(2):1–116.

[2] Gilbert WM, Nesbitt TS, Danielson B. The cost of prematurity: quantification by gestational age and birth weight. Obstet Gynecol 2003;102:488–92.

[3] Wang ML, Dorer DJ, Fleming MP, et al. Clinical outcomes of near-term infants. Pediatrics 2004;114:372–6.

[4] Sarici SU, Serdar MA, Korkmaz A, et al. Incidence, course, and prediction of hyperbilirubinemia in near-term and term newborns. Pediatrics 2004;113:775–80.

[5] Jones JS, Istwan NB, Jacques D, et al. Is 34 weeks an acceptable goal for a complicated singleton pregnancy? Manage Care 2002;11:42–7.

[6] Davidoff MJ, Dias T, Damus K, et al. Changes in the gestational age distribution among US singleton births: impact on rates of late preterm birth, 1992 to 2002. Semin Perinatol 2005:8–15.

[7] Battaglia FC, Lubchenco LO. A practical classification of newborn infants by weight and gestational age. J Pediatr 1967;71:159–63.

[8] Drillien CM. The low-birth-weight infants. In: Cockburn F, Drillien CM, editors. Neonatal medicine. Onsey Mead (Australia): Blackwell Scientific Publications; 1974. p. 51–61.

[9] World Health Organization. International statistical classification of diseases and related health problems. Geneva (Switzerland): World Health Organization; 1992.

[10] World Health Organization. Available at http://www.who.int/reproductive-health.

[11] American Academy of Pediatrics. ACOG: standard terminology for reporting of reproductive health statistics in the United States. In: Guidelines for perinatal care. 5th edition. Elk Grove (IL): American Academy of Pediatrics and American College of Obstetricians and Gynecologists; 2002. p. 377–94.

[12] Escobar GJ. Respiratory problems in near-term infants: is it TTN, RDS, pneumonia, or PPHN? Presented at the NIH Consensus Conference: Optimizing Care and Long-Term Outcome of Near-Term Pregnancy and Near-Term Newborn Infants. Bethesda (MD), July 18–19, 2005.

[13] Rubaltelli FF, Bonafe L, Tangucci M, et al. Epidemiology of neonatal acute respiratory disorders. A multi-center study on incidence and fatality rates of neonatal acute respiratory disorders according to gestational age, maternal age, pregnancy complications and type of delivery. Italian Group of Neonatal Pneumology. Biol Neonate 1998;74:7–15.

[14] Engle W. A recommendation for the definition of late preterm (near-term) and the birth weight–gestational age classification system. Semin Perinatol 2006;30(1):2–7.

[15] Mercer BM. Preterm premature rupture of the membranes. Obstet Gynecol 2003;101: 178–93.

[16] Lewis DF, Major CA, Towers CV, et al. Effects of digital cervical examination on expectantly managed preterm rupture of membranes. Obstet Gynecol 1992;80:630–4.

[17] Alexander JM, Mercer BM, Miodovnik M, et al. The impact of digital cervical examination on expectantly managed preterm rupture of membranes. Am J Obstet Gynecol 2000;183: 1003–7.

[18] Naef RW III, Allbert JR, Ross EL, et al. Premature rupture of membranes at 34 to 37 weeks' gestation: aggressive versus conservative management. Am J Obstet Gynecol 1998;178: 126–30.

[19] Ananth CV, Joseph KS, Smulian JC. Trends in twin neonatal mortality rates in the United States, 1989 through 1999: influence of birth registration and obstetric intervention. Am J Obstet Gynecol 2004;190:1313–21.

[20] Luke B. The changing pattern of multiple births in the United States: maternal and infant characteristics, 1973 and 1990. Obstet Gynecol 1994;84:101–6.

[21] Martin JA, Hammilton BE, Sutton PD, et al. Births: final data for 2002. Natl Vital Stat Rep 2002;52:1–113.

[22] Newman RB, Krombach RS, Myers MC, et al. Effect of cerclage on obstetric outcome in twin gestations with a shortened cervical length. Am J Obstet Gynecol 2002;186: 634–40.

[23] Crowther CA. Hospitalization and bed rest for multiple pregnancy. Cochrane Database Syst Rev 2001;1:CD000110.

[24] Norwitz ER, Valentine E, Park JS. Maternal physiology and complications of multiple pregnancy. Semin Perinatol 2005;29:338–48.

[25] Lee YM, Cleary-Goldman J, D'Alton ME. Multiple Gestations and Late preterm (near-term) deliveries. Semin Perinatol 2006:103–22.

[26] Norwitz ER, Valentine E, Park JS. Maternal physiology and complications of multiple pregnancy. Semi Perinatol 2005;29:338–48.

[27] Carr SR, Aronson MP, Coustan DR. Survival rates of monoamniotic twins do not decrease after 30 weeks' gestation. Am J Obstet Gynecol 1990;163:719–22.

[28] Rodis JF, McIlveen PF, Egan JF, et al. Monoamniotic twins: improved perinatal survival with accurate prenatal diagnosis and antenatal fetal surveillance. Am J Obstet Gynecol 1997;177:1046–9.

[29] Allen VM, Windrim R, Barrett J, et al. Management of monoamniotic twin pregnancies: a case series and systematic review of the literature. Br J Obstet Gynaecol 2001;108:931–6.

[30] Hecher K, Plath H, Bregenzer T, et al. Endoscopic laser surgery versus serial amniocenteses in the treatment of severe twin-twin transfusion syndrome. Am J Obstet Gynecol 1999;180: 717–24.

[31] Quintero RA, Dickinson JE, Morales WJ, et al. Stage-based treatment of twin–twin transfusion syndrome. Am J Obstet Gynecol 2003;188:1333–40.

[32] Senat MV, Deprest J, Boulvain M, et al. Endoscopic laser surgery versus serial amnioreduction for severe twin-to-twin transfusion syndrome. N Engl J Med 2004;351:136–44.

[33] Malone FD, Dalton ME. Anomalies peculiar to multiple gestations. Clin Perinatol 2000;27: 1033–46.

[34] Quintero RA, Morales WJ, Allen MH, et al. Staging of twin–twin transfusion syndrome. J Perinatol 1999;19:550–5.

[35] Kahn B, Lumey LH, Zybert PA, et al. Prospective risk of fetal death in singleton, twin, and triplet gestations: implications for practice. Obstet Gynecol 2003;102:685–92.

[36] Barigye O, Pasquini L, Galea P, et al. High risk of unexpected late fetal death in monochorionic twins despite intensive ultrasound surveillance: a cohort study. PloS Med 2005;2(6): e172.

[37] Lee YM, Cleary-Goldman J, D'Alton ME. Multiple Gestations and late preterm (near-term) deliveries. Semin Perinatol 2006:103–12.

[38] Sibai BM, Hauth J, Caritis S, et al. Hypertensive disorders in twins versus singleton gestations. National Institute of Child Health and Human Development Network of Maternal–Fetal Medicine Units. Am J Obstet Gynecol 2000;182:938–42.

[39] Demissie K, Ananth CV, Martin J, et al. Fetal and neonatal mortality among twin gestations in the United States: the role of intrapair birth weight discordance. Obstet Gynecol 2002;100: 474–80.

[40] Gonzalez-Quintero VH, Luke B, OSullivan MJ, et al. Antenatal factors associated with significant birth weight discordancy in twin gestations. Am J Obstet Gynecol 2003;189: 813–7.

[41] Blickstein I, Keith LG. Neonatal mortality rates among growth-discordant twins, classified according to the birth weight of the smaller twin. Am J Obstet Gynecol 2004;190: 170–4.

[42] Amaru RC, Bush MC, Berkowitz RL, et al. Is discordant growth in twins an independent risk factor for adverse neonatal outcome? Obstet Gynecol 2004;103(1):71–6.

[43] Sibai BM. Diagnosis and management of gestational hypertension-preeclampsia. Obstet Gynecol 2003;102:181–92.

[44] Sibai BM, Caritis S, Hauth J. What we have learned about preeclampsia. Semin Perinatol 2003;27:230–46.

[45] Sibai BM, Dekker G, Kupfermine M. Preeclampsia. Lancet 2005;365:785–99.

[46] Sibai BM. Preeclampsia as a cause of preterm and late preterm (near-term) births. Semin Perinatol 2006;30:16–9.

[47] Barton JR, O'Brien JM, Bergauer NK, et al. Mild gestational hypertension remote from term: progression and outcome. Am J Obstet Gynecol 2001;184:879–83.

[48] Knuist M, Bonsel GJ, Treffers PE. Intensification of fetal and maternal surveillance in pregnant women with hypertensive disorders. Int J Gynecol Obstet 1998;61:127–34.

[49] Sibai BM, Caritis S, Hauth J, et al. Hypertensive disorders in twin versus singleton gestations. Am J Obstet Gynecol 2000;182:934–42.

[50] Hnat MD, Sibai B, Caritis S, et al. Perinatal outcome in women with recurrent preeclampsia compared with women who develop preeclampsia as nulliparas. Am J Obstet Gynecol 2002; 186:422–6.

[51] Copper RL, Goldenberg RL, Dubard MB, et al, Collaborative Group on Preterm Birth Prevention, Risk factors for fetal death in white, black, and Hispanic women. Obstet Gynecol 1994;84:490–5.

[52] Froen F, Arnestad M, Frey K, et al. Risk factors for sudden intrauterine unexplained death epidemiologic characteristics of singleton cases in Oslo, Norway, 1986–1995. Am J Obstet Gynecol 2001;184:694–702.

[53] Hankins GD, Longo M. The role of stillbirth prevention and late preterm (near-term) births. Semin Perinatol 2006;30:20–3.

[54] Romero Gutierrez G, Martinez Ceja CA, Ponce Ponce de Leon AL, et al. Risk factors for stillbirth [Spanish]. Ginecol Obstet Mex

[55] Petersson K, Norbeck O, Westgren M, et al. Detection of parvovirus B19, cytomegalovirus and enterovirus infections in cases of intrauterine fetal death. J Perinat Med 2004; 32:516–21.

[56] American College of Obstetricians and Gynecologists. Delivery by vacuum extraction. ACOG Committee on Obstetric Practice. Committee Opinion. Number 208, September 1998.

[57] American College of Obstetricians and Gynecologists. Operative vaginal delivery. ACOG Practice Bulletin 2000;17.

[58] Modanlou HD. Neonatal subgaleal hemorrhage following vacuum extraction delivery. The Internet Journal of Pediatrics and Neonataology.

[59] Ezenagu LC, Kakaria R, Bofill JA. Sequential use of instruments at operative vaginal delivery: is it safe? Am J Obstet Gynecol 1999;180:1446–9.

[60] Castro MA, Hoey SD, Towner D. Controversies in the use of the vacuum extractor. Semin Perinatol 2003;27:46–53.

[61] Al-Kadri H, Sabr Y, Al-Saif S, et al. Failed individual and sequential instrumental vaginal delivery: contributing risk factors and maternal-neonatal complications. Acta Obstet Gynecol Scand 2003;82:642–8.

[62] Towner D, Castro MA, Eby-Wilkens E, et al. Effect of mode of delivery in nulliparous women on neonatal intracranial injury. N Engl J Med 1999;341:1709–14.

[63] Deulofeut R, Sola A, Lee B, et al. The impact of vaginal delivery in premature infants weighing less than 1251 grams. Obstet Gynecol 2005;105:525–31.

[64] Grant A, Glazener C. Elective cesarean section versus expectant management for delivery of the small baby. Cochrane Database Syst Rev 2004.

[65] American College of Obstetricians and Gynecologists. Diagnosis and management of preeclampsia and eclampsia. ACOG Practice Bulletin 2002;33.

[66] Hsieh HL, Lee KS, Knoshnood B, et al. Fetal death rate in the United States, 1979–1990: trend and racial disparity. Obstet Gynecol 1997;89:33–9.

[67] Martin JA, Hoyert DL. The national fetal death file. Semin Perinatol 2002;26:3–11.

[68] Goldenberg RL, Kirby R, Culhane JF. Stillbirth: a review. J Matern Fetal Neonatal Med 2004;16:79–94.
[69] Weersekera DS, Premaratne S. A randomized prospective trial of the obstetric forceps versus vacuum extraction using defined criteria. J Obstet Gynaecol 2002;22:344–5.
[70] Gardella C, Taylor M, Beneditti T, et al. The effect of sequential use of vacuum and forceps for assisted vaginal delivery on neonatal and maternal outcome. Am J Obstet Gynecol 2001; 185:896–902.

CLINICS IN
PERINATOLOGY

Clin Perinatol 33 (2006) 777–792

The Impact of Multiple Gestations on Late Preterm (Near-Term) Births

Young Mi Lee, MD*, Jane Cleary-Goldman, MD,
Mary E. D'Alton, MD

*Department of Obstetrics and Gynecology, Division of Maternal-Fetal Medicine, Columbia
University Medical Center, 622 West 168th Street, New York, NY 10032, USA*

Multiple pregnancies currently comprise 3% of all live births in the United States but are responsible for an estimated 17% of all preterm births, more than 25% of very low birth weight (VLBW) infants, and nearly 20% of neonatal deaths [1]. The high-risk nature of these gestations is reflected in this disparity. Recent decades have seen a rise in the number of twins and high-order multiple gestations, attributed in large part to the increasing numbers of older mothers and use of assisted conception. Most twins and high-order multiples deliver during the late preterm period between 34 $^{0/7}$ through 36 $^{6/7}$ weeks [2]. Neonates delivered in the late preterm gestation account for approximately 70% of all premature births and are the fastest growing subgroup of premature infants [3]. Infants born during these gestational ages remain exposed to risks such as respiratory complications, temperature instability, hypoglycemia, kernicterus, feeding problems, neonatal ICU admissions, and adverse neurologic sequelae including cerebral palsy [4]. The impact of multiples on late preterm prematurity is therefore an important public health challenge.

Multiple gestations and late preterm births

The twinning rate in 2003 was 31.5 twin births per 1000 total live births, a national record representing a 67% rise since 1980 [1]. More impressive, the numbers of triplets and high-order multiples have increased more than 500% over the same time period [1]. Preterm delivery at less than 37 completed weeks is presently the leading cause of hospitalization among

---

* Corresponding author.
E-mail address: yml2102@columbia.edu (Y.M. Lee).

0095-5108/06/$ - see front matter © 2006 Elsevier Inc. All rights reserved.
doi:10.1016/j.clp.2006.09.008 *perinatology.theclinics.com*

pregnant women and the second leading cause of infant death [5]. Multiple births contribute significantly to this problem of prematurity. Although the rate of late preterm births is uncertain, the incidence of preterm births from 32 through 36 completed weeks (often referred to as moderately premature) stratified by plurality is available from 2002 statistics (Fig. 1). The mean age at delivery for singletons is 38.8 weeks but 35.3 weeks for twins, 32.2 weeks for triplets, and 29.9 weeks for quadruplets (Table 1) [2]. The long-term outcomes for neonates born in the late preterm period are generally favorable, especially when compared with those born at the threshold of viability. Despite medical advances, however, a significant number of prematurity problems persist through late preterm period, including neonatal respiratory complications, low birth weight (LBW), and neurologic handicap [4]. In addition, conditions unique to multiples such as monochorionicity continue to place these fetuses at higher risk for adverse perinatal outcomes. Each pregnancy involves more than one fetus, and therefore delivery impacts more than one neonate. Finally, prematurity may result from either spontaneous preterm labor or iatrogenic intervention for obstetrical complications or a condition affecting one fetus.

Perinatal morbidity and mortality

In 2002, the latest year for which data are available, nearly one of every five neonatal deaths were born in a multiple delivery [1,2]. The two most important contributors to this increased mortality in twin gestations appear to be increased rates of prematurity and complications of monochorionicity. Some of the primary neonatal concerns seen in late preterm deliveries are

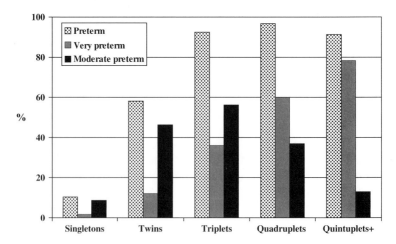

Fig. 1. Preterm birthrates by plurality. *Preterm* is less than 37 completed weeks of gestation. *Very preterm* is less than 32 completed weeks. *Moderate preterm* is 32 through 36 completed weeks. (*Adapted from* Martin JA, Hamilton BE, Sutton PD, et al. Births: final data for 2002. Natl Vital Stat Rep 2002;52(10):22.)

Table 1
Multiples and preterm births

Characteristic	Singletons	Twins	Triplets
Average gestational age at delivery (weeks) [2]	38.8	35.3	32.2
Preterm births from 32 through 36 completed weeks (%)[a] [2]	8.8	46.3	56.3
Low birthweight (%) [2]	6.1	55.4	94.4
Gestational age when prospective risk of fetal death intersects neonatal death rate (weeks)[b] [64]	—	39	36

Low birthweight is <2500 g.
[a] Compares with late preterm births (34 through 36 completed weeks).
[b] Not stratified by chorionicity.

respiratory complications such as transient tachypnea of the newborn, respiratory distress syndrome, and persistent pulmonary hypertension [6,7]. Monochorionic placentations are observed in approximately 20% of all twin pregnancies, and roughly 15% are affected by vascular anastomoses resulting in twin-twin transfusion syndrome (TTTS) [8]. In monochorionic twins, single intrauterine fetal demise (IUFD) can be associated with a coincident insult to the surviving cotwin, resulting in cerebral white matter damage. Triplets and high-order multiples present more complex clinical scenarios as the proportion and degree of premature births rise. Knowledge regarding these pregnancies remains limited, as much of the literature is limited by small sample sizes and noncontemporary data [9,10].

Low birth weight

LBW (less than 2500 g) is found more commonly in neonates of multiple pregnancies compared with singletons. This often becomes a concern antenatally during the late preterm period. Twenty-four percent of LBW infants are born from multiples [11]. The mean birth weight is 3332 g for singletons, 2347 g for twins, 1687 g for triplets, and 1309 g for quadruplets [2]. Matched by gestational age at delivery, plurality does not appear to alter birth weight significantly [12]. Average birth weights are similar for triplets, twins, and singletons until 29 weeks for triplets and 32 weeks for twins, when the differences observed are generally because of the smaller twin's weight [13]. Very LBW infants are 100 times more likely to die before 1 year of age than heavier infants weighing at least 2500 g at birth [1]. Therefore, LBW can contribute significantly to the neonatal morbidity and mortality associated with multiple births and late preterm prematurity, as lagging fetal growth often becomes a concern during this period.

Neurologic outcome

Fetal plurality has been associated with adverse neonatal neurologic outcomes. Infants from a multiple pregnancy have a 4 to 17 times higher risk of developing cerebral palsy compared with their singleton counterparts

[11,13,14]. Prematurity and plurality are independent risk factors for cerebral palsy, but the contribution of multiples appears more significant at higher birth weights. One epidemiologic study from Japan estimated the risks of producing at least one child with cerebral palsy were 1.5%, 8.0%, and 42.9% in twin, triplet, and quadruplet pregnancies, respectively [15]. Although a portion of these cases are because of higher rates of prematurity, other risk factors for cerebral palsy are seen with higher frequency in multiples including bleeding in pregnancy, maternal hypertensive disease, LBW infants, and congenital anomalies [14]. Current literature is conflicting on the correlation between birth order and gender with long-term neurologic impairment [14].

In utero fetal demise of one member of a monochorionic twin gestation may be associated with a greater than 20% risk for multi-cystic encephalomalacia in the surviving cotwin [16]. The incidence of cerebral palsy in cases of a cotwin IUFD ranges from 4 to 15 times higher than when both twins survive [14,17,18,]. A follow-up of 613 twin pregnancies with one IUFD found an overall 83 per 1000 prevalence of cerebral palsy in the live-born cotwin, a 40-fold increase over the background population prevalence [19]. Although neonatal gender was used as a surrogate for zygosity, the prevalence of cerebral palsy was 106 per 1000 in concordant sex twins and 29 per 1000 for discordant sex twins, thus suggesting a much greater risk for neurologic impairment with monochorionic placentation [19]. A recent systematic review of 28 studies by Ong and colleagues found the risk of cotwin demise following the death of one twin to be 12% (95% confidence interval [CI] 7% to 11%) and 4% (95% CI 2% to 7%) for monochorionic and dichorionic placentations, respectively [20]. The risk of neurologic abnormality in the surviving cotwin was 18% (95% CI 11% to 26%) for monochorionic pregnancies and 1% (95% CI 0% to 7%) for dichorionic gestations [20]. A higher risk for adverse neurologic outcomes has been observed in monochorionic twins unaffected by IUFD as compared with dichorionic twins, but this topic remains controversial [14]. Factors implicated include marginal cord insertion, intrauterine growth retardation (IUGR), fetal growth discordance, preterm rupture of membranes, and mode of delivery [14].

Potential indications for late preterm delivery

Of late preterm births in multiples, a considerable portion are iatrogenic because of interventions for maternal or fetal indications rather than spontaneous preterm labor. Expectant mothers of multiples are almost six times more likely to be hospitalized for obstetrical complications such as preterm labor, premature rupture of membranes, IUGR, or placental abruption, or maternal complications including preeclampsia and gestational hypertensive diseases [11]. Many of these problems manifest during the gestational weeks before term, thus serving as common indications for delivery during the late preterm period.

Maternal and obstetric complications

Compared with 25% of singleton gestations, over 80% of multiple pregnancies develop complications antenatally, including a substantial number of maternal conditions [21]. Examples of potential adverse complications affecting multi-fetal gestations include preeclampsia, gestational hypertension, and placental abruption [11,22–24]. Women carrying multi-fetal pregnancies seem prone to developing acute fatty liver of pregnancy, one of the most serious maternal obstetrical complications [25]. This disease is characterized by hepatic dysfunction, severe coagulopathy, hypoglycemia, and hyperammonemia, potentially resulting in fetal or maternal death.

Preeclampsia and its related spectrum of diseases occur in an estimated 5% to 8% of singleton pregnancies, but the incidence is higher in multiples and often manifests in the late preterm period [26,27]. Hypertensive diseases during pregnancy may manifest as hemolysis, elevated liver enzymes, and low platelets (HELLP) syndrome or eclampsia and can be associated with adverse sequelae such as IUGR, placental abruption, renal failure, disseminated intravascular coagulation, and IUFD. Fetal plurality increases the risk for hypertensive diseases of pregnancy, the severity of disease, and the risk for adverse perinatal outcomes such as preterm delivery [28]. In one study of comparing 9593 multiple gestations with 24,781 singleton gestations, the incidence of pregnancy-related hypertensive conditions was 6.5% for singletons, 12.7% for twins, 20% for triplets, and 19.6% for quadruplets [28]. The overall incidence of hypertensive diseases, however, more commonly is quoted higher, at 12% to 22% of pregnancies [26]. Overall for twins, the rates are estimated to be 2 to 2.6 higher compared with singletons and appear similar for monozygotic versus dizygotic gestations [27–29]. Preeclampsia in triplets and higher-order multiples occurs more often during the late preterm gestation, with more severity, and in an atypical presentation than singletons [22,30].

Fetal complications

Intrauterine growth retardation and growth discordance

A multitude of factors influence neonatal birth weight such as gestational age, ethnicity, nutrition, teratogenic exposure, and genetic composition. Uncomplicated twins appear to grow at the same rate as singletons up to 30 to 32 weeks and then somatic growth rate decreases. Long associated with perinatal morbidity and mortality, IUGR remains a statistical diagnosis consisting of a sonographically estimated fetal weight (EFW) no more than the 10th percentile for gestational age [31]. Adverse outcomes of IUGR appear limited primarily to neonates being severely growth-restricted with birth weights below the 5th percentile. Other adverse outcomes include hypoglycemia, hyperbilirubinemia, hypothermia, apneic episodes, seizures, sepsis, stillbirth, and neonatal death [31]. Long-term outcomes are related to the etiology of growth disturbance, and studies demonstrate a twofold increased incidence of cerebral dysfunction ranging from minor learning disability to cerebral palsy in IUGR infants delivered at term and an even higher incidence for preterm infants, a common occurrence for multiples [14]. Multifetal pregnancies present a dilemma in diagnosis and management of IUGR; for example, suspected normally grown fetuses may be affected by iatrogenic preterm delivery secondary to interventions for a growth-restricted cotwin. Current management of IUGR is focused on early diagnosis, efforts in determining the underlying cause, and fetal surveillance to aid in timing delivery, often occurring in the late preterm period.

Like IUGR, growth discordance frequently occurs in multiples. The exact threshold of discordant growth most strongly associated with adverse neonatal outcomes is debatable, but the term generally refers to at least a 20% difference in EFW between fetuses of the same pregnancy expressed as a percentage of the larger EFW [32]. Fetal growth discordance is diagnosed in approximately 15% of twins, and like IUGR, it is associated with an increased risk for perinatal complications [33]. Risk factors include monochorionicity, velamentous cord insertion, fetal malformations, and gestational hypertensive disease [34]. For multiple gestations, uteroplacental insufficiency or unequal sharing remains a commonly attributed factor for IUGR and growth discordance and accentuates the heightened concern when either is found in monochorionic twins. Of discordant twin pairs, approximately two thirds have a smaller twin with a birth weight of less than the 10th percentile [35]. The significance of growth discordant twins in the absence of IUGR remains debatable, with some studies demonstrating an increased risk for perinatal morbidity, while others not demonstrating an increased risk [35,36]. Because of the conflicting studies regarding growth discordance and adverse neonatal outcomes, multiple gestations should be followed closely with serial growth scans, as ultrasound is currently the most accurate method for assessing fetal growth.

Monoamnionicity

Less than one percent of monozygotic twins are monoamniotic [8]. Monoamniotic twins have been associated with a high rate of perinatal mortality, with some older studies reporting a rate greater than 50%, and more recent studies indicating a range of 10% to 21% [37–39]. Preterm delivery, IUGR, congenital anomalies, cord entanglement, and cord accidents are common in monoamniotic placentations. Because cord compression remains a primary concern and may be indicated by variable decelerations, the preferred method of testing is the nonstress test rather than the biophysical profile. Balancing the risk of IUFD at any gestational age and risks of prematurity, early delivery in the late preterm period is advocated by some experts and rejected by others [40,41]. The authors' current practice for monoamniotic twins includes routine hospitalization beginning at 24 to 26 weeks, daily nonstress tests, and if uncomplicated, offering delivery at 34 weeks after corticosteroids and thorough counseling of the risks and benefits of late preterm delivery (Box 1). The management of these pregnancies remains controversial, however, particularly regarding the optimal protocol for antenatal surveillance and timing of delivery.

Twin-twin transfusion syndrome

Almost exclusively found in monochorionic placentation, TTTS is characterized by an unequal distribution of the blood flow across the shared placenta of two fetuses. The net effect of this hemodynamic imbalance is a large, plethoric recipient twin and a small, anemic donor twin. Although all monochorionic twins share a portion of their vasculature, approximately 15% will develop this condition [8,42]. Left untreated, there can be up to 60% to 100% mortality rate for both twins.

Treatment options depend on the severity and gestational age at diagnosis [42,43]. Patients with early-onset TTTS may decide on selective termination of one twin (usually the donor twin) or voluntary termination of the entire pregnancy. Management in the late second or third trimesters may be less aggressive depending on disease severity and the proximity to term. Current treatments for severe cases include serial amnioreduction, septostomy, or selective fetoscopic laser coagulation of the communicating vessels. Advocates of laser ablation of the anastomotic vessels have argued that other interventions do not treat the underlying condition. At least three studies comparing both techniques have demonstrated endoscopic surgery

---

Box 1. Suggested protocol for the management of monoamniotic twins by trimester

First trimester
- Early identification of amnionicity, chorionicity, and number of fetuses
- Nuchal translucency at 10 to 14 weeks gestation (optimally at 11 weeks)

Second trimester
- Anatomical survey and fetal echocardiogram at approximately 20 weeks
- Hospital admission and intensive fetal surveillance from time of viability (24 to 26 weeks) including daily nonstress tests
- Serial ultrasounds for growth every 4 weeks (intensified if there is evidence of fetal growth abnormalities)

Third trimester
- Early counseling regarding risks of cord accidents and complications of late preterm birth
- If variable decelerations present, continuous fetal heart rate monitoring
- Deliver if fetal testing is nonreassuring

results in lower mortality rates (with the survival of at least one twin in 71% to 83% of procedures) and lower rates of neurologic complications than serial amnioreduction [44–46]. In the prospective Eurofetus trial, 142 women with severe TTTS identified before 26 weeks gestation were randomized to the two therapies and showed a significant benefit in the laser group with improved perinatal survival (76% versus 51% at 6 months of age, $P = .002$) and short-term neurologic outcome (52% versus 31%, $P = .003$) [46]. Many answers, however, remain elusive, such as which patients will benefit most from each therapy, the prediction of affected twins, the optimal therapy for mild disease, and the long-term cardiac and neurodevelopmental outcomes. In the absence of a clear therapy for conditions such as mild or late-onset TTTS, delivery in the late preterm period remains one option to avoid disease progression or fetal demise.

Prevention of preterm delivery in multiples

Spontaneous preterm birth remains the primary adverse outcome for multiples. A reliable and effective therapy to deter spontaneous preterm labor, however, has not been found. Cerclage, routine bed rest, prophylactic hospitalization, and ambulatory home uterine monitoring have had a disappointing impact on the problem. Many of the currently used management strategies have potentially serious maternal risks and contribute to the high costs of prenatal care. Although antenatal steroid administration has not been studied specifically in multiple gestations, the National Institutes of Health recommends that all women in preterm labor who have no contraindications be given one course of steroids regardless of the number of fetuses [47].

Prophylactic cervical cerclage has not been effective in preventing prematurity or improving outcomes in twins or triplets [48,49]. A recent meta-analysis of randomized control trials of cerclage placed for women with a sonographically short cervical length included three trials of 49 twins [50]. In this subgroup analysis, prophylactic cerclage was associated with higher rates of premature birth and perinatal mortality than those without a cerclage [50]. Although the findings are concerning, the small sample size limits any definitive conclusions. The surgical procedure does carry potential risks for the mother and her fetuses. Therefore, it should be reserved for those individuals with a history clearly consistent with or objectively determined to be cervical incompetence. More studies are needed, in particular a large prospective, randomized trial of cerclage focused on multiples.

Prophylactic bed rest and reduced physical activity are the most commonly prescribed therapies for multiples. That this may decrease uterine activity conceptually makes common sense to patients and their physicians. Studies, however, do not demonstrate any significant benefit from routine bed rest or early hospitalization in multiples [11,51]. A Cochrane database review of six randomized trials involving in-patient bed rest for over 600 multiples demonstrated a trend toward a decrease in LBW infants and a paradoxical increased risk of delivery at less than 34 weeks gestation [52]. These interventions are not without risks. Sedentary physical activity and an enlarged uterus mechanically obstructing venous return may contribute to theoretical increased risk for thromboembolic disease. In addition, prophylactic bed rest and early hospitalization are expensive and potentially disruptive to families.

Prophylactic administration of various tocolytic agents such as magnesium sulfate and beta adrenergic agents are common, but their futility has been frustrating. Enthusiasm for these medications should be tempered with caution and judiciousness as in any patient, but especially for women carrying multiples. These patients appear particularly prone to developing pulmonary edema and cardiovascular complications because of higher blood volume and lower colloid osmotic pressure [21,53]. As such, it is prudent to restrict the use of tocolytic medications in women confirmed to be in preterm labor.

Home monitoring of uterine contractions with a tocodynamometer was conceived in an attempt to predict early preterm labor in an ambulatory setting. A meta-analysis of six randomized trials, however, was unable to demonstrate a significant benefit in the reduction of preterm delivery for twins [54]. A prospective trial of over 2400 patients (including 844 twins) randomized women to weekly nurse contact, daily nurse contact, or daily nurse contact in addition to home uterine activity monitoring. The trial demonstrated no difference in preterm delivery before 35 weeks gestation [55].

The strategies mentioned previously have failed to prevent preterm delivery in multiples, but one therapy has demonstrated promise in singletons. In the singleton population at high risk for preterm birth, weekly injections of 17 alpha-hydroxyprogesterone caproate (17P) have been shown to reduce the rate of recurrent preterm delivery by approximately one third compared with those receiving placebo (36.3% versus 54.9%) [56]. Extrapolations have been theorized, as some have suggested that this supplementation could also prevent rates of preterm birth in multiple gestations. Therefore, a large, multi-center National Institute of Child Health and Human Development Maternal Fetal Medicine Units (MFMU) Network randomized trial was completed recently to test this hypothesis. Named STTARS for Seventeen alpha-hydroxyprogesterone caproate for Twins and Triplets A Randomized Study, the findings have not been released [57]. Whether the mechanism for preterm labor in multiples differs from that in singleton gestations remains uncertain. In addition, another on-going MFMU trial is investigating the role of Omega-3 supplementation in preventing preterm birth in singletons. If the results are promising, studies in multiples may be designed. Many questions surrounding 17P remain unanswered, including the optimal route and dose of drug administration and utility in other high-risk obstetrical scenarios such as short cervical length or positive cervicovaginal fetal fibronectin [58]. Whether progesterone has a role in the treatment rather than prevention of preterm labor remains unclear and represents a fertile area for potential future research.

Specialized twin clinics and transvaginal cervical length surveillance are two additional methods used in attempts to reduce the risk of adverse outcomes associated with multi-fetal pregnancies. In specialized clinics, patients have the opportunity to develop rapport with a small group of dedicated caregivers. Mothers are able to provide psychological support to one another, and an increased awareness can lead to increased compliance with therapeutic directives [59]. Premature cervical shortening detected by transvaginal ultrasound has good predictive capability for the development of preterm labor and delivery in multiples [60–63]. Studies suggest that a cervical length measurement of greater than or equal to 35 mm at 24 to 26 weeks identifies women with twins who are at low risk for delivery before 34 weeks gestation [60]. Conversely, a cervical length of 25 mm or less with or without funneling at 24 weeks gestation predicts a high risk for preterm labor and delivery [61]. Finally, at least four studies of fetal fibronectin in twins or triplets demonstrated high negative predictive values with one test and moderate positive predictive values with serial tests [11].

A role for elective late preterm delivery of multiples?

Prospective risk of fetal death

When managing multiples, there is a temptation to be reassured as the pregnancy progresses into the third trimester as the potential complications of prematurity diminish. Recent studies, however, suggest that twins may benefit from delivery in the late preterm gestation [64–66]. The theory underlying these concerns is that progressive uteroplacental insufficiency in multiples at advanced gestational ages may place the fetuses at risk for IUFD. In the literature, the optimal time of delivery for twins is controversial and ranges from 37 to 40 weeks gestation [11,64,65,67]. The current practice bulletin on multiples from the American College of Obstetricians and Gynecologists (ACOG) states that in the presence of normal fetal growth and amniotic fluid volumes, reassuring antenatal testing, and absence of maternal complications, pregnancy can be continued [11]. Most recently, Soucie and colleagues conducted a retrospective cohort study of 60,443 twin pairs in the United States using the Matched Multiple Birth File [67]. Stratified by week of gestation from 37 to at least 40 weeks gestation, the neonatal mortality and morbidity was calculated for twin A and twin B individually. The incidence of neonatal deaths increased significantly after 40 weeks, while a decreased risk of assisted ventilation was observed at 38 and 39 weeks for twin A and 39 and at least 40 weeks for twin B [67]. Thus, the authors concluded that the most favorable gestational age for the delivery of twin pregnancies should be equal to or greater than 38 but less than 40 weeks [67]. An important limitation of this study is that the effect of chorionicity was not investigated. Is there a role for elective late preterm delivery of multiples?

In attempts to determine the optimal gestational age of delivery for multiples, the concept of the prospective risk of fetal death has been proposed [64–67]. This statistic is calculated as the number of stillbirths occurring at a particular gestational age divided by the number of fetuses at risk (all fetuses in all ongoing pregnancies). This statistic articulates a more accurate impression for IUFD risk than the classic definition of fetal death rate (number of fetal deaths at a particular gestational age divided by the number of live births and fetal deaths during the same period). For twins, the prospective risk of fetal death is equivalent to that of post-term singletons at approximately 36 to 37 weeks gestation [65].

Because delivering these pregnancies in the late preterm period exposes neonates to complications from prematurity, gestational age-specific prospective risk of fetal death should be considered in the context of gestational specific neonatal death rates. If the prospective risk of fetal death if the pregnancy continues is greater than the rate of neonatal death at a given gestational age, then delivery may be rational. Plots of the prospective risk of fetal death and neonatal mortality cross at 39 weeks for twins and 36 weeks for triplets (Table 1) [64]. This model suggests that elective delivery of twins and triplets at the end of the late preterm period may be advantageous in improving perinatal outcome, but this area requires further investigation including consideration of the impact of chorionicity.

Uncomplicated monochorionic diamniotic twin gestations

When is the optimal time to deliver uncomplicated monochorionic diamniotic twins? Two recent studies have brought this question into the spotlight. Barigye and colleagues reported the high risk of unexpected fetal death in 151 monochorionic twins despite intensive ultrasound surveillance at a single tertiary care center [66]. After excluding pregnancies complicated by TTTS, IUGR, structural anomalies, twin reversed arterial perfusion (TRAP) sequence, and monoamnionicity, 10 IUFDs (three double IUFDs and four single IUFDs) occurred in seven (4.6%) previously uncomplicated monochorionic, diamniotic pregnancies. The gestational age of IUFD occurred predominantly during the late preterm period, at a median gestational age of 34 $^{1/7}$ weeks (range 28 $^{0/7}$ to 36 $^{3/7}$). Two of the five cases that underwent autopsy had features suggestive of acute, late-onset TTTS, although no antenatal indicators of IUGR or TTTS were appreciated. The prospective risk of unexpected antepartum stillbirth after 32 weeks was 4.3% (95% CI 1.6% to 9.1%) of monochorionic diamniotic pregnancies, and the authors concluded that this risk might be obviated by a policy of elective late preterm delivery [66].

Simões and colleagues recently repeated a similar investigation of 193 monochorionic diamniotic twins and found a lower prospective risk of fetal death [68]. The IUFD rate was 5 of 193 pregnancies (2.6%), and the prospective risk of stillbirth per pregnancy after 32 weeks gestation was 1.2% (95% CI 0.3% to 4.2%). Their study differed from Barigye and colleagues in two main areas [66,68]. First, cases with malformations, growth abnormalities, and TTTS were included. Despite this, the prospective risk of IUFD in their cohort was much lower per pregnancy and per fetus in each stratum of gestational ages compared with the risks previously reported by Barigye and colleagues. Secondly, a more intensive antenatal surveillance was used in frequency (biweekly versus weekly) and methods (cardiotocography and sonography versus sonography alone). Citing the risks of respiratory complications after late preterm twin delivery, the authors concluded that elective preterm birth after 36 completed weeks was a more reasonable compromise [68]. However, the prospective risk of stillbirth per pregnancy after 32 weeks' gestation remained concerning at 1.2% [66,68].

Although the knowledge gained from these two studies highlights the high-risk nature of these pregnancies, the investigations have multiple limitations, including small numbers, retrospective design, and lack of dichorionic twin comparative data [66,68,69]. Currently, there is no consensus on fetal surveillance or management of apparently normal monochorionic diamniotic twin gestations, including timing of delivery. Decisions regarding the management of these pregnancies therefore are scheduled empirically rather than according to evidence-based recommendations, which are not available (Box 2) [69]. The risks of prematurity are not negligible during the late preterm period. Balancing the risk of iatrogenic preterm birth in an apparently uncomplicated monochorionic twin pregnancy with the risk of double IUFD or single IUFD with the concomitant risk of multi-cystic encephalomalacia for the surviving cotwin remain challenging [69]. One option may be to offer delivery of these apparently uncomplicated monochorionic twins at the end of the late preterm gestation following antenatal corticosteroid administration and thorough counseling regarding the risks of expectant management versus elective preterm delivery [69]. This may be a reasonable approach to this dilemma until larger, prospective observational studies have been conducted to better elucidate the natural history of these complex pregnancies.

There is one randomized trial underway that may assist in clarifying the debate on the optimal date of delivery for twin pregnancies. A multi-center research trial named the Twins: Timing of Birth Trial is being conducted at 15 centers across Australia and New Zealand [70]. Patients are randomized to either delivery at 37 weeks gestation or standard prenatal care. Approximately 576 twins are targeted with a composite neonatal morbidity and mortality index chosen as the primary outcome for the trial. Information from this research and others like it hopefully will shed some light on this dilemma regarding the timing of delivery for twin gestations, particularly when stratified by chorionicity.

Box 2. Suggested protocol for the management of uncomplicated monochorionic diamniotic twins by trimester

First trimester
- Early identification of amnionicity, chorionicity, and number of fetuses
- Nuchal translucency at 10 to 14 weeks gestation (optimally at 11 weeks)

Second trimester
- Anatomical survey and fetal echocardiogram at approximately 20 weeks
- Serial ultrasounds assessing amniotic fluid volumes and growth
- Fetal surveillance (composed of nonstress tests, biophysical profiles, and Doppler velocimetry studies) intensified if there is evidence of twin-twin transfusion syndrome, fetal growth abnormalities, or discordant fluid volumes

Third trimester
- Early counseling regarding the risks of intrauterine fetal demise and potential neurologic sequelae and complications from late preterm birth

---

Summary

Multiple pregnancies present numerous, unique challenges in obstetrical diagnosis and management. Most twins and many high-order multiples deliver in the late preterm period between 34 and 36 completed weeks because of spontaneous preterm labor or iatrogenic intervention for maternal or fetal medical complications. Although perinatal outcomes from late preterm delivery of multiples are generally favorable, adverse complications remain a potential risk. Further research is needed to determine the optimal schedule for effective fetal surveillance and whether it is prudent to electively deliver certain uncomplicated multiple gestations in the late preterm period.

References

[1] Martin JA, Hamilton BE, Sutton PD, et al. Births: final data for 2003. Natl Vital Stat Rep 2003;54(2):1–116.
[2] Martin JA, Hamilton BE, Sutton PD, et al. Births: final data for 2002. Natl Vital Stat Rep 2002;52(10):1–114.
[3] The March of Dimes. The News Desk page. Cesarean sections may be contributing to the rise in late preterm births. March 29, 2006. Available at: http://www.marchofdimes.com/aboutus/15796_19306.asp. Accessed August 28, 2006.

[4] Raju TN, Higgins RD, Stark AR, et al. Optimizing care and outcome for late preterm (near-term) infants: a summary of the workshop sponsored by the NICHD. Pediatrics 2006;118(3):1207–14.

[5] Beato CV. Healthy people 2010 progress report: maternal, infant, and child health. Washington, DC: US Department of Health and Human Services; October 22, 2003.

[6] Lewis DF, Fontenot MT, Robichaux AG, et al. Respiratory morbidity in well-dated twins approaching term: what are the risks of elective delivery? J Reprod Med 2002;47:841–4.

[7] Chasen ST, Madden A, Chervenak FA. Cesarean delivery of twins and neonatal respiratory disorders. Am J Obstet Gynecol 1999;181:1052–6.

[8] D'Alton ME, Simpson LL. Syndromes in twins. Semin Perinatol 1995;19(5):375–86.

[9] Blickstein I, Keith LG. Outcome of triplets and high-order multiple pregnancies. Curr Opin Obstet Gynecol 2003;15(2):113–7.

[10] Newman RB, Hamer C, Miller MC. Outpatient triplet management: a contemporary review. Am J Obstet Gynecol 1989;161(3):547–53.

[11] American College of Obstetricians and Gynecologists. Multiple gestation: complicated twin, triplet, and high-order multi-fetal pregnancy. ACOG Practice Bulletin. Number 56. October 2004.

[12] Kaufman GE, Malone FD, Harvey-Wilkes KB, et al. Neonatal morbidity and mortality associated with triplet pregnancy. Obstet Gynecol 1998;91:342–8.

[13] Garite TJ, Clark RH, Elliott JP, et al. Twins and triplets: the effect of plurality and growth on neonatal outcome compared with singleton infants. Am J Obstet Gynecol 2004;191(3):700–7.

[14] Neonatal encephalopathy and cerebral palsy. Defining the pathogenesis and pathophysiology. Washington, DC: American College of Obstetricians and Gynecologists and American Academy of Pediatrics; 2003.

[15] Yokoyama Y, Shimizu T, Hayakawa K. Prevalence of cerebral palsy in twins, triplets and quadruplets. Int J Epidemiol 1995;24:943–8.

[16] Weiss JJ, Cleary-Goldman J, Budorick N, et al. Multi-cystic encephalomalacia after first trimester intrauterine fetal demise in monochorionic twins. Am J Obstet Gynecol 2004;90:563–5.

[17] Petterson B, Nelson KB, Watson L, et al. Twins, triplets, and cerebral palsy in births in western Australia in the 1980s. BMJ 1993;307:1239–43.

[18] Pharoah PO, Cooke T. Cerebral palsy and multiple births. Arch Dis Child Fetal Neonatal Ed 1996;75:F174–7.

[19] Pharoah PO, Adi Y. Consequences of in utero death in a twin pregnancy. Lancet 2000;355:1597–602.

[20] Ong S, Zamora J, Khan K, et al. Prognosis for the cotwin following single twin death: a systematic review. BMJ 2006;113:992–8.

[21] Norwitz ER, Valentine E, Park JS. Maternal physiology and complications of multiple pregnancy. Semin Perinatol 2005;29:338–48.

[22] Devine PC, Malone FD, Athanassiou A, et al. Maternal and neonatal outcome of 100 consecutive triplet pregnancies. Am J Perinatol 2001;18(4):225–35.

[23] Graham G, Simpson LL. Diagnosis and management of obstetrical complications unique to multiple gestations. Clin Obstet Gynecol 2004;47:163–80.

[24] Campbell DM, Templeton A. Maternal complications of twin pregnancy. Int J Gynaecol Obstet 2004;84(1):71–3.

[25] Davidson KM, Simpson LL, Knox TA, et al. Acute fatty liver of pregnancy in triplet gestation. Obstet Gynecol 1998;91:806–8.

[26] American College of Obstetricians and Gynecologists. Diagnosis and management of preeclampsia and eclampsia. ACOG Practice Bulletin Number 33. Washington, DC: American College of Obstetricians and Gynecologists; 2002.

[27] Sibai BM, Hauth J, Caritis S, et al. Hypertensive disorders in twin versus singleton gestations. National Institute of Child Health and Human Development Network of Maternal-Fetal Medicine Units. Am J Obstet Gynecol 2000;182:938–42.

[28] Day MC, Barton JR, O'Brien JM, et al. The effect of fetal number on the development of hypertensive conditions of pregnancy. Obstet Gynecol 2005;106:927–31.

[29] Maxwell CV, Lieberman E, Norton M, et al. Relationship of twin zygosity and risk of preeclampsia. Am J Obstet Gynecol 2001;185:819–21.

[30] Hardardottir H, Kelly K, Bork MD, et al. Atypical presentation of preeclampsia in high-order multi-fetal gestations. Obstet Gynecol 1996;87(3):370–4.

[31] American College of Obstetricians and Gynecologists. Intrauterine growth restriction. ACOG Practice Bulletin. Number 12. Washington, DC: American College of Obstetricians and Gynecologists; 2000.

[32] Rode ME, Jackson M. Sonographic considerations with multiple gestation. Semin Roentgenol 1999;34(1):29–34.

[33] Demissie K, Ananth CV, Martin J, et al. Fetal and neonatal mortality among twin gestations in the United States: the role of intrapair birth weight discordance. Obstet Gynecol 2002; 100(3):474–80.

[34] Gonzalez-Quintero VH, Luke B, O'sullivan MJ, et al. Antenatal factors associated with significant birth weight discordancy in twin gestations. Am J Obstet Gynecol 2003;189(3): 813–7.

[35] Blickstein I, Keith LG. Neonatal mortality rates among growth-discordant twins, classified according to the birth weight of the smaller twin. Am J Obstet Gynecol 2004;190(1):170–4.

[36] Amaru RC, Bush MC, Berkowitz RL, et al. Is discordant growth in twins an independent risk factor for adverse neonatal outcome? Obstet Gynecol 2004;103(1):71–6.

[37] Carr SR, Aronson MP, Coustan DR. Survival rates of monoamniotic twins do not decrease after 30 weeks' gestation. Am J Obstet Gynecol 1990;163:719–22.

[38] Rodis JF, McIlveen PF, Egan JF, et al. Monoamniotic twins: improved perinatal survival with accurate prenatal diagnosis and antenatal fetal surveillance. Am J Obstet Gynecol 1997;177:1046–9.

[39] Allen VM, Windrim R, Barrett J, et al. Management of monoamniotic twin pregnancies: a case series and systematic review of the literature. Br J Obstet Gynaecol 2001;108: 931–6.

[40] House M, Harney K, D'Alton ME, et al. Intensive management of monoamniotic twin pregnancies improves perinatal outcome. Am J Obstet Gynecol 2002;185:S113.

[41] Tessen JA, Zlatnik FJ. Monoamniotic twins: a retrospective controlled study. Obstet Gynecol 1991;77:832–4.

[42] Harkness UF, Crombleholme TM. Twin-twin transfusion syndrome: where do we go from here? Semin Perinatol 2005;29:296–304.

[43] Quintero RA, Morales WJ, Allen MH, et al. Staging of twin-twin transfusion syndrome. J Perinatol 1999;19:550–5.

[44] Hecher K, Plath H, Bregenzer T, et al. Endoscopic laser surgery versus serial amniocenteses in the treatment of severe twin-twin transfusion syndrome. Am J Obstet Gynecol 1999;180: 717–24.

[45] Quintero RA, Dickinson JE, Morales WJ, et al. Stage-based treatment of twin-twin transfusion syndrome. Am J Obstet Gynecol 2003;188:1333–40.

[46] Senat MV, Deprest J, Boulvain M, et al. Endoscopic laser surgery versus serial amnioreduction for severe twin-to-twin transfusion syndrome. N Engl J Med 2004;351(2):136–44.

[47] National Institutes of Health. National Institutes of Health Consensus Development Conference Statement. Effect of corticosteroids for fetal maturation on perinatal outcomes, February 28–March 2, 1994. Am J Obstet Gynecol 1995;173:246–52.

[48] Newman RB, Krombach RS, Myers MC, et al. Effect of cerclage on obstetric outcome in twin gestations with a shortened cervical length. Am J Obstet Gynecol 2002;186:634–40.

[49] Elimian A, Figueroa R, Nigam S, et al. Perinatal outcome of triplet gestation: does prophylactic cerclage make a difference? J Matern Fetal Med 1999;8:119–22.

[50] Berghella V, Odibo AO, To MS, et al. Cerclage for short cervix on ultrasonography: meta-analysis of trials using individual patient-level data. Obstet Gynecol 2005;106(1):181–9.

[51] Saunders MC, Dick JS, Brown IM, et al. The effects of hospital admission for bed rest on the duration of twin pregnancy: a randomized trial. Lancet 1985;2(8459):793–5.

[52] Crowther CA. Hospitalization and bed rest for multiple pregnancy. Cochrane Database Syst Rev 2001;1:CD000110.

[53] Katz M, Robertson PA, Creasy RK. Cardiovascular complications associated with terbutaline treatment for preterm labor. Am J Obstet Gynecol 1981;139(5):605–8.

[54] Colton T, Kayne HL, Zhang Y, et al. A meta-analysis of home uterine activity monitoring. Am J Obstet Gynecol 1995;173(5):1499–505.

[55] Dyson DC, Danbe KH, Bamber JA, et al. Monitoring women at risk for preterm labor. N Engl J Med 1998;338(1):15–9.

[56] Meis PJ, Klebanoff M, Thom E, et al. Prevention of recurrent preterm delivery by 17 alpha-hydroxyprogesterone caproate. N Engl J Med 2003;348(24):2379–85.

[57] The Biostatistics Center of George Washington University. The National Institute of Child Health and Human Development Maternal-Fetal Medicine Units Network page. Available at: http://www.bsc.gwu.edu/MFMU/index.html. Accessed August 28, 2006.

[58] American College of Obstetricians and Gynecologists. Use of progesterone to reduce preterm birth. ACOG Committee Opinion. Number 291. Washington, DC: American College of Obstetricians and Gynecologists; 2003.

[59] Luke B, Brown MB, Misiunas R, et al. Specialized prenatal care and maternal and infant outcomes in twin pregnancy. Am J Obstet Gynecol 2003;189(4):934–8.

[60] Imseis HM, Albert TA, Iams JD. Identifying twin gestations at low risk for preterm birth with a transvaginal ultrasonographic cervical measurement at 24 to 26 weeks gestation. Am J Obstet Gynecol 1997;177(5):1149–55.

[61] Goldenberg RL, Iams JD, Miodovnik M, et al. The preterm prediction study: risk factors in twin gestations. National Institute of Child Health and Human Development Maternal-Fetal Medicine Units Network. Am J Obstet Gynecol 1996;175:1047–53.

[62] Ramin KD, Ogburn PL Jr, Mulholland TA, et al. Ultrasonographic assessment of cervical length in triplet pregnancies. Am J Obstet Gynecol 1999;180:1442–5.

[63] Gibson JL, Macara LM, Owen P, et al. Prediction of preterm delivery in twin pregnancy: a prospective, observational study of cervical length and fetal fibronectin testing. Ultrasound Obstet Gynecol 2004;23:561–6.

[64] Kahn B, Lumey LH, Zybert PA, et al. Prospective risk of fetal death in singleton, twin, and triplet gestations: implications for practice. Obstet Gynecol 2003;102:685–92.

[65] Sairam S, Costeloe K, Thilaganathan B. Prospective risk of stillbirth in multiple-gestation pregnancies: a population based analysis. Obstet Gynecol 2002;100:638–41.

[66] Barigye O, Pasquini L, Galea P, et al. High risk of unexpected late fetal death in monochorionic twins despite intensive ultrasound surveillance: a cohort study. PloS Med 2005;2(6):e172.

[67] Soucie JE, Yang Q, Wen SW, et al. Neonatal mortality and morbidity rates in term twins with advancing gestational age. Am J Obstet Gynecol 2006;195:172–7.

[68] Simões T, Amaral N, Lerman R, et al. Prospective risk of intrauterine death of monochorionic-diamniotic twins. Am J Obstet Gynecol 2006;195:134–9.

[69] Cleary-Goldman J, D'Alton ME. Uncomplicated monochorionic diamniotic twins and the timing of delivery. PloS Med 2005;2(6):e180.

[70] The Science Navigation Group. The current controlled trials page. Available at: http://www.controlled-trials.com/isrctn/trial/|/0/15761056.html. Accessed August 28, 2006.

CLINICS IN
PERINATOLOGY

Clin Perinatol 33 (2006) 793–801

Elective Cesarean Section and Induction and Their Impact on Late Preterm Births

Karin Fuchs, MD, Ronald Wapner, MD*

*Division of Maternal-Fetal Medicine, Department of Obstetrics and Gynecology,
Columbia University Medical Center, Presbyterian Hospital, 16th Floor,
Room 16-66, New York, NY 11032, USA*

Complications of prematurity account for 85% of perinatal morbidity and mortality in the United States [1]. Although severely preterm infants are more likely to suffer consequences of prematurity, late preterm births account for the majority of preterm deliveries and experience significantly more morbidity than infants born at term [2]. Recent efforts have focused on further assessing the outcomes of these late preterm infants and understanding their etiologies. This article will explore incidence of elective cesarean section and induction of labor and their impact on the timing of delivery and the increasing incidence of late preterm births.

Definition and incidence of late preterm births

The American College of Obstetrics and Gynecology (ACOG) and the American Academy of Pediatrics define term pregnancy as one that has completed 37 weeks of gestation and that delivers after the first day of the 38th week of pregnancy. In contrast, preterm deliveries are those that occur before 37 completed weeks of gestation. The group of infants labeled "preterm" is, however, extremely heterogeneous, and is applied to infants born at a wide range of gestational ages, which are associated with vastly different outcomes. According to the consensus statement of the National Institute of Child Health and Human Development (NICHD) workshop entitled "Optimizing Care and Outcome of the Near-Term Pregnancy and the Near-Term Newborn Infant," infants born 34 weeks 0 days and 36 weeks 6 days gestation should be classified as "late preterm" infants [3]. Although these late preterm infants have also been referred to as "near

* Corresponding author.
E-mail address: rw2191@columbia.edu (R. Wapner).

0095-5108/06/$ - see front matter © 2006 Elsevier Inc. All rights reserved.
doi:10.1016/j.clp.2006.09.010 *perinatology.theclinics.com*

term" or "minimally preterm," these labels have fallen out of favor as they are inconsistently defined and may misleadingly imply fetal maturity [4].

In 2004, the premature birth rate in the United States was 12.5%, representing a more than 30% increase since 1981 [5]. Although the number of infants born at less than 32 weeks has declined slightly since 1990, the birth of infants born between 32 and 37 weeks has increased over the same time period [6]. Late preterm births accounted for 6.9% of singleton births in the United States in 1992 and increased to 7.4% of singleton deliveries in 2002 [6]. Data from the US National Center for Health Statistics demonstrate that 74% of the 394,996 preterm singleton deliveries in the United States in 2002 occurred at either 34, 35, or 36 weeks gestation [6].

Impact

Numerous studies have shown that late preterm infants face increased morbidity when compared with their term counterparts. Although meconium aspiration syndrome is less common in late preterm infants than in term infants [7], all other forms of respiratory morbidity (including transient tachypnea of the newborn, respiratory distress syndrome, pneumonia, and pulmonary hypertension) affect late preterm infants at a higher rate than infants of more advanced gestational ages [8,9]. Hypothermia is another consequence of late preterm delivery and has been shown to trigger unnecessary sepsis investigations and more frequent neonatal intensive care unit (NICU) admissions in the late preterm population [10]. The suck-swallow reflex and intestinal motility is also impaired in late preterm infants, and can lead to difficulty breastfeeding and a higher likelihood of poor weight gain and dehydration [11]. Among infants born between 34 and 37 weeks gestation, the incidence of hypoglycemia is also significantly higher than demonstrated in term infants [10]. The relative immaturity of the livers of late preterm infants makes hyperbilirubinemia and posticteric sequelae more common and more severe in infants born in the late preterm period than in infants born at term [12].

In addition to the increased morbidity faced by late preterm infants, several studies have also demonstrated an increased risk of infant mortality among infants born between 34 and 37 weeks gestation [7]. One study demonstrated a two- to fivefold increased risk of infant death among late preterm infants and a twofold higher risk of sudden infant death syndrome when late preterm infants were compared with infants delivered at term [13]. Although the majority of late preterm infants survive the neonatal period, recent evidence also suggests that preterm and low birth weight infants suffer from long-term behavioral and developmental morbidities. One study with long-term follow up of low-birth weight infants demonstrated clinically significant behavioral problems in almost 20% of the infants born between 34 and 37 weeks gestation [14]. Compared with children born at term, infants born between 34 and 36 weeks gestation have an 80% increased risk of childhood attention-deficit/hyperactivity disorder [15].

Because late preterm infants account for the majority of preterm infants in the United States and experience increased morbidity compared with their term counterparts, late preterm births impose an enormous impact on the health care system. Late preterm infants accrue increased hospital expenses during their delivery hospitalizations [2] and have a higher rate of rehospitalization than infants born after 37 weeks of gestation [16,17]. A population-based cohort study demonstrated a 4.8% rehospitalization rate among late preterm infants, even with no history of prior NICU admission during the delivery hospitalization [16]. It has also been demonstrated that late preterm infants are 1.8 times as likely as term infants to require readmission; breastfed late preterm infants are at even higher risk of requiring readmission [17]. One estimate suggests that over 49 million dollars could be saved if nonindicated deliveries between 34 and 37 weeks were avoided for 1 year in the state of California alone [18].

Causes of late preterm birth

Spontaneous preterm labor and preterm rupture of membranes

Although the overall rate of preterm birth is on the rise, the rate of preterm delivery resulting from spontaneous preterm labor (PTL) before 32 weeks decreased by 9% between 1992 and 2002 [5]. Paradoxically, the rate of spontaneous preterm delivery among late preterm infants increased during the same period. By 2002, more than 7% of deliveries resulting from PTL occurred between 34 and 37 weeks gestation; this represented a 12% increase in births resulting from spontaneous late PTL between 1992 and 2002 [6]. The rate of premature rupture of membranes (PROM) between 34 and 36 weeks gestation also increased from 1992 to 2002; by 2002, 21% of cases of PROM occurred in late preterm pregnancies [6].

Standard obstetric management of PTL and preterm PROM (PPROM) may influence the percentage of these cases that result in late preterm birth beyond 34 weeks. According to practice guidelines published by the ACOG, the management of PTL should involve the use of tocolysis and glucocorticoids up to 34 weeks gestation [19]. The management of PPROM remains controversial, but expert opinion generally recommends expectant management before 34 weeks [20]. However, beyond 34 weeks efforts are no longer directed at prolonging the pregnancy. These management strategies are based upon the fact that the survival rate of infants born at 34 weeks is within 1% of those born at term and prolongation of a pregnancy complicated by PTL or PPROM beyond 34 weeks may have unnecessary maternal and fetal risk [21].

The practice of not aggressively attempting to treat PTL after 34 weeks of gestation may have contributed to the increasing rate of late preterm births. In addition, many practitioners actively deliver pregnancies with ruptured membranes beyond 34 weeks, or even earlier if fetal lung maturity has been documented. Modification of current management strategies could potentially decrease the incidence of late preterm births and prevent neonatal morbidity. For example, might the proportion of late preterm births that result from spontaneous PTL be decreased with tocolysis administered between 34 and 37 weeks gestation? Would expectant management of preterm PROM until 37 weeks result in reduced neonatal morbidity compared with induction at 34 weeks? Future research should be aimed at identifying the best balance between in utero and neonatal management.

Some progress has been made in preventing idiopathic preterm delivery and specific interventions have been identified to reduce the incidence of recurrent preterm birth. A randomized placebo controlled study of weekly 17 alpha-hydroxyprogesterone caproate (17P) demonstrated a significant reduction in the rate of recurrent preterm delivery (up to 37 weeks) in women with a history of prior preterm birth or preterm PROM (relative risk [RR] 0.66, 95% confidence interval [CI] 0.54–0.81) [22]. Although this study does not apply to woman who have not had a previous preterm birth, additional studies are underway to investigate potential benefits of 17P in other populations at risk for preterm delivery such as those with a shortened cervix on ultrasound. Because of limited availability and lack of provider and patient education, 17P is only recently being introduced into clinical care. Improved utilization of this treatment may help to reduce the preterm birth rate and may reduce the incidence of spontaneous late preterm birth.

Indicated late preterm delivery

In addition to PTL and PPROM, other medical and obstetric complications can arise in late preterm gestations and may warrant delivery before term. National data confirms an increasing rate of intervention for medical indications in both term and preterm pregnancies. In 1992, 29% of deliveries resulted from intervention for medical indication (defined as pregnancies induced or delivered by cesarean section without evidence of premature rupture of the fetal membranes); in 2002, this had risen to 41% [6]. Over the same period of time, the rate of intervention in the late preterm group for medical indications increased by 12%. Of pregnancies delivered for medical indications, 6.4% occurred between 34 and 36 weeks in 1992 and 7.4% occurred between 34 and 36 weeks in 2002 [6].

Hypertensive disorders are the most common medical complication of pregnancy and complicate 6% to 10% of pregnancies in the United States [23]. Several studies have reported an increased incidence of late preterm birth among women with gestational hypertension [23–25] or preeclampsia. Observed rates of late preterm birth range from 4% to 6% among women with gestational hypertension, and range from 10% to 11% among women with preeclampsia [24,25]. Unfortunately, available data do not differentiate between rates of induced preterm deliveries and the rates of spontaneous preterm birth occurring simultaneously in this population of hypertensive women. Although is it feasible that some of the preterm births seen among women with hypertensive disorders stem from coexisting PTL or PPROM, expert opinion recommends delivery of mild preeclampsia at 37 weeks of gestation and severe preeclampsia as early as 34 weeks. Accordingly, labor inductions and cesarean deliveries performed between 34 and 37 weeks gestation in pregnancies complicated by preeclampsia iatrogenically increase the late preterm birth rate. Although worsening maternal or fetal status clearly justifies preterm delivery in cases of preeclampsia, many current obstetric practice guidelines, which suggest delivery at 34 weeks, may warrant revision as the risks of late preterm birth are better quantified.

Elective induction of labor and elective cesarean delivery

Published reports estimate that cesarean deliveries at maternal request account for 4% to 18% of cesarean deliveries in the United States. Unfortunately, US birth records do not allow more precise estimates because distinction between cesarean deliveries performed electively at maternal request and low-risk cesarean sections performed for unspecified indications are not differentiated [26]. Similarly, little data is available to determine the proportion of vaginal deliveries that result from elective induction at term versus those that result from spontaneous labor or indicated induction. Although birth records in other countries report the frequency and timing of elective deliveries, birth records in the United States do not track inductions performed at "maternal request" or cesarean sections done by "patient choice." Accordingly, it is impossible to accurately determine the proportion of births—term or preterm—that might result from elective delivery.

Although little data directly link elective labor induction and cesarean delivery at maternal request to the increased rate of late preterm births, there is ample evidence demonstrating that rates of induction of labor and cesarean delivery have increased over the same time period. In addition, data provided by the US National Center for Health Statistics demonstrates that singleton deliveries are occurring at earlier overall gestational ages. Although spontaneous and indicated late preterm births may account for some of this shift, an increasing incidence of deliveries between 37 and 39 weeks gestation could also account for the shift toward shorter average gestational lengths [6]. In fact, deliveries occurring between 37 and 39 weeks increased 19.4% between 1992 and 2002, while the percentage of pregnancies that continue beyond term decreased significantly [6]. By 2002, the average pregnancy was 38.9 weeks in length compared with 39.2 weeks in 1992 ($P < 0.001$) [6]. Over the same period of time, the rate of induction of labor has risen sharply to reach a rate of 20.6% in 2003 [27,28], and the cesarean section rate reached an all time high of 29.1% in 2004 [5]. Although many inductions and cesarean sections occur for valid indications, some are electively performed for maternal and/or practitioner convenience in the absence of medical or obstetric indication. Increasing elective intervention in term pregnancies could account for the increasing proportion of deliveries occurring at earlier gestational ages.

Another factor potentially contributing to the increase in late preterm birth is the trend away from vaginal birth after a previous cesarean section (VBAC) and toward repeat abdominal deliveries. After years of a slowly increasing rate of VBAC, it began to fall in the mid 1990s. The VBAC rate rose steadily from 1980 to a high of 28% in 1996 and then fell to 21% in 2000, and to 10.6% by 2003 [29]. This increase in the repeat cesarean section rate increased the opportunity for iatrogenic late preterm birth.

Assuming they were performed at term, elective deliveries may have contributed to the decreasing average gestational age at delivery, but should have had minimal impact on the increasing rate of late preterm births seen over the last decades. However, because of the inherent inaccuracy of pregnancy dating with margins of error of up to 3 weeks in the third trimester, inductions of labor and elective cesarean section performed at "presumed term" might inadvertently contribute to the increasing incidence of late preterm birth. In addition, recent research has demonstrated that elective delivery of even a well-dated pregnancy at term can lead to neonatal morbidity. One study found the rate of respiratory morbidity after elective cesarean section at 37 weeks to be three times higher than seen at 39 weeks. Another large trial of women planning elective cesarean birth found the probability of admission to a NICU at 37 weeks was 11.4% and 1.5% at 39 weeks [9].

To avoid iatrogenic prematurity and to minimize the morbidity associated with elective induction of labor and elective cesarean delivery, the ACOG recommends that elective delivery should not be performed before 39 weeks gestation. Because of the inaccuracy of pregnancy dating, criteria have been outlined to determine whether a pregnancy can be considered to be at term (Box 1) [30,31]. If gestational age cannot be accurately assessed before elective delivery at term, fetal lung maturity should be demonstrated by amniocentesis. In an attempt to further decrease the morbidity associated with elective inductions and cesarean sections at term, physicians and patients need to be counseled regarding the vulnerability of late preterm infants and the potential for iatrogenic prematurity. Hospital guidelines should also be developed and enforced to ensure that elective deliveries are not performed before gestational age of 39 weeks, and that fetal lung maturity should be demonstrated when pregnancy dating cannot be confirmed before elective delivery. Based on data demonstrating the benefit of antenatal corticosteroids beyond 34 weeks, antenatal corticosteroids should be considered if amniocentesis fails to confirm fetal lung maturity and delivery is required.

Reduction of morbidity in late preterm births

Administration of antenatal corticosteroids undoubtedly reduce a number of neonatal morbidities including respiratory distress and intraventricular

---

Box 1. Confirmation of term gestation

- Fetal heart tones have been documented for 20 weeks by nonelectronic fetoscope or for 30 weeks by Doppler.
- It has been 36 weeks since a positive serum or urine human gonadotropin pregnancy test was performed by a reliable laboratory.
- An ultrasound measurement of the crown–rump length, obtained at 6–12 weeks, supports a gestational age of at least 39 weeks.
- An ultrasound obtained at 13–20 weeks confirms the gestational age of at least 39 weeks determined by clinical history and physical examination.

Adapted from American College of Obstetricians and Gynecologists (ACOG). Induction of Labor. Washington DC; American College of Obstetricians and Gynecologists; 1999. (ACOG practice bulletin; no. 10).

---

hemorrhage. However, given the low baseline risks of these complications in neonates delivered after 34 weeks of gestation, both the National Institutes of Health and ACOG recommend antenatal corticosteroid administration only for women at risk for preterm delivery at less than 34 weeks gestation [32,33]. Recent research, however, has demonstrated that corticosteroids improved neonatal outcomes even when administered later in pregnancy. The Antenatal Steroids for Term Caesarean Section study randomized women to antenatal steroids or none at the time of elective cesarean section at or beyond 37 weeks gestation and demonstrated a significant reduction in overall respiratory morbidity (including respiratory distress syndrome (RDS) and transient tachypnea) in the exposed neonates (RR 0.46; 95% CI 0.23–0.93) [9]. Given the results of this study, future research should be given to evaluating the benefits and risks of administration of antenatal corticosteroids either for spontaneous PTL or indicated iatrogenic delivery between 34 and 37 weeks of gestation.

Summary

At all gestational ages, the risks of continuing a pregnancy must be carefully balanced against the risks of delivery and the associated risk of prematurity. This concept is of increasing importance in late preterm pregnancy when medical or obstetric complications frequently warrant delivery and the risk of prematurity persists. Given that morbidity exists for infants born between 34 and 37 weeks gestation, efforts should be focused on minimizing the late preterm birth rate and at improving the outcome of these infants. Published guidelines outlining the appropriate timing of elective induction of labor and elective cesarean section should be closely followed to avoid unintended iatrogenic prematurity. Research should continue to investigate the etiology of spontaneous preterm deliveries and aim to develop strategies of primary prevention. The incidence and etiology of iatrogenic late preterm birth should also be further investigated and alternative management strategies should be considered. To gain information about the impact of elective delivery on late preterm births, the data collected from birth records should reflect the changing obstetric practices in the United States and be revised to include specific information on elective deliveries.

References

[1] Arias E, MacDorman MF, Strobino DM, et al. Annual summary of vital statistics: 2002. Pediatrics 2003;112(6 Pt 1):1215–30.
[2] Wang ML, Dorer DJ, Fleming MP, et al. Clinical outcomes of near-term infants. Pediatrics 2004;114(2):372–6.
[3] Raju TN, Higgins RD, Stark AR, et al. Optimizing care and outcome for late-preterm (near-term) infants: a summary of the workshop sponsored by the National Institute of Child Health and Human Development. Pediatrics 2006;118(3):1207–14.
[4] Engle WA. A recommendation for the definition of "late preterm" (near-term) and the birth weight - gestational age classification system. Semin Perinatol 2006;30:2–7.
[5] Hoyert DL, Mathews TJ, Menacker F, et al. Annual summary of vital statistics: 2004. Pediatrics 2006;117:168–83.
[6] Davidoff MJ, Dias T, Damus K, et al. Changes in the gestational age distribution among US singleton births: impact on rates of late preterm birth, 1992 to 2002. Semin Perinatol 2006;30: 8–15.
[7] Escobar GJ, Clark RH, Greene JD. Short-term outcomes of infants born at 35 and 36 weeks gestation: we need to ask more questions. Semin Perinatol 2006;30:28–33.
[8] Clark RH. The epidemiology of respiratory failure in neonates born at an estimated gestational age of 34 weeks or more. J Perinatol 2005;25(4):251–7.
[9] Stutchfield P, Whitaker R, Russell I. Antenatal betamethasone and incidence of neonatal respiratory distress after elective cesarean section: pragmatic randomized trial. Br Med J 331(7518):662 [Epub 2005 Aug 22].
[10] Laptook A, Jackson DL. Cold stress and hypoglycemia in the late preterm ("near-term") infant: impact on nursery of admission. Semin Perinatol 2006;30:77–80.
[11] Neu J. Gastrointestinal maturation and feeding. Semin Perinatol 2006;30(1):24–7.
[12] Bhutani VK, Johnson L. Kernicterus in late preterm infants cared for as term healthy infants. Semin Perinatol 2006;30:89–97.
[13] Kramer MS, Demissie K, Yang H, et al. The contribution of mild and moderate preterm birth to infant mortality. Fetal and Infant Health Study Group of the Canadian Perinatal Surveillance System. JAMA 2000;284(7):843–9.
[14] Gray RF, Indurkhya A, McCormick MC. Prevalence, stability, and predictors of clinically significant behavior problems in low birth weight children at 3, 5, and 8 years of age. Pediatrics 2004;114:736–43.
[15] Linnet KM, Wisborg K, Agerbo E, et al. Gestational age, birth weight, and the risk of hyperkinetic disorder. Arch Dis Child 2006;91:655–60.
[16] Shapiro-Mendoza CK, Tomashek KM, Kotelchuck M, et al. Risk factors for neonatal morbidity and mortality among "healthy," late preterm infants. Semin Perinatol 2006;30:55–60.
[17] Tomashek KM, Shapiro-Mendoza CK, Weiss J, et al. Early discharge among late preterm and term newborns and risk of neonatal morbidity. Semin Perinatol 2006;30:61–8.

[18] Gilbert WM, Nesbitt TS, Danielson B. The cost of prematurity: quantification by gestational age. Obstet Gynecol 2003;102:488–92.

[19] American College of Obstetricians and Gynecologists. Management of preterm labor. Practice Bulletin No. 43, May 2003.

[20] Mercer BM. Preterm premature rupture of the membranes. Obstet Gynecol 2003;101: 178–93.

[21] American College of Obstetricians and Gynecologists. Preterm labor. Technical Bulletin No. 206, June 1995.

[22] Meis PJ, Klebanoff M, Thom E, et al. Prevention of recurrent preterm delivery by 17 alpha-hydroxyprogesterone caproate. N Engl J Med 2003;348:2379–85.

[23] Sibai BM. Preeclampsia as a cause of preterm and later preterm (near-term) births. Semin Perinatol 2006;30:16–9.

[24] Hauth JC, Ewell MG, Levine RJ, et al. Pregnancy outcome in healthy nulliparous women who subsequently developed hypertension. Obstet Gynecol 2000;95:24–8.

[25] Knuist M, Bonsel GJ, Treffers PE. Intensification of fetal and maternal surveillance in pregnant women with hypertensive disorders. Int J Gynecol Obstet 1998;61:127–34.

[26] NIH State-of-the-Science Conference. Cesarean delivery on maternal request. Available at: http://consensus.nih.gov

[27] Barros FC, Victora CG, Barros A, et al. The challenge of reducing neonatal mortality in middle-income countries: findings from three Brazilian birth cohorts in 1982, 1993, and 2004. Lancet 2005;365:847–54.

[28] Martin JA, Hamilton BE, Sutton PD, et al. Births: final data for 2003. Natl Vital Stat Rep 2005;54(2):1–25.

[29] National Vital Statistics Reports, 2002–2003 data. Vol 53 No 9, November 23, 2004. Births: preliminary data for 2003.

[30] Morrison J, Rennie JM, Milton PJ. Neonatal respiratory morbidity and mode of delivery at term: influence of timing of elective cesarean section. Br J Obstet Gynaecol 1995;102:101–6.

[31] American College of Obstetricians and Gynecologists. Induction of labor. Practice Bulletin No. 10, November 1999.

[32] Hnat MD, Sibai BM, Caritis S, et al. Perinatal outcome in women with recurrent preeclampsia compared with women who develop preeclampsia as nulliparas. Am J Obstet Gynecol 2002;186:422–6.

[33] American College of Obstetricians and Gynecologists. Antenatal corticosteroid therapy for fetal maturation. Committee Opinion No. 273, May 2002.

ELSEVIER
SAUNDERS

CLINICS IN
PERINATOLOGY

Clin Perinatol 33 (2006) 803–830

Hypoxic Respiratory Failure in the Late Preterm Infant

Golde G. Dudell, MD*, Lucky Jain, MD, MBA

Emory University School of Medicine, 2015 Uppergate Drive, Atlanta, GA 30322, USA

They have been aptly called the great imposters; late preterm infants (also called near-term) often are passed off as mature infants, but manifest signs of physiologic immaturity or delayed transition in the neonatal period [1]. Births between 34 and 37 weeks gestation (referred to herein as late preterm births) account for a significant proportion of preterm births in North America and elsewhere. Several studies have documented the high incidence of respiratory distress and neonatal ICU (NICU) admissions in this population [2–4]. These infants have a higher incidence of transient tachypnea of the newborn (TTNB), respiratory distress syndrome (RDS), persistent pulmonary hypertension of the newborn (PPHN), and respiratory failure than term infants [3]. Data about respiratory failure and outcomes in near-term infants are hard to obtain because of the lack of large databases such as those available for preterm infants. It is estimated, however, that 17,000 infants greater than or equal to 34 weeks are admitted to NICUs each year in the United States alone, and these represent up to 33% of all NICU admissions [5]. Nearly 50% of infants born at 34 weeks gestation require intensive care; this number drops to 15% at 35 weeks and 8% at 36 weeks gestation. In addition to respiratory distress, these infants often have other neonatal complications including hypoglycemia, hyperbilirubinemia, feeding difficulties, and difficulty in maintaining body temperature. Long-term morbidity information is even harder to gather; an estimated 9% of normal birth weight infants with respiratory failure die in the neonatal period [5]. Factors associated with high morbidity and mortality include delivery by cesarean section, presence of maternal complications, male gender, and intrauterine growth retardation.

In obstetric and pediatric practice, late preterm infants often are considered functionally mature and are managed based on protocols developed for

---

* Corresponding author.
E-mail address: gdudell@emory.edu (G.G. Dudell).

0095-5108/06/$ - see front matter © 2006 Elsevier Inc. All rights reserved.
doi:10.1016/j.clp.2006.09.006   *perinatology.theclinics.com*

full-term infants. The late preterm infant has been excluded from randomized controlled trials (RCTs) that focus on respiratory diseases of the
more vulnerable very preterm infant (eg, trials of surfactant replacement
for the treatment of RDS and antenatal steroids for the prevention of
RDS). Instead they have been included in large multi-center, RCTs designed
to assess the efficacy and safety of newer ventilatory strategies and rescue
therapies in neonates with hypoxemic respiratory failure (HRF) born at
34 weeks gestation or more. Unlike studies in the preterm population, studies in term and the late preterm populations uniformly fail to either stratify
by gestational age or use gestational age as a major confounder when analyzing outcomes. Therefore, the evidence that is used to treat HRF in the
late preterm is extrapolated from studies where most infants enrolled are either term or postdates, and the mean gestational age is 39 plus or minus 2
weeks [6–10]. Based on data from the Extracorporeal Life Support Organization (ELSO) Neonatal Registry, gestational age is a major determinant of
survival. Not only is prematurity associated with decreased survival in
infants born with congenital diaphragmatic hernia but early term birth
(37 to $39^{6/7}$ weeks) results in a higher mortality than late term birth (40 to
$42^{6/7}$ weeks) [11]. Similar information is not available for other respiratory
diagnoses, but overall survival of the late preterm population with neonatal
respiratory failure was 96% compared with 98% at term in a large cohort
study done in Italy in the mid 1990s [12].

Delayed respiratory transition in late preterm infants

The last few weeks of gestation are critical for fetal development and maturation, gradually preparing the fetus for a safe landing. Biochemical and
hormonal changes that accompany spontaneous labor and vaginal delivery
also play an important role in this transition. For effective gas exchange to
occur, alveolar spaces must be cleared of excess fluid and ventilated, and
pulmonary blood flow increased to match ventilation with perfusion. Failure of either of these events can jeopardize neonatal transition and cause
the infant to develop respiratory distress. Understanding of the mecha-
nisms(s) by which fetal lungs are able to clear themselves of excessive fluid
at birth remains far from complete. It is clear though, that traditional expla-
nations that relied on Starling forces and vaginal squeeze can account for
only a fraction of the fluid absorbed [13–18]. Amiloride-sensitive sodium
transport by lung epithelia through epithelial sodium channels (ENaC)
has emerged as a key event in the transepithelial movement of alveolar fluid
[19–27], and this appears to be a two-step process. The first step is passive
movement of Na^+ from lumen across the apical membrane into the cell
through Na^+-permeable ion channels. The second step is active extrusion
of Na^+ from the cell across the basolateral membrane into the serosal space.
The lung epithelium is believed to switch from a predominantly chloride-

secreting membrane at birth to a predominantly Na^+-absorbing membrane after birth. These changes also have been correlated with an increased production of the mRNA for amiloride-sensitive epithelial Na^+ channels (ENaC) in the developing lung [23]. Disruption of this process has been implicated in several disease states including TTNB [28] and RDS [29]. It is known now that the experience of vaginal delivery greatly enhances respiratory performance, and this effect is greater than that achieved by simple reduction of lung liquid volume to half in fetuses delivered without enduring labor. Removal of lung fluid starts before birth and continues postnatally with fluid being carried away by several possible pathways including pulmonary lymphatics [30,31], blood vessels [32], upper airway, mediastinum [33], and pleural space [33]. In later life, pulmonary edema can result either from excessive movement of water and solute across the alveolar capillary membrane, or from failure of reabsorption of lung fluid [34,35].

Respiratory morbidity in late preterm neonates born by cesarean section without trial of labor

A significant number of late preterm neonates are delivered by cesarean section, and this number has been steadily increasing in North America. Overall, cesarean births rose a seventh year in a row in 2003 to a record 27.6% of all deliveries (National Vital Statistics Report, 2004), [36–40]. This rate is 33% higher than the rate seen in 1996 and is accompanied by a 16% drop in women attempting vaginal birth after a previous cesarean section in 2003 over the previous year (National Vital Statistics Report, 2004). Among many reasons cited for this increase are more older women giving birth, a rise in multiple gestations, and physicians' concerns about risks of vaginal birth [41]; predictions are that continued increases are inevitable. Rates of cesarean section are considerably higher in some other parts of the world, especially in Latin America [42–43]. Although indications for the high rate of operative deliveries can vary by region and by maternal choice, up to 50% of these procedures may be performed because of a previous cesarean section [36,44].

A higher occurrence of respiratory morbidity in late preterm and term infants delivered by elective cesarean section has been observed by many investigators [45–53]. These infants have a higher incidence of TTNB [45–52,54], RDS resulting from iatrogenic prematurity [45–47,55,56], and severe PPHN or HRF [49,50]. Some of these reports also show higher rates of NICU admissions, mechanical ventilation, oxygen therapy, extracorporeal life support (ECMO), and death [49,50]. Madar and colleagues [55] showed that infants born by ECS at 37 to 38 weeks are 120 times more likely to receive ventilatory support for RDS than those born at 39 to 41 weeks. In contrast, a large population-based longitudinal study of 6138 women in Nova Scotia comparing trial of labor to repeat elective cesarean section failed to show an increase in

respiratory morbidity in infants born without enduring labor [44]. No neonatal data, however, were presented in this report, and it is not clear if the
overall occurrence of respiratory morbidity in the two groups studied was
higher than that of infants delivered by normal spontaneous vaginal delivery
[44].

It is also important to remember that the bulk of deliveries in the United
States occur at community hospitals (3024 community hospitals and 241 academic medical centers that deliver babies), and many serve rural populations. Multiple factors contribute to less rigorous dating and timing of
deliveries in these settings. Once born, late preterm infants often are cared
for in term nurseries by pediatricians. Transitional care in these infants,
however, often requires a higher level of monitoring and support [57].

Why do elective cesarean deliveries carry a higher risk for the neonate?
Because elective cesarean section is commonly performed between 37 and
40 weeks gestation [58], it was believed that much respiratory morbidity
in newborns delivered by elective cesarean section is secondary to iatrogenic
prematurity. Indeed, studies evaluating large series of patients have shown
a higher rate of prematurity [45–47] and surfactant deficiency [55] in these
patients. Morrison and colleagues [51] showed that respiratory morbidity
in elective cesarean section is related inversely to gestational age at the
time of surgery: 73.8/1000 in the 37 th week, 42.3/1000 in the 38 th week,
and 17.8/1000 in the 39 th week of gestation. To minimize the occurrence
of iatrogenic RDS, fetal lung maturity testing was recommended initially before elective cesarean section, but this is seldom done given the risks associated with amniocentesis. Delaying elective cesarean section to 38 to 40
weeks has been shown to decrease the risk of respiratory distress, but this
carries the risk of the patient going into spontaneous labor. Further, it is
clear that in addition to RDS, infants delivered by elective cesarean section
are at higher risk of developing TTNB and PPHN unrelated to their gestational age at the time of delivery. Although most of these neonates develop
transient respiratory distress and recover without any long-term consequences, a significant number progress to severe respiratory failure [50].
These infants not only require prolonged hospitalization, but also are at increased risk for chronic lung disease and death [50]. In addition, there is
a higher incidence of respiratory depression at birth (low Apgar scores)
[54], thought to be related to fluid-clogged lungs, making the transition to
air breathing more difficult.

In an effort to reduce the occurrence of iatrogenic prematurity associated
with elective cesarean section deliveries, the American College of Obstetrics
and Gynecology [59] recommends scheduling elective cesarean section at 39
weeks or later on the basis of menstrual dates, or waiting for the onset of
spontaneous labor. It also lays down the criteria for establishing fetal maturity before elective cesarean section. As alluded to earlier, however, the
safety of this approach in mothers with previous cesarean section deliveries
has not been established in rigorous trials. Some population-based studies

[60] point to an increased risk of uterine rupture and perinatal death in mothers with previous cesarean section who went into spontaneous labor after 39 weeks. Such findings, and factors related to the convenience of scheduled elective cesarean section deliveries for both families and providers, will continue to influence the timing of elective cesarean section.

Severe hypoxic respiratory failure in late preterm infants

The general impression among clinicians is that TTNB is a benign self-limited illness that requires minimal intervention. Although respiratory distress from TTNB and other causes is seen frequently in infants delivered by elective cesarean section, it is not known how many of these infants become seriously ill and require clinical intervention. It is not clear if the risk-to-benefit ratio of an intervention that is designed to reduce respiratory morbidity in infants delivered by ECS will justify its clinical application in a large number of mothers. One approach would be to evaluate the true occurrence of severe hypoxic respiratory failure in this population [61]. Heritage and Cunningham [49] and Keszler and colleagues [50] reported severe respiratory morbidity and resulting mortality in infants born by elective cesarean section who developed pulmonary hypertension, hence the term malignant transient tachypnea of newborn (TTN). A significant number of these infants required ECMO [50]. The etiology of pulmonary hypertension and HRF in late preterm is not entirely clear. Many of these infants are asymptomatic immediately after birth or have mild respiratory distress, low oxygen requirements, and radiographic findings suggestive of retained lung fluid or mild RDS. In a subset of infants, however, there is a gradual increase in oxygen requirements and subsequent evidence of PPHN. Oxygen often is provided by oxyhoods. There are studies, especially in the adult anesthesia literature, that document a high incidence of alveolar collapse because of oxygen absorption and denitrogenation (nitrogen washout) [62,63]. Rothen and colleagues [62,63] have shown that in the postoperative period, atelectasis is twice more common in patients ventilated with 100% oxygen as compared with 30% oxygen. Detailed study of late preterm infants who required ECMO is warranted to better understand the pathophysiology of HRF in this population and the influence of confounding variables.

The authors recently reviewed data from the ELSO Neonatal Registry to study the demographic characteristics, ECMO course, morbidity, and mortality in late preterm infants. Infants with congenital anomalies including congenital diaphragmatic hernia were excluded. From 1989 to 2006, 15,590 neonates treated with ECMO were registered with ELSO. Of these, 2258 (14.5%) neonates were late preterm. Their demographic characteristics are shown in Table 1. The mean gestational age and birth weight of late preterm infants were 35.3 plus or minus 0.9 weeks and 2.8 plus or minus 0.51 kg respectively. More late preterm infants treated with ECMO were

Table 1
Demographic characteristics of the late preterm and term extracorporeal membrane oxygenation population

	Late preterm (N = 2062)	Term (N = 12,336)	P
Birth weight	2.82 ± 0.50 kg	3.42 ± 0.56 kg	<.0001
Gestation	35.4 ± 0.8 wks	39.7 ± 1.5 wks	<.0001
Male	66%	57%	<.0001
Median apgar 1	6	5	<.0001
Median apgar 5	8	7	<.0001

Data expressed as mean ± SD or percentage.

non-Hispanic whites and were delivered by elective cesarean section. The primary etiology of hypoxic respiratory failure in late preterm infants was RDS or sepsis as compared with term infants who were more likely to have aspiration syndromes. Pulmonary hypertension was reported with equal frequency in both groups. Data related to the ECMO course are summarized in Table 2. Late preterm infants were older at cannulation and had a longer duration of ECMO support. Table 3 compares the major complications reported in late preterm and term infants. Late preterm infants were more likely to have intraventricular hemorrhage and other neurologic complications than term infants. They were also more likely to die on ECMO or have ECMO support discontinued before lung recovery. The overall survival rate was 74% for late preterm infants as compared with 87% for term infants (P < .0001). Survival in the late preterm neonatal ECMO population fell from 81.5% in 1989 to 65.2% in 2005 (Fig. 1). Gestational age continued to be an independent risk factor for mortality in neonates treated with ECMO after correction for race, diagnosis, mode of delivery, and 5-minute Apgar score.

Table 2
Extracorporeal membrane oxygenation course in late preterm and term infants

	Late preterm (N = 2062)	Term (N = 12,336)	P
Age on ECMO	2.6 ± 3.3 days	2.2 ± 2.8 days	<.0001
Hours on ECMO	145 ± 102 hrs	136 ± 86 hrs	<.0001
Lung support (%)	99	99	NS
Discontinuation or death on ECMO	28.2%	15.5%	<.0001
Survival	74%	87%	<.0001

Late preterm infants were older at cannulation, had a longer duration of ECMO support, and had a significantly lower survival rate when compared to term infants. Data expressed as mean ± SD or percentage.

Abbreviations: ECMO, extracorporeal membrane oxygenation; NS, not significant; SD, standard deviation.

Table 3
Extracorporeal membrane oxygenation complication rates in late preterm and term infants

Complication	Late preterm (%)	Term (%)	RR	95% CI
Hemorrhagic	6.4	8.4	0.76	0.68–0.84
Mechanical	1.4	1.5	0.94	0.87–1.00
Metabolic	8.8	7.1	1.25	1.14–1.37
Neurologic	12.4	8.2	1.51	1.40–1.63
IVH	4.4	1.9	2.33	2.02–2.69
Other	8.0	6.3	1.27	1.15–1.39
Hemofiltration/dialysis	7.3	5.6	1.31	1.18–1.45
Culture-proven infection	2.6	2.4	1.11	0.94–1.32
Major cardiovascular	4.1	3.7	1.06	0.95–1.18
PDA	1.8	1.9	0.93	0.76–1.14
Other	4.1	3.7	1.12	0.98–1.21
Pulmonary hemorrhage	1.5	1.4	1.12	0.90–1.40

Late preterm infants were more likely to have intraventricular hemorrhage and other neurologic complications than term infants.

Abbreviations: CI, confidence interval; IVH, intraventricular hemorrhage; PDA, patent ductus arteriosis; RR, relative risk.

Management strategies for late preterm infants with hypoxic respiratory failure

Approximately 30,000 late preterm and term infants in the United States require mechanical ventilation each year secondary to neonatal respiratory failure [5]. Eighty five percent of these infants will fail to respond to conventional ventilation with high fractional oxygen concentrations and will develop neonatal HRF, which will require adjunctive therapies [3]. These infants have a higher mortality than preterm infants with acute respiratory failure [64]. Respiratory insufficiency occurs in late preterm and term infants as a complication of perinatal asphyxia, elective cesarean birth, perinatal aspiration syndromes, pneumonia, sepsis, RDS, pulmonary hypoplasia, and

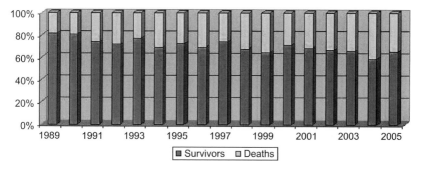

Fig. 1. Change in survival of late preterm infants treated with extracorporeal membrane oxygenation (ECMO) since 1989. Survival in this population fell from 81.5% in 1989 to 65.2% in 2005 in spite of improvements in ECMO.

other congenital anomalies of the lung. Maternal ingestion of nonsteroidal anti-inflammatory drugs [65] and late trimester use of selective serotonin re-uptake inhibitors [66] have also been implicated as possible causes of some cases of PPHN. The progression from respiratory insufficiency to neonatal HRF is accompanied by:

- Pulmonary artery hypertension with right-to-left shunting via fetal pathways
- Surfactant dysfunction with associated alveolar collapse
- Ventilator-induced lung injury

Newer techniques and adjuvant treatments have improved survival rates in this population by addressing the pathophysiology of HRF. These include administration of exogenous surfactant, iNO, high-frequency ventilation and ECMO. Liquid ventilation also has shown some promise in this regard [67].

Supportive care

Infants who have HRF require attention to detail. Continuous monitoring of oxygenation, blood pressure, and perfusion is critical. The oxygenation index (OI = Paw × FiO_2 × $100/Pao_2$) should be calculated for each arterial blood gas sample. The highest OI during the first 24 hours of life recently was found to be useful in predicting the outcome of HRF with results comparable to the SNAP II score [68]. Infants with PPHN frequently have right-to-left shunting across the patent ductus arteriosus. This can be demonstrated by pre- and postductal arterial blood gas sampling or placement of oximeter probes. Although it is a useful indicator of PPHN when present, a ductal shunt is frequently absent in late preterm and term infants who have PPHN.

Management of fluids and electrolytes is important. Normal values for glucose and ionized calcium should be maintained, because hypoglycemia and hypocalcemia tend to worsen PPHN. An adequate circulating blood volume is crucial to maintain right ventricular filling and cardiac output. Excessive volume administration, however, can lead to pulmonary edema and cardiac decompensation. Colloid infusions have not been shown to be superior to crystalloid solutions in restoring circulatory volume in hypotensive infants [69], children, and adults [14] and have been shown to worsen oxygenation in adult patients with acute respiratory distress syndrome (ARDS) [70] and renal function in neonatal ECMO patients [71]. Colloid infusions and blood products should be reserved for specific indications (eg, the correction of abnormal coagulation studies). The platelet count frequently is depressed in infants who have HRF regardless of the underlying disease; however, transfusion of platelets may result in increased pulmonary vasospasm or deposition of platelet thrombi in the pulmonary microcirculation [72]. Polycythemia can result in hyperviscosity syndrome and may cause or aggravate PPHN and anemia because acute blood loss can result in right-to-left shunting, hypotension, and systemic hypoperfusion. Both conditions require immediate treatment. Inotropic support with dopamine and dobutamine, alone or in combination, may be helpful in maintaining adequate cardiac output and systemic blood pressure [73]. Epinephrine and norepinephrine also have been used in this setting [74]. Infants who have vasopressor-resistant hypotension may benefit from steroid replacement [75].

A chest radiograph is useful for assessing underlying parenchymal lung disease, and it can exclude anomalies such as congenital diaphragmatic hernia. In infants who have idiopathic PPHN, the lung fields typically appear clear, with decreased vascular markings and a normal heart size. A two-dimensional echocardiogram is generally necessary to exclude cyanotic congenital heart disease. Defining the anatomy of the pulmonary veins can be extremely difficult if extrapulmonary right-to-left shunting of blood is present. Likewise, the diagnosis of coarctation of the aorta may be difficult in infants whose ductus arteriosus is widely patent. If the echocardiogram is not definitive, cardiac catheterization may be necessary to exclude these and other cardiac lesions. Color flow Doppler imaging can be used to determine if right-to-left shunting of blood across the ductus arteriosus, foramen ovale, or both is present. The peak velocity of the regurgitant flow across the tricuspid valve can be used to estimate right ventricular systolic pressure. The peak velocity of left-to-right or right-to-left flow in the ductus arteriosus can be used to estimate pulmonary artery pressure. Other echocardiographic findings suggestive of PPHN include right atrial dilation, right ventricular dilation, bowing of the interatrial or interventricular septum to the left, and flattening of the interventricular septum. The echocardiogram also can be helpful for assessing ventricular performance. Right ventricular dysfunction can cause right-to-left atrial shunting across the foramen ovale and decrease pulmonary blood flow in the absence of PPHN. Severe left ventricular dysfunction leads to right-to-left shunting at the ductal level, elevates left atrial pressure, and results in pulmonary edema and systemic hypoperfusion, acidosis, and multi-organ system dysfunction. Treatment with pulmonary vasodilators in this circumstance can result in cardiovascular collapse [76]. Cranial ultrasonography should be performed if the infant is being considered for extracorporeal life support. This is especially true in the late preterm infant who is at increased risk of intracranial hemorrhage on ECMO [77,78].

When caring for infants, the use of a protocol to minimize handling is imperative. Sedation and analgesia with opiates is often necessary to decrease sympathetic tone during stressful interventions and blunt the pulmonary vascular response to noxious stimuli. Fentanyl is the most frequently used opiate. Acute muscle rigidity, or chest wall syndrome, may occur following rapid infusion. Prolonged exposure leads to accumulation in fat and delays weaning. Tolerance develops rapidly, and significant withdrawal symptoms may develop if infusions are used for more than 5 days. Fentanyl has minimal effect on the cardiovascular system; however, the addition of benzodiazepines or other sedatives may decrease cardiac output and blood pressure [79]. The use of paralytic agents is controversial and reserved for the infant who cannot be treated with sedatives alone. The use of muscle relaxants may promote atelectasis of dependent lung regions and ventilation perfusion ratio (V/Q) mismatch. A review of 385 newborns with PPHN by Walsh-Sukys and colleagues suggests that paralysis may be associated with an increased risk of death [80].

Mechanical ventilation

Mechanical ventilation with high inspired oxygen concentration is the main support modality for the treatment of neonates with HRF. However, it has become apparent that mechanical ventilation can lead to numerous serious complications, including initiation or exacerbation of underlying lung injury. Mechanical ventilation with high fractions of inspired oxygen and high inspiratory pressures has been implicated in the pathogenesis of bronchopulmonary dysplasia [81]. In the late preterm and term infant, the pathophysiology of ventilation-induced lung injury is more akin to that of adult respiratory distress syndrome and involves factors such as complement, oxygen free radicals, proteases, endotoxin, eicosanoids, platelet activating factor, cytokines, growth factors and kallikreins [82–86]. Research over the past two decades has focused primarily on the mechanical forces producing ventilator-induced lung injury. Despite intense research and numerous innovations in ventilatory therapy aimed at minimizing such injury, the morbidity and mortality of acute respiratory failure remains high, and ventilator-induced lung injury remains a significant problem for the critically ill neonate [87]. In newborns developing HRF, only a small percentage goes on to die of respiratory failure. Rather, lung injury results in the development of a systemic inflammatory response that culminates in multi-organ dysfunction syndrome (MODS) and death [81].

One possible explanation for this observation is that mechanical ventilation initiates or potentiates an inflammatory response in the lung, which in turn results in a vicious cycle of inflammation leading to both local and systemic tissue injury. Although no studies have addressed whether mechanical ventilation is capable of altering lung cellular function leading to production of inflammatory mediators and lung injury, there is some evidence in the literature to support this concept. Clinical studies of adults developing ARDS have noted an association between lung inflammatory mediators and development of physiologic abnormalities [82]. Studies in a rabbit model of ARDS have found that conventional mechanical ventilation as opposed to high-frequency oscillatory ventilation (HFOV) led to increased neutrophil infiltration and activation, and increased lung lavage levels of platelet-activating factor and thromboxane [85]. Concurrent with these physiological studies, research over the past decade has shown that mechanotransduction (ie, the conversion of a mechanical stimulus such as cell deformation into biochemical and molecular alterations) plays a crucial role in determining the structure and function of numerous tissues, including the lung. Studies in vitro and in vivo have found that both the degree and the pattern of mechanical stretch are important in determining cell responses [87]. Given that mechanical ventilation alters both the pattern and magnitude of lung stretch, it is not unreasonable to postulate that alterations in gene expression or cellular metabolism may arise. Specific patterns of ventilation can produce or magnify the inflammatory response in the lung, and thus provide a mechanism whereby mechanical ventilation could lead to lung injury and contribute to the development of a systemic inflammatory response [85].

A tidal breath delivered to an injured lung preferentially will follow the path of least resistance and inflate the more compliant, nondependent alveoli. When large tidal volumes are delivered, this can lead to overdistension of such alveoli and aggravate injury, by a process termed volutrauma. Injury to alveoli in the poorly compliant dependent lung also can be aggravated by a suboptimal ventilation strategy. If insufficient peak end-expiratory pressure (PEEP) is applied, dependent alveoli are subjected to cyclic opening and closing, which leads to injury through a process termed atelectrauma. Therefore, an optimal lung protective strategy should use inspiratory volumes that avoid overinflation of nondependent alveoli, yet provide enough PEEP to prevent the atelectrauma caused by cyclic derecruitment of dependent alveoli [86,88]. When a conventional ventilator is used, such a protective strategy often will result in lower minute ventilation, higher levels of Pa_{CO_2}, and controlled respiratory acidosis or permissive hypercapnia. Although usually well tolerated in adults and pediatric patients with ARDS, permissive hypercapnia has not been well-studied in PPHN [88].

High-frequency ventilation can be used as a lung protective strategy in neonates who have HRF [88]. During HFOV, small tidal volumes are used at supraphysiologic rates to support gas exchange. If adequate mean airway pressure is used to recruit and maintain alveolar patency, the small magnitude of volume oscillations will neither cause overdistension of alveoli nor allow for derecruitment during expiration, thus avoiding the upper and lower limits of the pressure/volume curve. Because oxygenation and ventilation are not coupled directly during HFOV, it can be used as a lung protective strategy and achieve physiologic levels of Pa_{CO_2}, reducing concerns about the potentially deleterious effects of acidosis in neonates who have PPHN [7,89–91].

The relationship between ventilation strategy and the development and progression of lung injury recently was demonstrated by Rotta and colleagues in a small animal model of lung injury [85]. Compared with standard ventilation, two distinct lung protective strategies, low tidal volume with PEEP and HFOV, were associated with improved oxygenation, attenuation of inflammation as measured by tracheal fluid protein, elastase, tumor necrosis factor alpha and pulmonary leukostasis, and decreased lung injury. Animals treated with HFOV experienced less hemodynamic instability compared with the other experimental groups.

Ventilator settings should be adjusted to maintain normal expansion (ie, approximately 8 to 9 ribs) on chest radiograph. Monitoring of pulmonary mechanics may be helpful in avoiding overexpansion, which can contribute to elevated pulmonary vascular resistance and aggravate right-to-left shunting. In infants with severe pulmonary parenchymal disease who require high-peak inspiratory pressures, HFOV should be considered to reduce barotrauma [88]. Only two prospective randomized studies have compared HFOV with conventional ventilation in late preterm and term infants with acute HRF [7,92]. Neither showed a reduction in mortality or the need for ECMO, although HFOV, using a high volume strategy, can be used as an effective rescue therapy for some of these infants.

Of equal importance is determining the target arterial blood gas values. Pao_2 levels of 50 to 60 mm Hg typically provide for adequate oxygen delivery. Aiming for significantly higher Pao_2 concentrations may lead to increased ventilator support and lung injury. The use of hyperventilation first was described by Drummond and colleagues [93]. Forced alkalosis, using sodium bicarbonate, and hyperventilation became popular therapies because of their ability to produce acute pulmonary vasodilation and increases in Pao_2. Walsh-Sukys and colleagues [80] reviewed the management of PPHN and reported on unproven therapies (ie, hyperventilation, continuous infusion of alkali, sedation, paralysis, inotrope administration, and vasodilator drugs) used before widespread use of inhaled nitric oxide (iNO). No specific therapy was clearly associated with a reduction in mortality. Hyperventilation reduced the risk of ECMO without increasing the need for oxygen at 28 days of age. Hypocarbia, however, constricts the cerebral vasculature and reduces cerebral blood flow, and alkalosis and hypocarbia have been associated with later neurodevelopmental deficits, including a high rate of sensorineural hearing loss. The use of alkali infusion was associated with increased use of ECMO and an increased need for oxygen at 28 days of age. Successful management of infants with HRF without using alkalinization has been reported by Wung and colleagues [94] in a series of 15 neonates in whom a strategy designed to maintain Pao_2 at 50 to 70 and $Paco_2$ at less than 60 resulted in excellent outcome and a low incidence of chronic lung disease.

Surfactant replacement

Exogenous surfactant therapy is another promising adjunctive treatment for late preterm and term neonates who have severe HRF. There is evidence that surfactant deficiency contributes to decreased lung compliance and atelectasis in some patients who have PPHN [9,95–115]. Recent studies have suggested that exogenous surfactant therapy can cause sustained clinical improvement in late preterm and term infants with pneumonia and meconium aspiration syndrome and reduce the duration of ECMO [8,9,96,97,101,106, 108,110,115–118]. A randomized multi-center trial demonstrated that treatment with surfactant decreased the need for ECMO in late preterm and term newborns with respiratory failure. Subset analysis, however, showed that the decrease in ECMO use was limited to patients treated earlier in the course of their disease (OI less than or equal to 22) [8]. Surfactant treatment does not appear to be effective in patients who have advanced HRF; however, by improving lung inflation, surfactant treatment may augment the response to inhalational vasodilators such as iNO [116].

Management of pulmonary hypertension of the newborn

Persistent pulmonary hypertension of the newborn is associated with increased pulmonary vascular resistance and leads to hypoxemia secondary to right-to-left shunting by means of fetal pathways and V/Q mismatching. Numerous treatments have been advocated to reduce pulmonary vascular resistance, beginning with the use of tolazoline by Goetzman and colleagues [119].

The physiologic rationale for iNO therapy for treating neonatal HRF is based on its ability to achieve potent and sustained pulmonary vasodilation without decreasing systemic vascular tone. The use of intravenous vasodilator drugs such as tolazoline and sodium nitroprusside in PPHN has had limited success because of systemic hypotension and inability to achieve or sustain pulmonary vasodilation [120]. The ability of iNO therapy to selectively lower pulmonary vascular resistance (PVR) and decrease extrapulmonary right-to-left shunting accounts for the immediate improvement in oxygenation observed in newborns who have PPHN [121,122]. As described in children and adults with severe respiratory failure [123,124], oxygenation also can improve during iNO therapy in newborns who do not have extrapulmonary right-to-left shunting [10]. Low-dose iNO therapy can improve oxygenation by redirecting blood from poorly aerated or diseased lung regions to better-aerated distal air spaces, thereby improving V/Q matching [125].

In addition to its effects on vascular tone and reactivity, other physiologic targets for iNO therapy in HRF may include direct effects on lung inflammation, vascular permeability, thrombosis in situ and pulmonary remodeling [126]. Although laboratory studies initially suggested that NO can potentiate lung injury by promoting oxidative stress [127,128], surfactant inactivation, and stimulating inflammation, more recent studies have demonstrated striking antioxidant and anti-inflammatory effects in models of lung injury [129–133]. These findings suggest that low-dose iNO therapy may reduce lung inflammation and edema, as well as improve surfactant function in neonates with HRF, but these effects remain clinically unproven [126].

HRF in the late preterm and term newborn represents a heterogeneous group of disorders, and disease-specific responses have been described. Patients who have idiopathic PPHN show immediate improvement in oxygenation in response to iNO therapy, while patients with predominantly intrapulmonary shunting (eg, RDS) have less dramatic responses [91,134]. Several pathophysiologic disturbances contribute to hypoxemia in the newborn infant, including cardiac dysfunction, airway and pulmonary parenchymal abnormalities, and pulmonary vascular disorders. In some newborns who have HRF, only a single mechanism is operative, but in most, several of these mechanisms apply. The relative contribution of each mechanism may vary over time and dictate the use of different therapeutic modalities to reverse the hypoxemia [125].

Available evidence from clinical trials supports the use of iNO in late preterm (at least 34 weeks gestation) and term newborns with hypoxemic respiratory failure who require mechanical ventilation and high inspired oxygen concentrations [6,10,135,136]. A recent meta-analysis of six randomized controlled trials showed that about 50% of infants will have clinically significant increases in oxygenation within 60 minutes after initiating iNO [137]. Clinical trials of iNO in the newborn have incorporated ECMO treatment as an end point and have shown a 35% to 40% reduction in the need for ECMO in late preterm and term infants treated with iNO. Although one of the pivotal studies used to support the new drug application for iNO therapy included infants with a postnatal age up to 14 days, the average age at enrollment was 1.7 days. Currently, clinical trials support the use of iNO before treatment with ECMO, usually within the first week of life. Clinical experience, however, suggests that iNO may be of benefit as an adjuvant treatment after ECMO therapy in patients with sustained pulmonary hypertension (eg, congenital diaphragmatic hernia) [138]. Thus postnatal age alone should not define the duration of therapy in cases in which prolonged treatment could be beneficial.

Although clinical trials commonly used an OI greater than 25 for enrollment, the mean OI at study entry in multi-center trials approximated 40. A trial of the early institution of iNO in late preterm and term neonates with HRF at an OI of 15 to 25 resulted in improved oxygenation, with fewer iNO treated infants progressing to an OI greater than 40 [139]. There was no improvement in outcome, however (ie, mortality, morbidity, or the need for ECMO support) when compared with initiation of iNO at an OI greater than 25. Echocardiographic evidence of PPHN was a criteria for enrollment in all but the Neonatal Inhaled Nitric Oxide Study (NINOS) trial [6]. Echocardiography was performed before randomization in 97% infants of enrolled in the NINOS trial, and 78% had evidence of pulmonary hypertension. There was no difference in primary outcome or response to iNO based on the presence of echocardiographic evidence of pulmonary hypertension in this large series. Current multi-center studies suggest that indications for treatment with iNO include an OI greater than 25 even in the absence of echocardiographic evidence of extrapulmonary right-to-left shunting.

The first studies of iNO treatment in late preterm and term newborns reported initial doses that ranged from 80 to 20 ppm. The rationale for doses used in these clinical trials was based on concentrations that had previously been found to be effective in animal experiments. Roberts and colleagues reported that brief inhalation of nitric oxide (NO) at 80 ppm improved oxygenation in patients who had PPHN, but this response was sustained in only one patient after NO was discontinued [140]. In the second report, rapid improvement in oxygenation in neonates who had severe PPHN also was demonstrated, but this was achieved at lower doses (20 ppm) for 4 hours [121]. This study also reported that decreasing the iNO dose to 6 ppm for the duration of treatment provided sustained improvement in oxygenation. The relative effectiveness of low-dose iNO in improving oxygenation in newborns with severe PPHN was corroborated in a dose–response study by Finer and colleagues [141]. Immediate improvement in oxygenation during treatment was not different with doses of iNO ranging from 5 to 80 ppm. These laboratory and clinical studies established the iNO dosing protocols for subsequent randomized clinical trials in newborns. The initial dose in the NINOS trial was 20 ppm, but the dose was increased to 80 ppm if the improvement in Pao_2 was < 20 mm Hg. In this study, only 3 of 53 infants (6%) who failed to response to 20 ppm had an increase in Pao_2 > 20 mm Hg when treated with 80 ppm iNO [6]. Whether a progressive increase in Pao_2 would have occurred with continued exposure to 20 ppm could not be determined with this study design. Roberts et al initiated treatment with 80 ppm iNO and subsequently decreased the iNO concentration if oxygenation improved; thus, the effects of lower initial iNO doses could not be evaluated, and the effects on ECMO use were not evaluated [10]. Only one trial evaluated the effects of sustained exposure to different doses of iNO in separate treatment groups of newborns. Davidson and colleagues [136] reported the results of a randomized controlled dose–response trial in late preterm and term newborns with PPHN. In their study, patients randomly were assigned to treatment with placebo or 5, 20, or 80 ppm NO. Each iNO dose improved oxygenation compared with placebo, but there was no difference in responses between groups. In the 37 patients treated with 80 ppm, however, methemoglobinemia levels greater than 7% occurred in 35% of patients, and inspired nitrogen dioxide concentrations greater than 3 ppm were reported in 19% of patients. Therefore, the available evidence supports initiation of iNO at a dose of 20 ppm in late preterm and term newborns who have HRF. Finer and colleagues [142] reported their experience with very low-dose iNO (1 to 2 ppm) in a small series of late preterm and term neonates who had HRF. There was no significant difference in the initial response to low-dose versus high-dose iNO, although dose increases were required more often in the low-dose group. Among patients who did not respond to the initial iNO dose, 100% and 83% responded at higher doses of iNO for the low- and high-dose groups, respectively. No differences in mortality, PPHN-associated morbidity, or the need for ECMO were demonstrated between treatment groups.

In multi-center clinical trials of iNO therapy, the typical duration of iNO treatment has been less than 5 days, which parallels the clinical resolution of PPHN. Individual exceptions occur, however, particularly in cases of pulmonary hypoplasia. If iNO is required for longer than 5 days, investigations into other causes of pulmonary hypertension should be considered (eg, alveolar capillary dysplasia, pulmonary alveolar proteinosis, or undiagnosed congenital heart disease), particularly if discontinuation of iNO results in suprasystemic elevations of pulmonary artery pressure as determined by echocardiography. No controlled data are available to determine the maximal safe duration of iNO therapy.

After improvement in oxygenation occurs with the initiation of iNO therapy, strategies for weaning the iNO dose become important. Numerous approaches have been used. Generally, oxygenation does not decrease significantly until discontinuation of iNO treatment. In one study, iNO was reduced from 20 to 6 ppm after 4 hours of treatment without acute changes in oxygenation [135]. In another trial, iNO was reduced in a stepwise fashion to as low as 1 ppm without changes in oxygenation [6,136]. Weaning iNO is a different process than discontinuation of iNO therapy. Early clinical studies reported rapid and sometimes dramatic decreases in oxygenation and increases in PVR after abrupt cessation of iNO [136]. These responses are often mild and transient, and many patients with decreased oxygenation after iNO withdrawal will respond to brief elevations of FiO_2 and careful observation [143,144]. Discontinuation of iNO, however, can be associated with life-threatening elevations of PVR, profound desaturation, and systemic hypotension caused by decreased cardiac output even in those neonates whose oxygenation failed to improve on iNO [145]. In patients who deteriorate after withdrawal of iNO, restarting iNO treatment generally will cause rapid clinical improvement. Several possible mechanisms contribute to the rebound effect. First, iNO may downregulate endogenous NO production, which contributes directly to the severity of vasospasm after iNO withdrawal. Second, decreased vascular sensitivity to NO caused by alterations in other components of the NO-cyclic guanosine monophosphate (cGMP) pathway, such as decreased soluble guanylate cyclase or enhanced phosphodiesterase 5 activities, may contribute to vasospasm after NO withdrawal. In a prospective study of patients who had undergone heart surgery with marked hemodynamic changes after iNO withdrawal, sildenafil (cGMP-specific phosphodiesterase-type V inhibitor) inhibited the adverse effects of acute iNO withdrawal [146]. These findings led to the speculation that sildenafil may sustain smooth muscle cGMP content and that persistent phosphodiesterase type V activity may contribute to the rebound pulmonary hypertension after iNO withdrawal. Alternatively, the rise in PVR and drop in oxygenation after iNO withdrawal simply may represent the presence of more severe underlying pulmonary vascular disease with loss of treatment effect of iNO. The sudden increase in pulmonary artery pressure after rapid withdrawal of vasodilator therapy is not unique to iNO and has been observed in other clinical settings, such as prostacyclin withdrawal in patients who have primary pulmonary hypertension [147].

Pharmacologic augmentation of the iNO response also may prove to be effective in some patients who have PPHN. Inhaled NO causes pulmonary vasodilation by stimulating soluble guanylate cyclase and increasing cGMP content in vascular smooth muscle. Smooth muscle cGMP content is regulated further by cGMP-specific phosphodiesterase type V, which inactivates cGMP by hydrolysis. Whether the inability to sustain cGMP contributes to the failure of some patients with PPHN to respond or to sustain improved oxygenation during iNO therapy is uncertain. Early clinical experience with dipyrdamole, which has phosphodiesterase type V inhibitory activity, has been variable [148–150]. Although dipyridamole may enhance the response to iNO in some patients, its effects are variable and are not selective for the pulmonary circulation. Recent studies with sildenafil, a more selective phosphodiesterase type V antagonist, appear more promising and may lead to novel clinical strategies to enhance the treatment of pulmonary hypertension [151–153].

Considering the important role of parenchymal lung disease in this condition, pharmacologic pulmonary vasodilation alone would not be expected to cause sustained clinical improvement in many cases. Moreover, patients not responding to iNO can show marked improvement in oxygenation with adequate lung inflation alone. High success rates in early studies were achieved by withholding iNO treatment until attempts were made to optimize ventilation and lung inflation with mechanical ventilation [6,10,135,136]. These early studies demonstrated that the effects of iNO may be suboptimal when lung volume is decreased in association with pulmonary parenchymal disease. Atelectasis and air space disease may decrease the effective delivery of iNO to its site of action in terminal lung units. In cases complicated by severe lung disease and underinflation, pulmonary hypertension may be the result of the adverse mechanical effects of underinflation on pulmonary vascular resistance. Aggressive ventilation may result in overinflation because of inadvertent PEEP and gas trapping and may elevate pulmonary vascular resistance caused by vascular compression. This commonly complicates the treatment of infants with asymmetric lung disease or airway obstruction, as observed in meconium aspiration syndrome. In newborns with severe lung disease, HFOV frequently is used to optimize lung inflation and minimize lung injury. A randomized multi-center trial demonstrated that treatment with HFOV plus iNO was often successful in patients with severe PPHN who did not respond to HFOV or iNO alone and that differences in responses were related to the underlying diagnosis [92]. For patients with PPHN complicated by severe lung disease, response rates for HFOV plus iNO were better than those for HFOV or iNO alone.

In contrast, for patients who have idiopathic PPHN, both iNO and HFOV plus iNO were more effective than HFOV alone. This response to combined treatment with HFOV plus iNO is likely because of improvement in both intra- and extrapulmonary right-to-left shunting based on maneuvers that simultaneously recruit and sustain lung volume and augment NO delivery to its site of action.

Published reports on the use of iNO in ECMO centers have not substantiated early concerns that iNO would affect outcome adversely by delaying ECMO use [3,6,135,136,139]. Decreased ECMO use with iNO treatment in multi-center RCTs has not been associated with an increase in mortality, neurologic injury, or bronchopulmonary dysplasia. Indeed, in one trial, iNO treatment was associated with improved pulmonary outcomes [135]. In another study, the median time from randomization to treatment with ECMO was 4.4 and 6.7 hours for the control and iNO groups, respectively [136]. Although this difference was statistically significant, there were no apparent adverse consequences caused by the delay. More recently, the use of iNO before initiation of ECMO was shown to improve ECMO outcomes by decreasing the need for cardiopulmonary resuscitation before ECMO cannulation [154]. Although marked improvement in oxygenation occurs in many late preterm and term newborns with severe PPHN, sustained improvement may be compromised in some patients by progressive worsening of pulmonary compliance or cardiovascular function necessitating referral for ECMO support. Withdrawal of iNO during transport to an ECMO center may lead to acute decompensation [136,145]. In such cases, iNO provides an important therapeutic bridge, ensuring stability during transport. When progressive deterioration in oxygenation occurs during iNO treatment in institutions that cannot offer more advanced rescue therapy, provisions must be in place to accomplish transport to the ECMO center without interruption of iNO treatment.

Other vasodilators that have not yet been shown to have selective or clinically beneficial effects when given systemically are being studied for use by inhalation. They include tolazoline, prostaglandin derivatives, and nitrosodilators [155–159]. The most appropriate drug would have a direct immediate effect on the pulmonary vasculature and be degraded rapidly by circulating enzymes to prevent systemic effects even after prolonged treatment. The vasodilating actions of prostacyclin are dependent on a receptor-mediated increase in intracellular cyclic adenosine monophosphate. This suggests that there may be synergy with iNO, whose actions are mediated through cGMP. Combined treatment with iNO and prostacyclin therefore may have even greater benefits, and isolated reports and small case series of successful combined treatment of refractory PPHN have been published [157,160].

Extracorporeal membrane oxygenation

Recent data from the ELSO Neonatal Registry show a decrease in the use of ECMO support, presumably because of the effectiveness of the previously described treatments such as lung protective ventilation, iNO, and exogenous surfactant administration in late preterm and term infants [161]. Not all infants will respond to these new treatments, however. Extracorporeal life support is used to treat acute respiratory failure when other treatment modalities have failed. ECMO was shown to improve the survival in late preterm and term infants with severe respiratory failure in at least two single institution RCTs [162,163]. Subsequently, the United Kingdom collaborative randomized trial of neonatal ECMO and follow-up studies reported that ECMO significantly reduced the risk of death without an increase in severe disabilities [164]. In this study, 30 of 93 infants in the ECMO group died, compared with 54 of 92 in the conventional care group.

Infants with diaphragmatic hernia had a poorer outcome than other patients receiving extracorporeal membrane oxygenation, with a survival rate of 62% compared with 83% in infants with other diagnoses. Venovenous ECMO, which is used less frequently, is preferable to venoarterial ECMO in acute respiratory failure, as it avoids cannulation of the carotid artery and seems to have fewer complications [165,166]. Newer techniques for extracorporeal gas exchange, such as the single lumen cannula push-pull method, known as AREC (assistance respiratoire extracorporelle), provides effective support in smaller neonates, is faster to apply since the cannulation is generally percutaneous, and is simpler to operate [167].

Consideration of ECMO therapy should include an evaluation of risks versus benefits because of the invasive nature of the therapy and the need for heparinization. Usual criteria for ECMO support include:

- 34 weeks gestation or greater
- Weight 2000 g or more
- No major intracranial hemorrhage
- Reversible lung disease, on mechanical ventilation for no more than 14 days
- No lethal congenital anomalies
- Refractory hypoxemia
- Circulatory collapse

Prematurity is associated with increased morbidity and mortality rates related to ECMO and has led to the exclusion of very premature infants from consideration for bypass support. In 1992, Revenis and colleagues [78] reported their experience with lower birth weight infants (2000 to 2500 gm) treated with ECMO at a single center. Mortality was significantly higher in the lower birth weight infants (relative risk [RR] 3.45, confidence interval [CI] 1.68 to 5.79) compared with infants with normal birth weights. For infants who had RDS, mortality was 56% for the lower birth weight versus

8% for the normal birth weight group ($P < .01$). The most frequent cause of death was intracranial hemorrhage. The overall incidence of any neuroimaging abnormality and the risk of developmental delay among survivors was significantly greater among the lower birth weight infants. More recently, the role of postconceptual age as an independent predicator of intracranial hemorrhage in premature neonates treated with ECMO has been published [80]. These results were corroborated further by the authors' recent review of data from the ELSO Neonatal Registry detailed earlier.

The late preterm infant with refractory hypoxemia should be referred for bypass support if he or she fails to respond to other rescue therapies. The timing of referral to an ECMO center is critical. As recently as 10 to 15 years ago, mortality for neonatal HRF was 40% to 60%, with an incidence of major neurologic handicap of 15% to 60% [164,168]. If all available rescue therapies including ECMO are used, mortality is currently less than 20% to 25%, and the incidence of major neurologic handicap for surviving infants is approximately 15% to 20%. Early consultation and discussion with the ECMO center is recommended strongly. Guidelines for consultation are available at: http://www.elso.med.umich.edu/.

Summary

In the United States, a significant number of babies each year are delivered at late preterm gestations, and up to 50% of these deliveries occur by cesarean section. Of these, a significant number of infants develop severe hypoxic respiratory failure, resulting in need for additional treatments like ventilation, surfactant, inhaled nitric oxide, and ECMO. There is an urgent need for preventive and therapeutic interventions that can help in optimizing the outcome of this vulnerable population.

References

[1] Buus-Frank ME. The great imposter. Adv Neonatal Care 2005;5(5):233–6.
[2] Escobar GJ, Greene JD, Hulac P, et al. Rehospitalisation after birth hospitalisation: patterns among infants of all gestations. Arch Dis Child 2005;90(2):125–31.
[3] Clark RH. The epidemiology of respiratory failure in neonates born at an estimated gestational age of 34 weeks or more. J Perinatol 2005;25(4):251–7.
[4] Roth-Kleiner M, Wagner BP, Bachmann D, et al. Respiratory distress syndrome in near-term babies after caesarean section. Swiss Med Wkly 2003;133:283–8.
[5] Angus DC, Linde-Zwirble WT, Clermont G, et al. Epidemiology of neonatal respiratory failure in the United States: projections from California and New York. Am J Respir Crit Care Med 2001;164(7):1154–60.
[6] Inhaled nitric oxide in full-term and nearly full-term infants with hypoxic respiratory failure. The Neonatal Inhaled Nitric Oxide Study Group. N Engl J Med 1997;336(9):597–604.
[7] Clark RH, Yoder BA, Sell MS. Prospective, randomized comparison of high-frequency oscillation and conventional ventilation in candidates for extracorporeal membrane oxygenation. J Pediatr 1994;124(3):447–54.

[8] Lotze A, Mitchell BR, Bulas DI, et al. Multi-center study of surfactant (beractant) use in the treatment of term infants with severe respiratory failure. Survanta in Term Infants Study Group. J Pediatr 1998;132(1):40–7.

[9] Halliday HL, Speer CP, Robertson B. Treatment of severe meconium aspiration syndrome with porcine surfactant. Collaborative Surfactant Study Group. Eur J Pediatr 1996; 155(12):1047–51.

[10] Roberts JD Jr, Fineman JR, Morin FC III, et al. Inhaled nitric oxide and persistent pulmonary hypertension of the newborn. The Inhaled Nitric Oxide Study Group. N Engl J Med 1997;336(9):605–10.

[11] Stevens TP, Chess PR, McConnochie KM, et al. Survival in early- and late-term infants with congenital diaphragmatic hernia treated with extracorporeal membrane oxygenation. Pediatrics 2002;110(3):590–6.

[12] Rubaltelli FF, Bonafe L, Tangucci M, et al. Epidemiology of neonatal acute respiratory disorders. A multi-center study on incidence and fatality rates of neonatal acute respiratory disorders according to gestational age, maternal age, pregnancy complications and type of delivery. Italian Group of Neonatal Pneumology. Biol Neonate 1998;74(1): 7–15.

[13] Jain L. Alveolar fluid clearance in developing lungs and its role in neonatal transition. Clin Perinatol 1999;26(3):585–99.

[14] Baines DL, Folkesson HG, Norlin A, et al. The influence of mode of delivery, hormonal status and postnatal O2 environment on epithelial sodium channel (ENaC) expression in perinatal guinea-pig lung. J Physiol 2000;522:147–57.

[15] Berger PJ, Kyriakides MA, Smolich JJ, et al. Massive decline in lung liquid before vaginal delivery at term in the fetal lamb. Am J Obstet Gynecol 1998;178(2):223–7.

[16] Berger PJ, Smolich JJ, Ramsden CA, et al. Effect of lung liquid volume on respiratory performance after caesarean delivery in the lamb. J Physiol 1996;492:905–12.

[17] Berthiaume Y, Broaddus VC, Gropper MA, et al. Alveolar liquid and protein clearance from normal dog lungs. J Appl Physiol 1988;65(2):585–93.

[18] Berthiaume Y, Staub NC, Matthay MA. Beta-adrenergic agonists increase lung liquid clearance in anesthetized sheep. J Clin Invest 1987;79(2):335–43.

[19] Jain L, Chen XJ, Ramosevac S, et al. Expression of highly selective sodium channels in alveolar type II cells is determined by culture conditions. Am J Physiol Lung Cell Mol Physiol 2001;280(4):L646–58.

[20] Bland RD. Lung epithelial ion transport and fluid movement during the perinatal period. Am J Physiol 1990;259:L30–7.

[21] Bland RD. Loss of liquid from the lung lumen in labor: more than a simple squeeze. Am J Physiol Lung Cell Mol Physiol 2001;280(4):L602–5.

[22] O'Brodovich H. Epithelial ion transport in the fetal and perinatal lung. Am J Physiol 1991; 261:C555–64.

[23] O'Brodovich H, Canessa C, Ueda J, et al. Expression of the epithelial Na + channel in the developing rat lung. Am J Physiol 1993;265(2 Pt 1):C491–6.

[24] O'Brodovich H. When the alveolus is flooding, it's time to man the pumps [editorial]. Am Rev Respir Dis 1990;142:1247–8.

[25] O'Brodovich HM. The role of active Na + transport by lung epithelium in the clearance of airspace fluid. New Horiz 1995;3(2):240–7.

[26] O'Brodovich HM. Immature epithelial Na + channel expression is one of the pathogenetic mechanisms leading to human neonatal respiratory distress syndrome. Proc Assoc Am Physicians 1996;108(5):345–55.

[27] O'Brodovich HM. Respiratory distress syndrome: the importance of effective transport. J Pediatr 1997;130(3):342–4.

[28] Gowen CW Jr, Lawson EE, Gingras J, et al. Electrical potential difference and ion transport across nasal epithelium of term neonates: correlation with mode of delivery, transient tachypnea of the newborn, and respiratory rate. J Pediatr 1988;113:121–7.

[29] Barker PM, Gowen CW, Lawson EE, et al. Decreased sodium ion absorption across nasal epithelium of very premature infants with respiratory distress syndrome. J Pediatr 1997; 130(3):373–7.

[30] Bland RD, Hansen TN, Haberkern CM, et al. Lung fluid balance in lambs before and after birth. J Appl Physiol 1982;53(4):992–1004.

[31] Humphreys PW, Normand IC, Reynolds EO, et al. Pulmonary lymph flow and the uptake of liquid from the lungs of lamb at the start of breathing. J Physiol 1967;193:1.

[32] Raj JU, Bland RD. Lung luminal liquid clearance in newborn lambs. Effect of pulmonary microvascular pressure elevation. Am Rev Respir Dis 1986;134(2):305–10.

[33] Cummings JJ, Carlton DP, Poulain FR, et al. Lung luminal liquid is not removed via the pleural space in health newborn lambs. Physiologist 1989;32:202.

[34] Matthay MA, Berthiaume Y, Staub NC. Long-term clearance of liquid and protein from the lungs of unanesthetized sheep. J Appl Physiol 1985;59(3):928–34.

[35] Matthay MA, Landolt CC, Staub NC. Differential liquid and protein clearance from the alveoli of anesthetized sheep. J Appl Physiol 1982;53(1):96–104.

[36] Office of Vital and Health Statistics. Rates of cesarean delivery–United States, 1991. MMWR Morb Mortal Wkly Rep 1993;42(15):285–9.

[37] Eskew PN Jr, Saywell RM Jr, Zollinger TW, et al. Trends in the frequency of cesarean delivery. A 21-year experience, 1970–1990. J Reprod Med 1994;39(10):809–17.

[38] Taffel SM, Placek PJ, Kosary CL. US cesarean section rates 1990: an update. Birth 1992; 19(1):21–2.

[39] Taffel SM, Placek PJ, Moien M, et al. 1989 US cesarean section rate steadies—VBAC rate rises to nearly one in five. Birth 1991;18(2):73–7.

[40] Soliman SR, Burrows RF. Cesarean section: analysis of the experience before and after the National Consensus Conference on Aspects of Cesarean Birth. CMAJ 1993;148(8):1315–20.

[41] Groom K, Brown SP. Caesarean section controversy. The rate of caesarean sections is not the issue. BMJ 2000;320(7241):1072–3 [discussion 1074].

[42] Abitbol MM, Taylor-Randall UB, Barton PT, et al. Effect of modern obstetrics on mothers from third-world countries. J Matern Fetal Med 1997;6(5):276–80.

[43] Belizan JM, Althabe F, Barros FC, et al. Rates and implications of caesarean sections in Latin America: ecological study. BMJ 1999;319(7222):1397–400.

[44] McMahon MJ, Luther ER, Bowes WA Jr, et al. Comparison of a trial of labor with an elective second cesarean section. N Engl J Med 1996;335(10):689–95.

[45] Goldenberg RL, Nelson K. Iatrogenic respiratory distress syndrome. An analysis of obstetric events preceding delivery of infants who develop respiratory distress syndrome. Am J Obstet Gynecol 1975;123(6):617–20.

[46] Hack M, Fanaroff AA, Klaus MH, et al. Neonatal respiratory distress following elective delivery. A preventable disease? Am J Obstet Gynecol 1976;126(1):43–7.

[47] Maisels MJ, Rees R, Marks K, et al. Elective delivery of the term fetus. An obstetrical hazard. JAMA 1977;238(19):2036–9.

[48] Parilla BV, Dooley SL, Jansen RD, et al. Iatrogenic respiratory distress syndrome following elective repeat cesarean delivery. Obstet Gynecol 1993;81(3):392–5.

[49] Heritage CK, Cunningham MD. Association of elective repeat cesarean delivery and persistent pulmonary hypertension of the newborn. Am J Obstet Gynecol 1985;152:627–9.

[50] Keszler M, Carbone MT, Cox C, et al. Severe respiratory failure after elective repeat cesarean delivery: a potentially preventable condition leading to extracorporeal membrane oxygenation. Pediatrics 1992;89:670–2.

[51] Morrison JJ, Rennie JM, Milton PJ. Neonatal respiratory morbidity and mode of delivery at term: influence of timing of elective caesarean section. Br J Obstet Gynaecol 1995;102(2): 101–6.

[52] Annibale DJ, Hulsey TC, Wagner CL, et al. Comparative neonatal morbidity of abdominal and vaginal deliveries after uncomplicated pregnancies. Arch Pediatr Adolesc Med 1995; 149(8):862–7.

[53] van den Berg A, van Elburg RM, van Geijn HP, et al. Neonatal respiratory morbidity following elective caesarean section in term infants. A 5-year retrospective study and a review of the literature. Eur J Obstet Gynecol Reprod Biol 2001;98(1):9–13.

[54] Hook B, Kiwi R, Amini SB, et al. Neonatal morbidity after elective repeat cesarean section and trial of labor. Pediatrics 1997;100:348–53.

[55] Madar J, Richmond S, Hey E. Surfactant-deficient respiratory distress after elective delivery at term. Acta Paediatr 1999;88(11):1244–8.

[56] Schreiner RL, Stevens DC, Smith WL, et al. Respiratory distress following elective repeat cesarean section. Am J Obstet Gynecol 1982;143(6):689–92.

[57] Medoff-Cooper B, Ratcliffe SJ. Development of preterm infants: feeding behaviors and Brazelton neonatal behavioral assessment scale at 40 and 44 weeks' postconceptional age. ANS Adv Nurs Sci 2005;28(4):356–63.

[58] Hales KA, Morgan MA, Thurnau GR. Influence of labor and route of delivery on the frequency of respiratory morbidity in term neonates. Int J Gynaecol Obstet 1993;43(1): 35–40.

[59] Guidelines for Perinatal Care, 5th edition. Kearneysville (WV): American College of Obstetricians and Gynecology; 2002. p. 148.

[60] Smith GC, Pell JP, Cameron AD, et al. Risk of perinatal death associated with labor after previous cesarean delivery in uncomplicated term pregnancies. JAMA 2002;287(20): 2684–90.

[61] Halliday HL. Elective delivery at term: implications for the newborn. Acta Paediatr 1999; 88(11):1180–1.

[62] Rothen HU, Sporre B, Engberg G, et al. Influence of gas composition on recurrence of atelectasis after a re-expansion maneuver during general anesthesia. Anesthesiology 1995; 82(4):832–42.

[63] Rothen HU, Sporre B, Engberg G, et al. Prevention of atelectasis during general anaesthesia. Lancet 1995;345(8962):1387–91.

[64] Gnanaratnem J, Finer NN. Neonatal acute respiratory failure. Curr Opin Pediatr 2000; 12(3):227–32.

[65] Alano MA, Ngougmna E, Ostrea EM Jr, et al. Analysis of nonsteroidal antiinflammatory drugs and its relation to persistent pulmonary hypertension of the newborn. Pediatrics 2001;107(3):519–23.

[66] Chambers CD, Hernandez-Diaz S, Van Marter LJ, et al. Selective serotonin reuptake inhibitors and risk of persistent pulmonary hypertension of the newborn. N Engl J Med 2006; 354(6):579–87.

[67] Barrington KJ, Finer NN. Recent advances. Care of near-term infants with respiratory failure. BMJ 1997;315(7117):1215–8.

[68] Kumar D, Super DM, Fajardo RA, et al. Predicting outcome in neonatal hypoxic respiratory failure with the score for neonatal acute physiology (SNAP) and highest oxygen index (OI) in the first 24 hours of admission. J Perinatol 2004;24(6):376–81.

[69] Greenough A. Use and misuse of albumin infusions in neonatal care. Eur J Pediatr 1998; 157(9):699–702.

[70] Banerjee RR. Interactions between hematological derivatives and dipalmitoyl phosphatidyl choline: implications for adult respiratory distress syndrome. Colloids Surf B Biointerfaces 2004;34(2):95–104.

[71] Vrancken SL, Heijst AF, Zegers M, et al. Influence of volume replacement with colloids versus crystalloids in neonates on venoarterial extracorporeal membrane oxygenation on fluid retention, fluid balance, and ECMO runtime. ASAIO J 2005;51(6): 808–12.

[72] Humbert M, Morrell NW, Archer SL, et al. Cellular and molecular pathobiology of pulmonary arterial hypertension. J Am Coll Cardiol 2004;43:13S–24S.

[73] Evans N. Which inotrope for which baby? Arch Dis Child Fetal Neonatal Ed 2006;91(3): F213–20.

[74] Schindler MB, Hislop AA, Haworth SG. Postnatal changes in response to norepinephrine in the normal and pulmonary hypertensive lung. Am J Respir Crit Care Med 2004;170(6): 641–6.

[75] Fernandez E, Schrader R, Watterberg K. Prevalence of low cortisol values in term and near-term infants with vasopressor-resistant hypotension. J Perinatol 2005;25(2):114–8.

[76] Kinsella JP, Abman SH. Controversies in the use of inhaled nitric oxide therapy in the newborn. Clin Perinatol 1998;25(1):203–17.

[77] Hardart GE, Hardart MK, Arnold JH. Intracranial hemorrhage in premature neonates treated with extracorporeal membrane oxygenation correlates with conceptional age. J Pediatr 2004;145(2):184–9.

[78] Revenis ME, Glass P, Short BL. Mortality and morbidity rates among lower birth weight infants (2000 to 2500 grams) treated with extracorporeal membrane oxygenation. J Pediatr 1992;121(3):452–8.

[79] Gruber EM, Laussen PC, Casta A, et al. Stress response in infants undergoing cardiac surgery: a randomized study of fentanyl bolus, fentanyl infusion, and fentanyl-midazolam infusion. Anesth Analg 2001;92(4):882–90.

[80] Walsh-Sukys MC, Tyson JE, Wright LL, et al. Persistent pulmonary hypertension of the newborn in the era before nitric oxide: practice variation and outcomes. Pediatrics 2000; 105:14–20.

[81] Clark RH, Gerstmann DR, Jobe AH, et al. Lung injury in neonates: causes, strategies for prevention, and long-term consequences. J Pediatr 2001;139(4):478–86.

[82] Chollet-Martin S, Gatecel C, Kermarrec N, et al. Alveolar neutrophil functions and cytokine levels in patients with the adult respiratory distress syndrome during nitric oxide inhalation. Am J Respir Crit Care Med 1996;153(3):985–90.

[83] Brower RG, Ware LB, Berthiaume Y, et al. Treatment of ARDS. Chest 2001;120(4): 1347–67.

[84] Luce JM. Acute lung injury and the acute respiratory distress syndrome. Crit Care Med 1998;26(2):369–76.

[85] Rotta AT, Gunnarsson B, Fuhrman BP, et al. Comparison of lung protective ventilation strategies in a rabbit model of acute lung injury. Crit Care Med 2001;29(11):2176–84.

[86] Royall JA, Levin DL. Adult respiratory distress syndrome in pediatric patients. I. Clinical aspects, pathophysiology, pathology, and mechanisms of lung injury. J Pediatr 1988;112(2): 169–80.

[87] Auten RL, Vozzelli M, Clark RH. Volutrauma. What is it, and how do we avoid it? Clin Perinatol 2001;28(3):505–15.

[88] Clark RH, Slutsky AS, Gerstmann DR. Lung protective strategies of ventilation in the neonate: what are they? Pediatrics 2000;105:112–4.

[89] Clark RH, Gerstmann DR. Controversies in high-frequency ventilation. Clin Perinatol 1998;25(1):113–22.

[90] Kinsella JP, Abman SH. Clinical approaches to the use of high-frequency oscillatory ventilation in neonatal respiratory failure. J Perinatol 1996;16:S52–5.

[91] Paranka MS, Clark RH, Yoder BA, et al. Predictors of failure of high-frequency oscillatory ventilation in term infants with severe respiratory failure. Pediatrics 1995; 95(3):400–4.

[92] Kinsella JP, Truog WE, Walsh WF, et al. Randomized, multi-center trial of inhaled nitric oxide and high-frequency oscillatory ventilation in severe, persistent pulmonary hypertension of the newborn. J Pediatr 1997;131:55–62.

[93] Drummond WH, Gregory GA, Heymann MA, et al. The independent effects of hyperventilation, tolazoline, and dopamine on infants with persistent pulmonary hypertension. J Pediatr 1981;98(4):603–11.

[94] Wung JT, James LS, Kilchevsky E, et al. Management of infants with severe respiratory failure and persistence of the fetal circulation, without hyperventilation. Pediatrics 1985; 76(4):488–94.

[95] Brown DL, Pattishall EN. Other uses of surfactant. Clin Perinatol 1993;20(4):761–89.

[96] Auten RL, Notter RH, Kendig JW, et al. Surfactant treatment of full-term newborns with respiratory failure. Pediatrics 1991;87(1):101–7.

[97] Blanke JG, Jorch G. Surfactant therapy in severe neonatal respiratory failure—multi-center study—II. Surfactant therapy in 10 newborn infants with meconium aspiration syndrome. Klin Padiatr 1993;205(2):75–8 [in German].

[98] Chen CT, Toung TJ, Rogers MC. Effect of intra-alveolar meconium on pulmonary surface tension properties. Crit Care Med 1985;13(4):233–6.

[99] Cochrane CG, Revak SD, Merritt TA, et al. Bronchoalveolar lavage with KL4-surfactant in models of meconium aspiration syndrome. Pediatr Res 1998;44(5):705–15.

[100] Clark DA, Nieman GF, Thompson JE, et al. Surfactant displacement by meconium free fatty acids: an alternative explanation for atelectasis in meconium aspiration syndrome. J Pediatr 1987;110(5):765–70.

[101] Findlay RD, Taeusch HW, Walther FJ. Surfactant replacement therapy for meconium aspiration syndrome. Pediatrics 1996;97(1):48–52.

[102] Hallman M, Kankaanpaa K. Evidence of surfactant deficiency in persistence of the fetal circulation. Eur J Pediatr 1980;134(2):129–34.

[103] Holm BA, Notter RH, Finkelstein JN. Surface property changes from interactions of albumin with natural lung surfactant and extracted lung lipids. Chem Phys Lipids 1985;38(3):287–98.

[104] Holm BA, Notter RH. Effects of hemoglobin and cell membrane lipids on pulmonary surfactant activity. J Appl Physiol 1987;63(4):1434–42.

[105] Ibara S, Ikenoue T, Murata Y, et al. Management of meconium aspiration syndrome by tracheobronchial lavage and replacement of Surfactant-TA. Acta Paediatr Jpn 1995;37(1):64–7.

[106] Khammash H, Perlman M, Wojtulewicz J, et al. Surfactant therapy in full-term neonates with severe respiratory failure. Pediatrics 1993;92(1):135–9.

[107] Lotze A, Whitsett JA, Kammerman LA, et al. Surfactant protein A concentrations in tracheal aspirate fluid from infants requiring extracorporeal membrane oxygenation. J Pediatr 1990;116(3):435–40.

[108] Lotze A, Knight GR, Martin GR, et al. Improved pulmonary outcome after exogenous surfactant therapy for respiratory failure in term infants requiring extracorporeal membrane oxygenation. J Pediatr 1993;122(2):261–8.

[109] Lotze A, Stroud CY, Soldin SJ. Serial lecithin/sphingomyelin ratios and surfactant/albumin ratios in tracheal aspirates from term infants with respiratory failure receiving extracorporeal membrane oxygenation. Clin Chem 1995;41:1182–8.

[110] Marks SD, Nicholl RM. The reduction in the need for ECMO by using surfactant in meconium aspiration syndrome. J Pediatr 1999;135:267–8.

[111] Moses D, Holm BA, Spitale P, et al. Inhibition of pulmonary surfactant function by meconium. Am J Obstet Gynecol 1991;164(2):477–81.

[112] Seeger W, Stohr G, Wolf HR, et al. Alteration of surfactant function due to protein leakage: special interaction with fibrin monomer. J Appl Physiol 1985;58(2):326–38.

[113] Sun B, Curstedt T, Robertson B. Surfactant inhibition in experimental meconium aspiration. Acta Paediatr 1993;82(2):182–9.

[114] Sun B, Curstedt T, Song GW, et al. Surfactant improves lung function and morphology in newborn rabbits with meconium aspiration. Biol Neonate 1993;63(2):96–104.

[115] Soll RF, Dargaville P. Surfactant for meconium aspiration syndrome in full-term infants. Cochrane Database Syst Rev 2000;(2):CD002054.

[116] Abman SH, Kinsella JP. Surfactant use in the term neonate with hypoxemic respiratory failure. J Pediatr 1998;133(5):716–7.

[117] Paranka MS, Walsh WF, Stancombe BB. Surfactant lavage in a piglet model of meconium aspiration syndrome. Pediatr Res 1992;31(6):625–8.

[118] Lam BC, Yeung CY. Surfactant lavage for meconium aspiration syndrome: a pilot study. Pediatrics 1999;103:1014–8.

[119] Goetzman BW, Sunshine P, Johnson JD, et al. Neonatal hypoxia and pulmonary vasospasm: response to tolazoline. J Pediatr 1976;89(4):617–21.

[120] Stevenson DK, Kasting DS, Darnall RA Jr, et al. Refractory hypoxemia associated with neonatal pulmonary disease: the use and limitations of tolazoline. J Pediatr 1979;95(4): 595–9.

[121] Kinsella JP, Neish SR, Shaffer E, et al. Low-dose inhalation nitric oxide in persistent pulmonary hypertension of the newborn. Lancet 1992;340(8823):819–20.

[122] Kinsella JP, Neish SR, Ivy DD, et al. Clinical responses to prolonged treatment of persistent pulmonary hypertension of the newborn with low doses of inhaled nitric oxide. J Pediatr 1993;123(1):103–8.

[123] Gerlach H, Rossaint R, Pappert D, et al. Time-course and dose-response of nitric oxide inhalation for systemic oxygenation and pulmonary hypertension in patients with adult respiratory distress syndrome. Eur J Clin Invest 1993;23(8):499–502.

[124] Abman SH, Griebel JL, Parker DK, et al. Acute effects of inhaled nitric oxide in children with severe hypoxemic respiratory failure. J Pediatr 1994;124(6):881–8.

[125] Kinsella JP, Abman SH. Efficacy of inhalational nitric oxide therapy in the clinical management of persistent pulmonary hypertension of the newborn. Chest 1994;105(Suppl 3): 92S–4S.

[126] Kinsella JP, Abman SH. Inhaled nitric oxide: current and future uses in neonates. Semin Perinatol 2000;24(6):387–95.

[127] Beckman JS, Beckman TW, Chen J, et al. Apparent hydroxyl radical production by peroxynitrite: implications for endothelial injury from nitric oxide and superoxide. Proc Natl Acad Sci U S A 1990;87(4):1620–4.

[128] Ekekezie II, Thibeault DW, Garola RE, et al. Monocyte chemoattractant protein-1 and its receptor CCR-2 in piglet lungs exposed to inhaled nitric oxide and hyperoxia. Pediatr Res 2001;50(5):633–40.

[129] Hallman M. Molecular interactions between nitric oxide and lung surfactant. Biol Neonate 1997;71(Suppl 1):44–8.

[130] Issa A, Lappalainen U, Kleinman M, et al. Inhaled nitric oxide decreases hyperoxia-induced surfactant abnormality in preterm rabbits. Pediatr Res 1999;45(2):247–54.

[131] O'Donnell VB, Chumley PH, Hogg N, et al. Nitric oxide inhibition of lipid peroxidation: kinetics of reaction with lipid peroxyl radicals and comparison with alpha-tocopherol. Biochemistry 1997;36(49):15216–23.

[132] Robbins CG, Davis JM, Merritt TA, et al. Combined effects of nitric oxide and hyperoxia on surfactant function and pulmonary inflammation. Am J Physiol 1995;269: L545–50.

[133] Weigand MA, Snyder-Ramos SA, Mollers AG, et al. Inhaled nitric oxide does not enhance lipid peroxidation in patients with acute respiratory distress syndrome. Crit Care Med 2000; 28(10):3429–35.

[134] Goldman AP, Tasker RC, Haworth SG, et al. Four patterns of response to inhaled nitric oxide for persistent pulmonary hypertension of the newborn. Pediatrics 1996;98: 706–13.

[135] Clark RH, Kueser TJ, Walker MW, et al. Low-dose nitric oxide therapy for persistent pulmonary hypertension of the newborn. Clinical Inhaled Nitric Oxide Research Group. N Engl J Med 2000;342(7):469–74.

[136] Davidson D, Barefield ES, Kattwinkel J, et al. Inhaled nitric oxide for the early treatment of persistent pulmonary hypertension of the term newborn: a randomized, double-masked, placebo-controlled, dose-response, multi-center study. The I-NO/PPHN Study Group. Pediatrics 1998;101:325–34.

[137] Finer NN, Barrington KJ. Nitric oxide for respiratory failure in infants born at or near term. Cochrane Database Syst Rev 2000;(2):CD000399.

[138] Kinsella JP, Parker TA, Ivy DD, et al. Noninvasive delivery of inhaled nitric oxide therapy for late pulmonary hypertension in newborn infants with congenital diaphragmatic hernia. J Pediatr 2003;142(4):397–401.

[139] Konduri GG, Solimano A, Sokol GM, et al. A randomized trial of early versus standard inhaled nitric oxide therapy in term and near-term newborn infants with hypoxic respiratory failure. Pediatrics 2004;113:559–64.

[140] Roberts JD, Polaner DM, Lang P, et al. Inhaled nitric oxide in persistent pulmonary hypertension of the newborn. Lancet 1992;340(8823):818–9.

[141] Finer NN, Etches PC, Kamstra B, et al. Inhaled nitric oxide in infants referred for extracorporeal membrane oxygenation: dose response. J Pediatr 1994;124(2):302–8.

[142] Finer NN, Sun JW, Rich W, et al. Randomized, prospective study of low-dose versus high-dose inhaled nitric oxide in the neonate with hypoxic respiratory failure. Pediatrics 2001; 108(4):949–55.

[143] Aly H, Sahni R, Wung JT. Weaning strategy with inhaled nitric oxide treatment in persistent pulmonary hypertension of the newborn. Arch Dis Child Fetal Neonatal Ed 1997; 76(2):F118–22.

[144] Carriedo H, Rhine W. Withdrawal of inhaled nitric oxide from nonresponders after short exposure. J Perinatol 2003;23(7):556–8.

[145] Davidson D, Barefield ES, Kattwinkel J, et al. Safety of withdrawing inhaled nitric oxide therapy in persistent pulmonary hypertension of the newborn. Pediatrics 1999;104:231–6.

[146] Atz AM, Wessel DL. Sildenafil ameliorates effects of inhaled nitric oxide withdrawal. Anesthesiology 1999;91(1):307–10.

[147] Badesch DB, Abman SH, Ahearn GS, et al. Medical therapy for pulmonary arterial hypertension: ACCP evidence-based clinical practice guidelines. Chest 2004;126(Suppl 1): 35S–62S.

[148] Ivy DD, Kinsella JP, Ziegler JW, et al. Dipyridamole attenuates rebound pulmonary hypertension after inhaled nitric oxide withdrawal in postoperative congenital heart disease. J Thorac Cardiovasc Surg 1998;115(4):875–82.

[149] Kinsella JP, Torielli F, Ziegler JW, et al. Dipyridamole augmentation of response to nitric oxide. Lancet 1995;346(8975):647–8.

[150] Ziegler JW, Ivy DD, Wiggins JW, et al. Effects of dipyridamole and inhaled nitric oxide in pediatric patients with pulmonary hypertension. Am J Respir Crit Care Med 1998;158: 1388–95.

[151] Baquero H, Soliz A, Neira F, et al. Oral sildenafil in infants with persistent pulmonary hypertension of the newborn: a pilot randomized blinded study. Pediatrics 2006;117(4): 1077–83.

[152] Chaudhari M, Vogel M, Wright C, et al. Sildenafil in neonatal pulmonary hypertension due to impaired alveolarisation and plexiform pulmonary arteriopathy. Archives of Disease in Childhood Fetal and Neonatal Edition 2005;90(6):F527–8.

[153] Ladha F, Bonnet S, Eaton F, et al. Sildenafil improves alveolar growth and pulmonary hypertension in hyperoxia-induced lung injury. American Journal of Respiratory and Critical Care Medicine 2005;172(6):750–6.

[154] Fliman PJ, deRegnier RA, Kinsella JP, et al. Neonatal extracorporeal life support: impact of new therapies on survival. J Pediatr 2006;148(5):595–9.

[155] Fattouch K, Sbraga F, Bianco G, et al. Inhaled prostacyclin, nitric oxide, and nitroprusside in pulmonary hypertension after mitral valve replacement. J Card Surg 2005;20(2):171–6.

[156] Hartigan D. Is nebulised tolazoline an effective treatment for persistent pulmonary hypertension of the newborn? Arch Dis Child 2003;88(1):84.

[157] Kelly LK, Porta NF, Goodman DM, et al. Inhaled prostacyclin for term infants with persistent pulmonary hypertension refractory to inhaled nitric oxide. J Pediatr 2002;141(6): 830–2.

[158] Max M, Rossaint R. Inhaled prostacyclin in the treatment of pulmonary hypertension. Eur J Pediatr 1999;158(Suppl 1):S23–6.

[159] Sood BG, Delaney-Black V, Aranda JV, et al. Aerosolized PGE1: a selective pulmonary vasodilator in neonatal hypoxemic respiratory failure results of a Phase I/II open-label clinical trial. Pediatr Res 2004;56(4):579–85.

[160] Parker TA, Ivy DD, Kinsella JP, et al. Combined therapy with inhaled nitric oxide and intravenous prostacyclin in an infant with alveolar-capillary dysplasia. Am J Respir Crit Care Med 1997;155(2):743–6.

[161] Roy BJ, Rycus P, Conrad SA, et al. The changing demographics of neonatal extracorporeal membrane oxygenation patients reported to the Extracorporeal Life Support Organization (ELSO) Registry. Pediatrics 2000;106(6):1334–8.

[162] Bartlett RH, Roloff DW, Cornell RG, et al. Extracorporeal circulation in neonatal respiratory failure: a prospective randomized study. Pediatrics 1985;76(4):479–87.

[163] O'Rourke PP, Crone RK, Vacanti JP, et al. Extracorporeal membrane oxygenation and conventional medical therapy in neonates with persistent pulmonary hypertension of the newborn: a prospective randomized study. Pediatrics 1989;84(6):957–63.

[164] UK collaborative randomised trial of neonatal extracorporeal membrane oxygenation. UK Collaborative ECMO Trail Group. Lancet 1996;348(9020):75–82.

[165] Cornish JD, Heiss KF, Clark RH, et al. Efficacy of venovenous extracorporeal membrane oxygenation for neonates with respiratory and circulatory compromise. J Pediatr 1993; 122(1):105–9.

[166] Knight GR, Dudell GG, Evans ML, et al. A comparison of venovenous and venoarterial extracorporeal membrane oxygenation in the treatment of neonatal respiratory failure. Crit Care Med 1996;24(10):1678–83.

[167] Durandy Y, Chevalier JY, Lecompte Y. Single-cannula venovenous bypass for respiratory membrane lung support. J Thorac Cardiovasc Surg 1990;99(3):404–9.

[168] Morin FC 3rd, Stenmark KR. Persistent pulmonary hypertension of the newborn. Am J Respir Crit Care Med 1995;151(6):2010–32.

ELSEVIER
SAUNDERS

CLINICS IN
PERINATOLOGY

Clin Perinatol 33 (2006) 831–837

Feeding Problems in the Late Preterm Infant

David H. Adamkin, MD

*Department of Pediatrics, University of Louisville School of Medicine, University of
Louisville, 571 South Floyd Street, Suite 342, Louisville, KY 40201, USA*

Prematurity is the major determinant of neonatal mortality and morbidity. Much of the neonatal nutrition literature has focused on the management of very low birth weight infants, a group of infants usually less than 33 weeks gestation [1]. Much less attention has been paid to nutritional management issues in preterm infants at higher gestations.

Replacing near-term with late preterm is useful, because it better reflects the higher risk for complications of preterm birth experienced by this subgroup of preterm infants. This article reviews nutritional issues that exist from the 239th day (34 0/7 weeks gestation) and ending on the 259th day (36 6/7 weeks gestation) since the first day of the mother's last normal menstrual period.

The 34- to 37-week neonate presents a nutritional challenge to health care providers beginning from the decision where the appropriate level of care should be provided immediately following birth. Triage of the late preterm may vary among hospitals; some infants may be directly admitted to a newborn nursery whereas others may be cared for in the neonatal intensive care units. Additionally, such differences in initial care are more apparent for infants in the 34 to 35 week strata compared with the 36 to 37 week strata.

A recent study [2] selecting infants from the previously published Moderately Premature Infant Project [3,4] with gestational ages at the lower end of the 34 0/7 to 36 6/7 week range included only infants admitted to neonatal ICUs (NICUs) in the same hospitals of their birth. They found striking variations in nutritional practices, which might have influenced rates of weight gain [2]. About 17% of infants received total parenteral nutrition (TPN), but the range was 5% to 66%. Likewise, there was a range in the type of formula recommended at discharge [2]. Although nearly half (46%) of

E-mail address: david.adamkin@lousiville.edu

0095-5108/06/$ - see front matter © 2006 Elsevier Inc. All rights reserved.
doi:10.1016/j.clp.2006.09.003   *perinatology.theclinics.com*

infants were discharged with advice to be fed with a formula containing more than 20 calories per ounce, this practice ranged from 4% to 72%.

Late preterm infants are born only a few weeks early, and most often they are only slightly smaller than full-term infants; however, these late preterm infants have a wide spectrum of nutritional needs. The needs may vary from timely lactation support in the inpatient and outpatient setting to providing TPN for the late preterm infant receiving inhaled nitric oxide for respiratory failure.

Breast-feeding the late preterm infant

The advantages of breast milk feeding for premature infants appear to be even greater than those for term infants. Establishing breastfeeding in the late preterm infant, however, is frequently more problematic than in the full-term infant. Because of their immaturity, late preterm infants may be sleepier and have less stamina. They may have more difficulty with latch, suck, and swallow; more difficulty maintaining body temperature; increased vulnerability to infection; greater delays in bilirubin excretion, and more respiratory instability than the full-term infant. The sleepiness and inability to suck vigorously often is misinterpreted as sepsis, leading to unnecessary separation and treatment. Alternatively, the late preterm infant may appear deceptively vigorous at first glance. Physically large newborns often are mistaken for being more developmentally mature than their actual gestational age. (Remember the 3.84 kg baby born at 40 weeks was 3.0 kg at 36 weeks of gestation.) Late preterm infants are more likely to be separated from their mother as a result of the infant being ill or requiring a screening procedure such as evaluation for sepsis, intravenous placement for antibiotics, and phototherapy.

Mothers who deliver near but not at term are more likely to deliver multiples, or they may have a medical condition such as diabetes, pregnancy-induced hypertension, prolonged rupture of membranes, chorioamnionitis, oxytocin induction, or a cesarean section delivery that may affect the success of breast-feeding. Any one or a combination of these conditions places these mothers and infants at risk for difficulty in establishing successful lactation or for breast-feeding failure.

The potential maternal and infant problems place the late preterm breast-feeding infant at increased risk for hypothermia, hypoglycemia, excessive weight loss, slow weight gain, failure to thrive, prolonged artificial milk supplementation, exaggerated jaundice, kernicterus, dehydration, fever secondary to dehydration, rehospitalization, and breast-feeding failure. In places where early discharge is the norm, these infants will be sent home soon after delivery. Discussion and parental education become crucial in the proper management of breast-feeding.

Most of the acute problems encountered in the newborn are managed on the postpartum floor in the first few hours and days after parturition;

however, there are times that an infant's condition deteriorates in the interval between discharge and the first office visit. Therefore, timely evaluation of the late preterm infant after discharge is critical. Just as many hospitals are becoming breast-feeding friendly, the outpatient office or clinic needs to be not only supportive of the breast-feeding mother, but also able to assist mothers with uncomplicated problems or questions related to breast-feeding. In addition, it is essential to be able to refer mothers and infants in a timely manner to a trained lactation professional for more complicated breast-feeding problems. A lactation referral should be viewed with the same medical urgency as any other acute medical referral.

Specific protocols for managing breast-feeding are beyond the scope of this article. Resources are available including protocols from the Academy of Breastfeeding Medicine [5–7].

Feeding problems in late preterm infants

A recent study demonstrated that 27% of all late preterm infants had a clinical condition whereby intravenous fluid was given, compared with only 5% of all term infants [8]. Various clinical problems including hypoglycemia and poor feeding precipitated this treatment [8]. This same study also linked delayed discharge home with more clinical problems in late preterm infants than in term infants. Feeding problems were the dominant reason for delay in discharge [8]. Given that immature infants are less able to achieve effective sucking and swallowing, this is not entirely unexpected. In the author's clinical experience, many late preterm infants require repeated assistance and support before achieving consistent, nutritive breast-feeding; initially, supplementation with expressed breast milk or formula often is required.

Successful enteral feeding of these infants demands creativity and flexibility. An infant may need multiple feeding methods during the transition to oral feedings. The team approach, including input of the nutritionist, nurse, occupational therapist, speech pathologist, lactation consultant, and physician can facilitate choosing successful feeding regimens for infants at different stages in their development and clinical course.

Nutritional considerations

Nutrition in respiratory disease

Respiratory distress, defined as sustained distress more than 2 hours after birth accompanied by grunting, flaring, tachypnea, retractions, or supplemental oxygen requirement, was observed more often in late preterm infants (28.9% versus 4.2%) than in term newborns [8]. The rate of occurrence of any form of respiratory distress increases dramatically among infants born at less than 37 weeks [9,10]. In addition, compared with babies with a gestational age of 38 to 40 weeks, babies born at 37 weeks were five times as likely, and babies born at 35 weeks, nine times as likely, to have respiratory distress [11].

Therefore, TPN may become an important therapy in late preterm infants. TPN usually is indicated when a sufficient nutrient supply cannot be provided enterally to prevent or correct malnutrition. Until full enteral feeding can be established, these preterm infants can be supported with TPN. In the late preterm infant with respiratory disease, the indication for TPN is critical illness. Infants with a functioning gastrointestinal system should begin enteral feeds as soon as clinically possible in combination with TPN.

For the late preterm infant with respiratory disease, energy balance during the first several days usually is equated to absorption of sufficient energy to match energy expenditure. Most studies show that energy expenditure of nongrowing low birth weight infants (less than 2500 g birth weight) is 45 to 55 cal/kg/d [12–14].

These infants are very capable of catabolizing amino acids. Parenteral protein including about 2 g/kg/d can be initiated immediately and with regimens delivering as few as 35 cal/kg/d result in positive nitrogen balance [15,16]. Protein intakes of 2.5 to 3.0 g/kg/d will achieve similar weight gain as a term infant fed human milk if these infants require longer periods of exclusive TPN [17].

The most controversial nutrient to be considered in the late preterm infant with respiratory disease is the use of intravenous lipids (IVL). Two different populations within the group of late preterm infants with respiratory disease emerge for this discussion: those without increased pulmonary vascular resistance (PVR) and those with signs consistent with persistent pulmonary hypertension (PPHN) or increased PVR.

Concerns have been raised regarding the possible adverse effect of IVL on pulmonary function [18], especially in premature neonates and those with acute lung injury. A potential hazard of hyperlipidemia resulting from failure to clear infused lipid is the adverse effect on gas exchange in the lungs. This was demonstrated in adult volunteers after a large dose of soybean emulsion [19]. Preterm neonates randomized to different lipid infusion rates, however, did not demonstrate any effect on alveolar–arterial oxygen gradient or arterial blood pH [20]. Similarly, the author found no difference in oxygenation in preterm infants randomly assigned to modest doses of lipids (0.6 to 1.4 g/kg/d) over the first week of life. These infants had received surfactant and were on intermittent mechanical ventilation [21].

For the late preterm infant with increased PVR and respiratory disease, however, it appears a more prudent approach with IVL should be taken. Significant concerns have been raised because of the high polyunsaturated fatty acid content (PUFA) of lipid emulsions as excessive omega 6 (linoleic acid, 18:2ω6) acids are required substrates for arachidonic acid pathways, which lead to synthesizing prostaglandins and leukotrienes (Fig. 1). It is speculated that IVL infusion may enhance thromboxane synthetase activity,

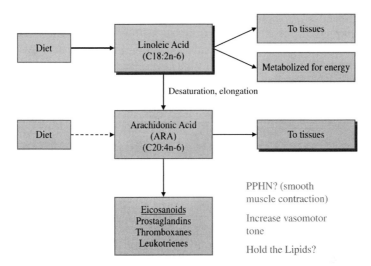

Fig. 1. Metabolic derivatives of linoleic acid and arachidonic acid (ARA).

which increases thromboxane production [22]. The prostaglandins may cause changes in vasomotor tone with resultant hypoxemia [18,23,24]. In addition, the production of hydroperoxides in the lipid emulsion also might contribute to untoward effects by increasing prostaglandin levels [25–27].

Although there is no firm evidence of the effects of lipid emulsions in infants with severe acute respiratory failure with or without pulmonary hypertension, it appears prudent to avoid high dosages in these patients. The author's opinion is to provide those with respiratory diseases without increased PVR lipid at a dosage to prevent essential fatty acid deficiency. For those with elements of PPHN, avoidance of lipids during the greatest lability and critical stages of their illness should be considered. Once more stable, hopefully within 48 hours, IVL at a modest dosage can be initiated.

Nutrition in late preterm infants after discharge

The establishment of feeding guidelines in these infants is complicated by the range of chronologic and gestation-corrected ages of near preterm infants at the time of hospital discharge. The strategy after discharge also is impacted by whether these infants have developed chronic conditions that may impact feeding and long-term growth. The first year of life may provide an important opportunity for human somatic and brain growth to compensate for earlier deprivation for these late preterm infants who suffered critical illness.

Generally speaking, the 34- or 35-week late preterm infant is a candidate for a nutrient-enriched strategy after discharge. The 36- or 37-week late preterm infant who has an uncomplicated neonatal course probably does not require nutrient enrichment after discharge.

Preterm infants generally are discharged from the hospital on standard term formula, specialized postdischarge formula, or unfortified breast milk. Nutrient-enriched postdischarge formulas that provide 22 kcal/oz have been marketed in the United States since the mid-1990s. The formulas provide levels of nutrients between those of preterm and term infant formulas. The main differences between the formulas are a higher protein content (approximately 1.9 versus 1.4 g/dL), a modest increase in energy (22 versus 20 kcal/oz), and additional calcium, phosphorous, zinc, trace elements, and vitamins in the postdischarge formulas. Because they are fortified with iron and vitamins, no other supplements are needed.

Few studies have compared the growth of infants fed term formula versus the postdischarge formulas. The available evidence, however, indicates that catch-up growth is increased with the feeding of the enriched formulas.

Provision of enriched feedings after hospital discharge may be particularly beneficial for infants who have a chronic condition such as bronchopulmonary dysplasia (BPD), which often is associated with growth failure. A study randomly assigned preterm infants with BPD to a 90 kcal/dL formula but with differing protein-to-energy ratio (0.026 versus 0.017). Infants fed the enriched formula had significantly greater nitrogen retention at 38 weeks postmenstrual age. At 3 months corrected age, the infants fed the enriched formula had greater length and lean mass. Energy intakes and volumes of formula were similar; however, protein and mineral intakes were greater with formula enriched with protein and minerals. The authors concluded that in infants recovering from BPD, growth failure is related to inadequate nutrient intake and not to malabsorption of nutrients.

Summary

Important differences in clinical outcomes become apparent when hospital courses of late preterm infants are compared with those of full-term infants. Differences in feeding issues and strategies mirror those differences in outcomes.

Late preterm infants may masquerade as term infants on the basis of their relatively large size and mature, chubby appearance. This masquerading infant, however, may be at risk for breast-feeding failure with dehydration and feeding difficulties delaying discharge. The critically ill late preterm infant requires unique considerations with TPN and a nutrient-enriched postdischarge strategy.

References

[1] Adamkin DH. Feeding the preterm infant. In: Bhatia JB, editor. Perinatal nutrition: optimizing infant health and development. New York: Marcel Dekker; 2005. p. 165–90.
[2] McCormick MC, Escobar GJ, Zheng Z, et al. Place of birth and variations in management of late preterm (near-term) infants. Semin Perinatol 2006;30(1):44–7.

[3] Richardson DK, Zupancic JAF, Escobar GJ, et al. The moderately premature infant project: interinstitutional practice variations. Pediatr Res 2003;53:382A.

[4] Eichenwald EC, Escobar GJ, Zupancic JAF, et al. Inter-NICU variation in discharge timing of moderately premature infants: earlier discharge does not affect three-month outcome. Pediatr Res 2004;55:372A.

[5] Jensen D, Wallace S, Kelsay P. LATCH: a breastfeeding charting system and documentation tool. J Obstet Gynecol Neonatal Nurs 1994;23:27–32.

[6] Matthews MK. Developing an instrument to assess infant breastfeeding behaviour in the early neonatal period. Midwifery 1988;4:154–65.

[7] Mulford C. The mother–baby assessment (MBA): an Apgar score for breastfeeding. J Hum Lact 1992;8:79–82.

[8] Wang ML, Dorer DJ, Fleming MP, et al. Clinical outcomes of near-term infants. Pediatrics 2004;114:2.

[9] Hjalmarson O. Epidemiology and classification of acute, neonatal respiratory disorders. A prospective study. Acta Paediatr Scand 1981;70:773–83.

[10] Dani C, Reali MF, Bertini G, et al. Risk factors for the development of respiratory distress syndrome and transient tachypnoea in newborn infants. Italian Group of Neonatal Pneumology. Eur Respir J 1999;14:155–9.

[11] Escobar GJ, Clark RH, Greene JD. Short-term outcomes of infants born at 35 and 36 weeks gestation: we need to ask more questions. Semin Perinatol 2006;30(1):28–33.

[12] Brooke OG. Energy balance and metabolic rate in preterm infants fed with standard and high-energy formulas. Br J Nutr 1980;44:13–23.

[13] Freymond D, Yves S, Decombaz J, et al. Energy balance, physical activity, and thermogenic effect of feeding in premature infants. Pediatr Res 1989;20:638–45.

[14] Marks KH, Nardis EE, Derr JA. Day-to-day energy expenditure variability in low birth-weight neonates. Pediatr Res 1987;21:66–71.

[15] Anderson TL, Muttart CR, Bieber MA, et al. A controlled trial of glucose versus glucose and amino acids in premature infants. J Pediatr 1979;94:947–51.

[16] Kashyap S. Nutritional management of the extremely low birth-weight infant. In: Cowett RM, Hay WW, editors. The micropreemie: the next frontier. Report of the ninety-ninth Ross Conference on Pediatric Research. Columbus (OH): Ross Laboratories; 1990. p. 115–22.

[17] Zlotkin SH. Intravenous nitrogen intake requirements in full-term newborns undergoing surgery. Pediatrics 1984;73:493–6.

[18] Hageman JR, Hunt CE. Fat emulsions and lung function. Clin Chest Med 1986;7:69–77.

[19] Greene HL, Hazlett D, Demare R. Relationship between intralipid-induced hyperlipemia and pulmonary function. Am J Clin Nutr 1976;29:127.

[20] Brans YW, Dutton EB, Drew DS, et al. Fat emulsion tolerance in very low birthweight neonates: effect on diffusion of oxygen in the lungs and on blood pH. Pediatrics 1986;78(1):79.

[21] Adamkin DH, Gelke KN, Wilkerson SA. Clinical and laboratory observations: influence of intravenous fat therapy on tracheal effluent phospholipids and oxygenation in severe respiratory distress syndrome. J Pediatr 1985;106:122.

[22] Hunt CE, Pachman LM, Hageman JR, et al. Liposyn infusion increases prostaglandin concentrations. Pediatr Pulmonol 1986;2:154.

[23] Shulman RJ, Phillips S. Parenteral nutrition in infants and children. J Pediatr Gastroenterol Nutr 2003;36:557–60.

[24] Hammerman C, Aramburo MJ, Hill V. Intravenous lipids in newborn lungs: thromboxane-mediated effects. Crit Care Med 1989;17:430–6.

[25] Pitkanen O, Hallman M, Andersson S. Generation of free radicals in lipid emulsion used in parenteral nutrition. Pediatr Res 1991;29:56–9.

[26] Helbock HJ, Motchnik PA, Ames BN. Toxic hydroperoxides in intravenous lipid emulsions used in preterm infants. Pediatrics 1993;91:83–7.

[27] Lavoie JC, Chessex P. The increase in vasomotor tone induced by a parenteral lipid emulsion is linked to an inhibition of prostacyclin production. Free Radic Biol Med 1994;16:795–9.

ELSEVIER
SAUNDERS

CLINICS IN
PERINATOLOGY

Clin Perinatol 33 (2006) 839–852

Hyperbilirubinemia and Bilirubin Toxicity in the Late Preterm Infant

Jon F. Watchko, MD[a,b,*]

[a]*Division of Newborn Medicine, Department of Pediatrics, University
of Pittsburgh School of Medicine, Pittsburgh, PA 15213, USA*
[b]*Magee-Womens Research Institue, Magee-Womens Hospital,
300 Halket Street, Pittsburgh, PA 15213, USA*

Hyperbilirubinemia is the most common clinical condition requiring evaluation and treatment in the newborn [1] and the most common cause for hospital readmission during the first week of postnatal life [2–5]. Although generally a benign transitional phenomenon of no overt clinical significance, in a select few, the total serum bilirubin (TSB) may rise to hazardous levels that pose a direct threat of brain damage. Acute bilirubin encephalopathy, an uncommon disorder [4], may ensue, frequently evolving into kernicterus, a devastating, chronic and disabling condition characterized by the clinical tetrad of:

- Choreoathetoid cerebral palsy
- High-frequency central neural hearing loss
- Palsy of vertical gaze
- Dental enamel hypoplasia, the result of bilirubin-induced cell toxicity [6]

Originally described in newborns with Rh hemolytic disease, kernicterus more recently has been reported in apparently healthy term and late preterm gestation breast-fed infants without documented hemolysis [4,7,8]. Late preterm gestation ($34^{0/7}$ to $36^{6/7}$ weeks [9,10]) is one of the most prevalent identified risk factors for the development of severe hyperbilirubinemia (TSB at least 20 mg/dL [342 μmol/L]) [11] and kernicterus [4,12], and is the focus of this article.

Late preterm infants frequently are cared for in normal newborn nurseries, wherein caretakers may be lured into thinking they are as mature as term

---

* Division of Newborn Medicine, Department of Pediatrics, Magee-Womens Hospital, 300 Halket Street, Pittsburgh, PA 15213.
E-mail address: jwatchko@mail.magee.edu

0095-5108/06/$ - see front matter © 2006 Elsevier Inc. All rights reserved.
doi:10.1016/j.clp.2006.09.002
perinatology.theclinics.com

(at least $37^{0/7}$ weeks) neonates. Indeed, late preterm infants often can be managed in many respects like their more mature term counterparts for:

- They are typically large enough to maintain their temperature in an open crib
- They often have an established suck–swallow reflex and can take their feedings by mouth (although not necessarily breast-feed vigorously)
- They generally have a strong respiratory drive and are thus not prone to periodic breathing or apnea of prematurity (although the author's hospital monitors all neonates born between $34^{0/7}$ and $34^{6/7}$ weeks gestation on a cardiorespiratory monitor for the first 24 hours of postnatal life to ensure they are apnea-free) [13].

In contrast, the late preterm infant remains relatively immature compared with term newborns in their capacity to handle unconjugated bilirubin, placing them at risk for marked neonatal jaundice [12]. Indeed, as in preterm infants [14], neonatal hyperbilirubinemia in late preterm newborns is more prevalent, more pronounced, and more protracted in nature than it is in their term counterparts. Underscoring the singular importance of late preterm gestational age are:

- The approximately eightfold increased risk of developing a TSB of greater than 20 mg/dL (342 µmol/L) in infants born at 36 weeks gestational age (5.2%) as compared with those born at 41 or 42 or more weeks gestation (0.7% and 0.6% respectively) [11]
- The over-representation of late preterm infants in the US Pilot Kernicterus Registry [4,12], a database of voluntarily reported cases of kernicterus

Pathobiology

Late preterm and full-term infants become jaundiced by similar mechanisms. There is:

- An increased bilirubin load on the hepatocyte as a result of decreased erythrocyte survival, increased erythrocyte volume, and increased enterohepatic circulation of bilirubin
- Decreased hepatic uptake of bilirubin from plasma
- Defective bilirubin conjugation

The imbalance between bilirubin production and elimination in neonates is illustrated by the unitless bilirubin production–conjugation index described by Kaplan and colleagues [15]. This index is given by the numeric ratio of the blood carboxyhemoglobin corrected for ambient carbon monoxide (COHbc) and the serum total conjugated bilirubin [15]. The former is a measure of heme catabolism and therefore bilirubin production (the rate-limiting step in bilirubin production is the conversion of heme to biliverdin by heme-oxygenase, an enzymatic reaction that produces an equimolar amount of carbon monoxide), whereas the latter is an indirect measure of hepatic bilirubin conjugation capacity [15]. Late preterm infants evidence a similar degree of red blood cell (RBC) turnover and heme degradation as indexed by comparable COHbc levels as their term counterparts. They differ from their term counterparts, however, in how effectively they handle the resultant bilirubin load, demonstrating a significantly lower conjugated bilirubin fraction and resultant increased bilirubin production–conjugation index (Table 1 [16]). Moreover, late preterm neonates demonstrate a slower postnatal maturation of hepatic bilirubin uptake and bilirubin conjugation as compared with their term counterparts. This exaggerated hepatic immaturity [16,17] contributes to the greater prevalence, severity, and duration of neonatal jaundice in late preterm infants.

Kernicterus

Compared with term neonates, infants born prematurely are considered to be at an increased risk for developing kernicterus [18,19]. It may be that late preterm neonates are also at a higher risk compared with their term counterparts. Indeed, late preterm infants are represented disproportionately in the US Pilot Kernicterus Registry [4,12]. Moreover, the registry demonstrates that late preterm neonates evidence signs of bilirubin neurotoxicity at an earlier postnatal age than term newborns, indirectly suggesting a greater vulnerability to bilirubin-induced brain injury [12]. Clinical hyperbilirubinemia management guidelines for preterm [20,21] and late preterm [22] infants therefore recommend treatment at lower total serum bilirubin thresholds than term newborns, a distinction that is an important component of the most current American Academy of Pediatrics (AAP) practice parameter on neonatal jaundice [22].

Table 1
Comparison of values for the production-conjugation index for neonates ≤ 37 weeks gestation and those > 37 weeks

Variable	≤37 weeks gestation	>37 weeks gestation	p value
Production-conjugation index (unitless)	2.31 (2.12–3.08)	1.05 (0.53–1.81)	0.003
COHbc (% tHb)	0.88 (0.21)	0.82 (0.20)	0.46
TCB (% TSB)	0.39 (0.31–0.42)	0.74 (0.44–1.69)	0.009
STB (μmol/L)	160 (35)	141 (72)	0.48

Values are mean (SD) or median (interquartile range), as appropriate.
Abbreviations: COHbc, carboxyhemoglobin corrected for inspired carbon monoxide; TCB, total conjugated bilirubin; tHb, total hemoglobin; TSB, Total serum bilirubin.
From Kaplan M, Muraca M, Vreman HJ, et al. Neonatal bilirubin production-conjugation imbalance: effect of glucose-6-phosphate dehydrogenase deficiency and borderline prematurity. Arch Dis Child Fetal Neonatal Ed 2005;90:F125; reproduced with permission from the BMJ Publishing Group.

The mechanisms that potentially could account for an increased susceptibility to bilirubin-induced central nervous system (CNS) injury in late preterm newborns have not been defined. Theoretically, however, they include a diminished serum bilirubin binding capacity, an enhanced permeability of the blood–brain or blood–CSF barriers to unconjugated bilirubin influx, or an immaturity of neuronal protective mechanisms, among others. In this regard, the serum albumin level is low in premature neonates and increases significantly with increasing gestational age [23], but increases only minimally between 34 and 35 weeks gestation (3.02 plus or minus 0.21 g/dL) and term (3.57 plus or minus 0.37 g/dL) [23]. In addition, there is little to suggest the existence of developmental differences in serum's actual bilirubin binding capacity between the late preterm and term neonate [24]. With respect to the anatomy and function of the blood–brain and blood–CSF barriers, there has been considerable controversy regarding their relative maturity in neonates [25]. Although gestational age may be an important variable in modulating blood–brain and blood–CSF permeability to selected substrates in experimental animals (eg, ontogenic decreases in ovine blood–brain barrier permeability [26]), clinical and morphologic data on people are less convincing, at least from the gestational age of viability onward [25,27]. Similarly, virtually nothing is known about potential developmental differences in human neuronal vulnerability to unconjugated bilirubin (UCB) in vivo. It has, however, been shown repeatedly that UCB-induced toxicity in vitro in murine-derived CNS primary cell cultures is modulated by culture age (ie, younger presumably less mature neurons and astrocytes are more susceptible to bilirubin-induced apoptosis and necrosis than their older presumably more mature counterparts) [28–31]. Whether these findings are reflective of a clinically relevant in vivo phenomenon is unclear, but they collectively suggest that CNS cellular maturity may be a factor in modulating UCB-induced injury. Purportedly these in vitro cell culture models reflect ontogenic changes in brain development (ie, differentiation) [32], as opposed to postnatal maturational effects. The importance of postnatal maturation on reducing susceptibility to bilirubin-induced CNS injury is documented in experimental animals [25,33,34] and presumably operational in human newborns also.

Breast-feeding and late preterm gestation neonates

Several clinical risk factors for marked hyperbilirubinemia and kernicterus have been identified in late preterm neonates and are shown in Box 1. Of these, breast milk feeding has been identified the most consistently (almost uniformly) and therefore appears to be of paramount importance. Indeed, late preterm infants who are breast-fed may be at greatest risk for severe neonatal hyperbilirubinemia and merit close postbirth hospitalization discharge follow-up and lactation support. Late preterm neonates, because of their immaturity, often demonstrate less effective sucking and swallowing

---

Box 1. Clinically associated risk factors for marked hyperbilirubinemia and/or kernicterus in late preterm neonates

Breast milk feeding
- J Perinatol 2004;24:650–62 [4]
- Semin Perinatol 2006;30:89–97 [12]

Large for gestational age status
- Semin Perinatol 2006;30:89–97 [12]

Male sex
- J Perinatol 2004; 24:650–62 [4]
- Semin Perinatol 2006;30:89–97 [12]

Glucose-6-phosphate dehydrogenase deficiency and breast-feeding
- J Pediatr 2006; 149:83–8 [62]

---

and may have difficulties achieving consistent nutritive breastfeeding [35], phenomena that may predispose to varying degrees of lactation failure. Suboptimal feeding was the leading reason for discharge delay during birth hospitalization in late preterm neonates in one recent study [35]. This propensity may be compounded in primiparous women [36] who are known to produce significantly less milk than multiparous women during the first several days after giving birth, some with markedly low volumes [37].

Inadequate breast milk intake, in addition to contributing to varying degrees of dehydration, can enhance hyperbilirubinemia by increasing the enterohepatic circulation of bilirubin and resultant hepatic bilirubin load. The enterohepatic circulation of bilirubin already is exaggerated in the neonatal period, in part because the newborn intestinal tract is not colonized yet with bacteria that convert conjugated bilirubin to urobilinogen, and because intestinal β-glucuronidase activity is high [38,39]. Earlier studies in newborn humans and primates confirmed that the enterohepatic circulation of bilirubin accounts for up to 50% of the hepatic bilirubin load in newborns [40, 41]. Moreover, fasting hyperbilirubinemia is largely due to intestinal reabsorption of unconjugated bilirubin [42,43] suggesting an additional mechanism by which inadequate lactation or poor enteral intake may contribute to the genesis of marked hyperbilirubinemia in some neonates. A recent study confirmed that early breast-feeding-associated jaundice is associated with a state of relative caloric deprivation [44] and resultant enhanced enterohepatic circulation of bilirubin [44,45]. In the context of the exaggerated hepatic immaturity of the late preterm neonate, any further increase in hepatic bilirubin load likely will result in more marked hyperbilirubinemia. Breast-feeding-related jaundice, however, is not associated with increased bilirubin production [46,47].

It is notable that almost every reported case of kernicterus over the past two decades has been in breast-fed infants and that suboptimal lactation was the most frequent experience in late preterm infants who developed acute bilirubin encephalopathy [12]. Pediatricians need to be alert to the potential of suboptimal breast milk feeding in late preterm neonates and not be misled by the seemingly satisfactory breastfeeding efforts of late preterm newborns during the birth hospitalization when limited colostrum volumes make it a challenge to adequately assess the effectiveness of breast milk transfer [48]. While recognizing the relationship between breast milk feeding and jaundice in late-preterm neonates, it is important to emphasize that the benefits of breast milk feeds far outweigh the related risk of hyperbilirubinemia.

Large for gestational age status and risk

In addition to the almost uniform prevalence of breast milk feedings, another salient clinical feature of kernicterus risk in late preterm neonates in the US Pilot Kernicterus Registry is a large for gestational age (LGA) categorization. Indeed, more than a third of kernicteric late preterm infants were LGA [12]. Not surprisingly, prevalent birth-related risk factors for hyperbilirubinemia in this LGA subgroup included oxytocin induction, vacuum or forceps delivery, and cutaneous bruising [12]. No other specific underlying mechanisms for hyperbilirubinemia were identified. Whether the LGA status of late preterm neonates (ie, birth weight comparable to a typical term neonate) served to mask their immaturity is not clear, nor is it known if antecedent or concomitant hypoglycemia occurred in the hyperbilirubinemic LGA cohort and possibly contributed to the risk for injury [12].

Male sex and risk

Another clinical feature of affected neonates in the US Pilot Kernicterus Registry is the predominance of males (n = 84) to females (n = 38) [12]. This approximately twofold greater prevalence of kernicteric males is also evident in the late preterm subgroup in the registry [4]. Previous observations demonstrated that males have higher bilirubin levels than females [2,49,50], and not surprisingly, they are over represented in that cohort of infants readmitted to the hospital for evaluation and management of neonatal jaundice, with an odds ratio of 2.89 (confidence interval [CI] 1.46 to 5.74) as compared with their female counterparts [2]. Taken together, these findings suggest an increased risk for marked jaundice and an increased susceptibility to bilirubin-induced injury in male neonates. Regarding the former, it is of interest that the prevalence of the Gilbert's syndrome is reportedly more than twofold higher in males (12.4%) than in females (4.8%). Additionally, within this cohort, male TSB levels are significantly higher than female TSB levels [51]. Gilbert's syndrome, an inherited disorder of impaired bilirubin conjugation capacity, would be expected to enhance the risk of neonatal hyperbilirubinemia, particularly when coexpressed with other icterogenic conditions [52,53]. Regarding the susceptibility to bilirubin-induced injury, early studies on neonates who had hemolytic disease demonstrated a male pre-dominance in neonatal mortality attributable to kernicterus [54–56], a find-ing also reported in hyperbilirubinemic premature neonates [57]. Studies in the hyperbilirubinemic Gunn rat model of kernicterus are also consistent with the notion of an increased male susceptibility to bilirubin-induced in-jury, demonstrating an increased prevalence of kernicterus [58] and higher cerebellar brain bilirubin contents in jaundiced male pups [59] as contrasted with their jaundiced female counterparts. The similar total serum bilirubin and serum albumin levels in hyperbilirubinemic male and female Gunn rat pups in the latter study suggest sex-specific differences in:

- Blood–brain barrier permeability to unbound bilirubin
- Neuronal plasma membrane bilirubin passage
- CNS bilirubin binding, metabolism, or clearance [59]

A potential role for sex hormones in this process remains unexplored but merits study, as surges in gonadotropin secretion during late embryonic and early postnatal life impact CNS development in rodents [60].

Glucose-6-phosphate dehydrogenase deficiency and risk

Of additional note regarding male sex and risk of neonatal hyperbilirubi-nemia is the cohort of newborns who are glucose-6-phosphate dehydroge-nase (G-6-PD) deficient. Given that G-6-PD deficiency is an X-linked condition, affected males predominate (although as a result of X chro-mosome inactivation [lyonization] female heterozygotes have two red cell populations, normal and G-6-PD deficient, and can be affected when inactivation is non-random, in addition to homozygous deficient females). Of clinical note, many affected neonates in the US Pilot Kernicterus registry are G-6-PD deficient (20.8% of all cases [4]); most of those being African American males [4]. A recent report assessing risk factors for the prediction of hyperbilirubinemia in term and late preterm African American male ne-onates demonstrated that G-6-PD deficient males who were also late pre-term and breast-feeding represented the subgoup at highest risk for hyperbilirubinemia (defined as any bilirubin values greater than 95% on the hour-of-life-specific bilirubin nomogram of Bhutani and colleagues [61]), affecting approximately 60% of such newborns (odds ratio 10.2, 1.35 to 76.93 95% CI) [62].

Treatment guidelines

The current management guidelines of the AAP Subcommittee on Hyper-bilirubinemia outline hour-specific phothotherapy (Fig. 1) and exchange transfusion (Fig. 2) treatment thresholds for three separate groups of neonates:

- Infants at lower risk (at least 38 weeks gestation and well)

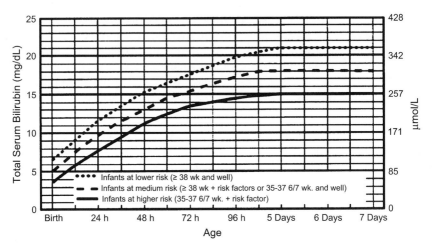

Fig. 1. Phototherapy guideline from the 2004 practice parameter of the American Academy of Pediatrics Subcommittee on Hyperbilirubinemia. Use total bilirubin. Do not subtract direct reacting or conjugated bilirubin. Risk factors include isoimmune hemolytic disease, G6PD deficiency, asphyxia, significant lethargy, temperature instability, sepsis, acidosis, or albumin less than 3.0g/dL (if measured). For well infants ($35^{0/7}$–$37^{6/7}$ wks), can adjust TSB levels for intervention around the medium risk line. It is an option to intervene at lower TSB levels for infants closer to 35 wks and at higher TSB levels for those closer to $37^{6/7}$ wks. (*From* American Academy of Pediatrics Subcommittee on Hyperbilirubinemia. Management of hyperbilirubinemia in the newborn infant 35 or more weeks of gestation. Pediatrics 2004;114:304; with permission. © Copyright 2004 by the American Academy of Pediatrics.)

- Infants at medium risk (at least 38 weeks gestation with risk factors [defined as isoimmune hemolytic disease, G-6-PD deficiency, asphyxia, significant lethargy, temperature instability, acidosis, or albumin less than 3.0 g/dL (if measured)] or $35^{0/7}$ to $37^{6/7}$ weeks gestation and well)
- Infants at higher risk ($35^{0/7}$ to $37^{6/7}$ weeks gestation with risk factors) [22]

These three risk groups, lower, medium, and higher, are identified in Figs. 1 and 2 and in Table 2, which shows the bilirubin to albumin (B/A) ratios that can be used as an additional risk factor, but not in lieu of the TSB in determining the need for exchange transfusion (see Fig. 2 legend). Because the AAP guidelines are hour-, gestational age-, and risk-specific it is often helpful to use instruments such as BiliTool (access at www.bilitool.org), which are designed to assist the clinician in characterizing an individual patient's risk toward the development of hyperbilirubinemia and in accurately identifying relevant phototherapy treatment and exchange transfusion thresholds. Such tools can be accessed online or downloaded to personal hand-held computer devices. Of note, the AAP guideline treatment thresholds are lower in well late preterm neonates than in healthy term neonates and lower still if the late preterm neonate also evidences risk factors [22]. Of additional note, the management of late preterm newborns born between

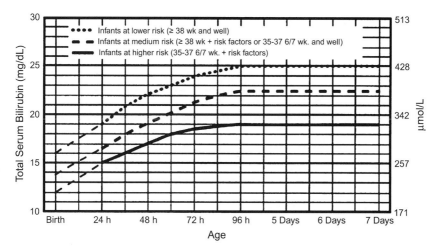

Fig. 2. Exchange transfusion guideline from the 2004 practice parameter of the American Academy of Pediatrics subcommittee on hyperbilirubinemia. The dashed lines for the first 24 hours indicate uncertainty caused by a range of clinical circumstances and a range of responses to phototherapy. Immediate exchange transfusion is recommended if infant shows signs of acute bilirubin encephalopathy (hypertonia, arching, retrocollis, opisthotonos, fever, high-pitched cry [functional immaturity of the late preterm neonate may mask these signs of acute bilirubin encephalopathy [12]]) or if TSB is ≥ 5 mg/dL (85 μmol/L above these lines). Risk factors include isoimmune hemolytic disease, G6PD deficiency, asphyxia, significant lethargy, temperature instability, sepsis, and acidosis. Measure serum albumin and calculate B/A ratio (see Table 2). Use total bilirubin. Do not subtract direct reacting or conjugated bilirubin. If infant is well and $35^{0/7}$–$37^{6/7}$ wks (median risk), can individualize TSB levels for exchange based on actual gestational age. (*From* American Academy of Pediatrics Subcommittee on Hyperbilirubinemia. Management of hyperbilirubinemia in the newborn infant 35 or more weeks of gestation. Pediatrics 2004;114:305; with permission. © Copyright 2004 by the American Academy of Pediatrics.)

$34^{0/7}$ and $34^{6/7}$ weeks gestation is not addressed by the 2004 AAP clinical practice guideline [22]. Also, infants born between $37^{0/7}$ and $37^{6/7}$ weeks gestation, although strictly defined as term. are characterized in the AAP guideline as medium to higher risk and are to be managed as late preterm regarding phototherapy and exchange thresholds [22]. The latter underscores the importance of maturity in defining risk and reflects a consensus that even $37^{0/7}$ to $37^{6/7}$ weeks gestation newborns are predisposed to develop hyperbilirubinemia and bilirubin-induced CNS injury. The management of late preterm neonates born between $34^{0/7}$ and $34^{6/7}$ weeks gestation is akin to guidelines for preterm neonates, the framing of which has proven to be a capricious exercise at best and one for which no claim of evidence base can be made [20]. Nevertheless, it seems prudent in the absence of additional data to apply treatment thresholds that approximate those of the AAP higher risk group to this cohort of late preterm neonates, even when they are clinically well, commensurate with several other published management guidelines for premature newborns [21].

WATCHKO

Table 2
The following B/A ratios can be used together with, but not in lieu of, the total serum bilirubin level as an additional factor in determining the need for exchange transfusion

Risk category	B/A ratio at which exchange transfusion should be considered	
	TSB mg/dL/Alb, g/dL	TSB μmol/L/Alb, μmol/L
Infants $\geq 38^{0/7}$ wks	8.0	0.94
Infants $35^{0/7}$–$37^{6/7}$ wks and well or $\geq 38^{0/7}$ wk if higher risk or isoimmune hemolytic disease or G6PD deficiency	7.2	0.84
Infants $35^{0/7}$–$37^{6/7}$ wks if higher risk or isoimmune hemolytic disease or G6PD deficiency	6.8	0.80

From American Academy of Pediatrics Subcommittee on Hyperbilirubinemia. Management of hyperbilirubinemia in the newborn infant 35 or more weeks of gestation. Pediatrics 2004; 114:305; with permission. © Copyright 2004 by the American Academy of Pediatrics.

Intravenous immune globulin

In addition to phototherapy and exchange transfusion, several studies have demonstrated the effectiveness of early high-dose (500–1000 mg/kg) intravenous immune globulin (IVIG) therapy in attenuating hemolysis and resultant hyperbilirubinemia associated with Coombs-positive hemolytic disease (Rh isoimmunization and ABO in compatibility) [63–65]. Indeed, IVIG significantly decreased blood carboxyhemoglobin levels by 24 hours after IVIG, a sensitive marker of neonatal hemolysis [63]. Additionally, a recent systematic review reported that the number needed to treat with IVIG to prevent one exchange transfusion was low, at 2.7, attesting to the efficacy of this intervention [65]. IVIG should be given slowly (over at least 2 hours), and it can be repeated at 12-hour intervals until the bilirubin stabilizes [64]. This effective means of attenuating hemolysis should be considered strongly in late preterm neonates who have Coombs-positive hemolytic disease to reduce their risk of hyperbilirubinemia reaching exchange levels.

Prevention

Ultimately, the best clinical strategy to avoid the development of marked hyperbilirubinemia and attendant risk of acute bilirubin encephalopathy in the late preterm neonate is preventive and includes screening for jaundice in the newborn nursery, the provision of lactation support, parental education, timely postdischarge follow-up, and appropriate treatment when clinically indicated. Screening for neonatal jaundice before birth hospitalization discharge is critical in late preterm neonates, and it is the author's current practice to obtain either a TSB or transcutaneous bilirubin measurement to accurately assess their risk for hyperbilirubinemia using the hour-specific Bhutani nomogram [22,61]. The provision of lactation support during the birth hospitalization and during the early postdischarge period, coupled with regular neonatal weight checks, is helpful in averting lactation difficulties and in the early identification of those mother–infant pairs prone to suboptimal lactation or lactation failure. This practice is encouraged for all breast-feeding primiparous mothers. Parental education about neonatal jaundice and counseling regarding when to call the pediatrician is also important. A shortened hospital stay (less than 48 hours after delivery), although permitted for selected healthy term neonates [66], is not recommended for late preterm neonates. The AAP recommends close postdischarge follow-up for all newborns [66], a recommendation strongly reinforced in the current 2004 practice parameter, and one that is particularly relevant to the late-preterm neonate [22]. Indeed, timely post-discharge follow-up should identify many infants at risk in time to initiate appropriate treatment. Finally, when significant hyperbilirubinemia occurs, attention to phototherapy and exchange transfusion treatment thresholds as a function of gestational age and risk is a critical component in efforts to prevent brain injury.

References

[1] Watchko JF. Indirect hyperbilirubinemia in the neonate. In: Maisels MJ, Watchko JF, editors. Neonatal jaundice. Monographs in clinical pediatrics. Amsterdam (Netherlands): Harwood Academic; 2000. p. 51–66.

[2] Maisels MJ, Kring E. Length of stay, jaundice, and hospital readmission. Pediatrics 1998; 101:995–8.

[3] Brown AK, Damus K, Kim MH, et al. Factors relating to readmission of term and near term neonates in the first two weeks of life. Early Discharge Survey Group of the Health Professional Advisory Board of the Greater New York Chapter of the March of Dimes. J Perinat Med 1999;27:263–75.

[4] Bhutani VK, Johnson LH, Maisels MJ, et al. Kernicterus: epidemiological strategies for its prevention through systems-based approaches. J Perinatol 2004;24:650–62.

[5] Escobar GJ, Greene JD, Hulac P, et al. Rehospitalization after birth hospitalization: patterns among infants of all gestations. Arch Dis Child 2005;90:125–31.

[6] Perlstein MA. The late clinical syndrome of posticteric encephalopathy. Pediatr Clin North Am 1960;7:665–87.

[7] Maisels MJ, Newman TB. Kernicterus in otherwise healthy, breast-fed term newborns. Pediatrics 1995;96:730–3.

[8] Ip S, Chung M, Kulig J, et al. An evidence-based review of important issues concerning neonatal hyperbilirubinemia. Pediatrics 2004;114:e130–53.

[9] Engle WA. A recommendation for the definition of late preterm (near-term) and the birth weight–gestational age classification system. Semin Perinatol 2006;30:2–7.

[10] Raju TN, Higgins RD, Stark AR, et al. Optimizing care and outcome for late preterm (near-term) infants: a summary of the workshop sponsored by the NICHD. Pediatrics 2006;118: 1207–14.

[11] Newman TB, Escobar GJ, Gonzales VM, et al. Frequency of neonatal bilirubin testing and hyperbilirubinemia in a large health maintenance organization. Pediatrics 1999;104: 1198–203.

[12] Bhutani VK, Johnson L. Kernicterus in late preterm infants cared for as term healthy infants. Semin Perinatol 2006;30:89–97.

[13] Watchko JF. The clinical sequelae of hyperbilirubinemia. In: Maisels MJ, Watchko JF, editors. Neonatal jaundice. Amsterdam (Netherlands): Harwood Academic Publishers; 2000. p. 115–35.

[14] Billing BH, Cole PG, Lathe GH. Increased plasma bilirubin in newborn infants in relation to birth weight. BMJ 1954;2:1263–5.

[15] Kaplan M, Muraca M, Hammerman C, et al. Imbalance between production and conjugation of bilirubin: a fundamental concept in the mechanism of neonatal jaundice. Pediatrics 2002;110:e47.

[16] Kaplan M, Muraca M, Vreman HJ, et al. Neonatal bilirubin production-conjugation imbalance: effect of glucose-6-phosphate dehydrogenase deficiency and borderline prematurity. Arch Dis Child Fetal Neonatal Ed 2005;90:F123–7.

[17] Kawade N, Onish S. The prenatal and postnatal development of UDP-glucuronyltransferase activity towards bilirubin and the effect of premature birth on this activity in the human liver. Biochem J 1981;196:257–60.

[18] Gartner LM, Snyder RN, Chabon RS, et al. Kernicterus: high incidence in premature infants with low serum bilirubin concentrations. Pediatrics 1970;45:906–17.

[19] Watchko JF, Oski FA. Kernicterus in preterm newborns: past, present, and future. Pediatrics 1992;90:707–15.

[20] Maisels MJ, Watchko JF. Treatment of jaundice in low-birth weight infants. Arch Dis Child Fetal Neonatal Ed 2003;88:F459–63.

[21] Watchko JF, Maisels MJ. Management of jaundice in preterm infants. In: David TJ, editor. Recent advances of paediatrics. London: Royal Society of Medicine Press Limited; 2005. p. 121–34.

[22] American Academy of Pediatrics Subcommittee on Hyperbilirubinemia. Management of hyperbilirubinemia in the newborn infant 35 or more weeks of gestation. Pediatrics 2004; 114:297–316 [Erratum, Pediatrics 2004;114:1138].

[23] Hyvarinen M, Zelter P, Oh W, et al. Influence of gestational age on serum levels of alpha-1 fetoprotein, IgG globulin, and albumin in newborn infants. J Pediatr 1973;82:430–7.

[24] Ritter DA, Kenny JD. Influence of gestational age on cord serum bilirubin binding studies. J Pediatr 1985;106:118–21.

[25] Wennberg RP. The blood–brain barrier and bilirubin encephalopathy. Cell Mol Neurobiol 2000;20:97–109.

[26] Stonestreet BS, Patlak CS, Pettigrew KD, et al. Ontogeny of blood-brain barrier function in ovine fetuses, lambs, and adults. J Appl Physiol 1996;271:R1594–601.

[27] Virgintino D, Errede M, Robertson D, et al. Immunolocalization of tight junction proteins in the adult and developing human brain. Histochem Cell Biol 2004;122:51–9.

[28] Amit Y, Brenner T. Age-dependent sensitivity of cultured rat glial cells to bilirubin toxicity. Exp Neurol 1993;121:248–55.

[29] Rhine WD, Schmitter SP, Yu ACH, et al. Bilirubin toxicity and differentiation of cultured astrocytes. J Perinatol 1999;19:206–11.

[30] Rodrigues CMP, Sola S, Silva RFM, et al. Aging confers different sensitivity to the neurotoxic properties of unconjugated bilirubin. Pediatr Res 2002;51:112–8.

[31] Falcao AS, Fernandes A, Brito MA, et al. Bilirubin-induced inflammatory response, glutamate release, and cell death in rat cortical astrocytes are enhanced in younger cells. Neurobiol Dis 2005;20:199–206.

[32] Abney ER, Bartlett PP, Raff M. Astrocytes, ependymal cells, and oligodendrocytes develop on schedule in dissociated cell cultures of embryonic rat brain. Dev Biol 1981; 83:301–10.

[33] Ahlfors CE, Bennett SH, Shoemaker CT, et al. Changes in the auditory brainstem response associated with intravenous infusion of unconjugated bilirubin into infant rhesus monkeys. Pediatr Res 1986;20:511–5.

[34] Hansen TWR, Allen JW. Oxidation of bilirubin by brain mitochondrial membranes – dependence on cell type and postnatal age. Biochem Mol Med 1997;60:155–60.

[35] Wang ML, Dorer DJ, Fleming MP, et al. Clinical outcomes of near-term infants. Pediatrics 2004;114:372–6.

[36] Edmonson MB, Stoddard JL, Owens LM. Hospital readmission with feeding-related problems after early postpartum discharge of normal newborns. JAMA 1997;278:299–303.

[37] Ingram J, Woolridge M, Greenwood R. Breastfeeding: it is worth trying with the second baby. Lancet 2001;358:986–7.

[38] Takimoto M, Matsuda I. β-glucuronidase activity in the stool of newborn infant. Biol Neonate 1972;18:66–70.

[39] Gourley GR. Perinatal bilirubin metabolism. In: Gluckman PD, Heymann MA, editors. Perinatal and pediatric pathophysiology. A clinical perspective. Boston: Hodder and Stoughton; 1993. p. 437–9.

[40] Poland RD, Odell GB. Physiologic jaundice: the enterohepatic circulation of bilirubin. N Engl J Med 1971;284:1–6.

[41] Gartner LM, Lee KS, Vaisman S, et al. Development of bilirubin transport and metabolism in the newborn rhesus monkey. J Pediatr 1977;90:513–31.

[42] Gartner U, Goeser T, Wolkoff AW. Effect of fasting on the uptake of bilirubin and sulfobromophthalein by the isolated perfused rat liver. Gastroenterology 1997;113:1707–13.

[43] Fevery J. Fasting hyperbilirubinemia: unraveling the mechanism involved. Gastroenterology 1997;113:1798–9.

[44] Bertini G, Carlo C, Tronchin M, et al. Is breastfeeding really favoring early neonatal jaundice? Pediatrics 2001;107:e41.

[45] Maisels MJ. Epidemiology of neonatal jaundice. In: Maisels MJ, Watchko JF, editors. Neonatal jaundice. Amsterdam: (Netherlands): Harwood Academic Publishers; 2000. p. 37–49.

[46] Stevenson DK, Bortoletti AL, Ostrander CR, et al. Pulmonary excretion of carbon monoxide in the human infant as an index of bilirubin production. IV: Effects of breast feeding and caloric intake in the first postnatal week. Pediatrics 1980;65:1170–2.

[47] Hintz SR, Gaylord TD, Oh W, et al. Serum bilirubin levels at 72 hours by selected characteristics in breastfed and formula-fed term infants delivered by cesarean section. Acta Paediatr 2001;90:776–81.

[48] Neifert MR. Prevention of breastfeeding tragedies. Pediatr Clin North Am 2001;48:273–97.

[49] Maisels MJ, Gifford K, Antle CE, et al. Jaundice in the healthy newborn infant: a new approach to an old problem. Pediatrics 1988;81:505–11.

[50] Gale R, Seidman DS, Dollberg S, et al. Epidemiology of neonatal jaundice in the Jerusalem population. J Pediatr Gastroenterol Nutr 1990;10:82–6.

[51] Sieg A, Arab L, Schlierf G, et al. Prevalence of Gilbert's syndrome in Germany. Dtsch Med Wochenschr 1987;112:1206–8.

[52] Watchko JF. Vigintiphobia revisited. Pediatrics 2005;115:1747–53.

[53] Kaplan M, Hammerman C. Bilirubin and the genome: the hereditary basis of unconjugated neonatal hyperbilirubinemia. Current Pharmacogenomics 2005;3:21–42.

[54] Diamond LK, Vaughn VC, Allen FH Jr. Erythroblastosis fetalis III. Prognosis in relation to clinical and serologic manifestations at birth. Pediatrics 1950;6:630–7.

[55] Armitage P, Mollison PL. Further analysis of controlled trials of treatment of haemolytic disease of the newborn. J Obstet Gynaecol Brit Emp 1953;60:605–20.

[56] Walker W, Mollison PL. Haemolytic disease of the newborn: deaths in England and Wales during 1953 and 1955. Lancet 1957;1:1309–14.

[57] Crosse VM. The incidence of kernicterus (not due to haemolytic disease) among premature babies. In: Sass-Kortsak A, editor. Kernicterus. Toronto: University of Toronto Press; 1961. p. 4–9.

[58] Johnson L, Garcia ML, Figueroa E, et al. Kernicterus in rats lacking glucuronyl transferase. Am J Dis Child 1961;101:322–49.

[59] Cannon C, Daood MJ, Watchko JF. Sex specific regional brain bilirubin content in hyper-bilirubinemic Gunn rat pups. Biol Neonate 2006;90:40–5.

[60] Becu-Villabos D, Gonzalez Iglesias A, Diaz-Torga G, et al. Brain sexual differentiation and gonadotropins secretion in the rat. Cell Mol Neurobiol 1997;17:699–715.

[61] Bhutani VK, Johnson L, Sivieri EM, et al. Predictive ability of a predischarge hour-specific serum bilirubin for subsequent significant hyperbilirubinemia in healthy term and near-term newborns. Pediatrics 1999;103:6–14.

[62] Kaplan M, Herschel M, Hammerman C, et al. Neonatal hyperbilirubinemia in African American males: the importance of glucose-6-phosphate dehydrogenase deficiency. J Pediatr 2006;149:83–8.

[63] Hammerman C, Vreman HJ, Kaplan M, et al. Intravenous immune globulin in neonatal immune hemolytic disease: does it reduce hemolysis. Acta Paediatr 1996;85:1351–3.

[64] Hammerman C. Recent developments in the management of neonatal hyperbilirubinemia. NeoReviews 2000;1:e19–24.

[65] Gottstein R, Cooke RWI. Systematic review of intravenous immunoglobulin in haemolytic disease of the newborn. Arch Dis Child Fetal Neonatal Ed 2003;88:F6–10.

[66] American Academy of Pediatrics. Care of the newborn. In: Gilstrap LC, Oh W, editors. Guidelines for perinatal care. 5th edition. Elk Grove Village (IL): American Academy of Pediatrics, American College of Obstetrics and Gynecology; 2002. p. 211–5.

CLINICS IN
PERINATOLOGY

Clin Perinatol 33 (2006) 853–870

Glucose Metabolism in the Late Preterm Infant

Meena Garg, MD, Sherin U. Devaskar, MD*

*Division of Neonatology & Developmental Biology, Department of Pediatrics,
David Geffen School of Medicine at University of California Los Angeles and
Mattel Children's Hospital at University of California Los Angeles, 10833 LeConte Avenue,
Room B2-377 MDCC, Los Angeles, CA 90095, USA*

"The questions that arise at the bedside are, (1) How low a glucose concentration is too low? (2) Which glucose concentration causes brain damage? (3) How long should it be low before we encounter irreversible brain damage"

Prematurity and low birth weight are important determinants of neonatal morbidity and mortality. A rising trend of preterm births is caused by an increase in the birth rate of near-term infants [1]. Near-term infants are defined as infants of 34 to 36 6/7 weeks gestation. The term "near-term" recently was renamed as the "late preterm" to alert health care providers to anticipate increased potential problems that may present in labor and delivery, in the nursery, and beyond [2–4]. Demands on limited acute care beds in neonatal ICUs, along with established clinical practices, often result in early transition of these infants to the well baby nursery and to the mother's room to honor the rooming in practice. This transition takes place once spontaneous respirations and adequate oxygenation are established. This is exacerbated further by early discharge of the mother and baby resulting in increased rehospitalizations. Treating these infants as term well babies serves as a distinct disadvantage to this subgroup. Transitional problems persist and consist of poor thermoregulation, inability to adequately establish feeding, unrecognized hypoglycemia, and subsequent issues with hyperbilirubinemia. It is dangerous to assume that the incidence of hypoglycemia in the late preterm infant is similar to the infant born at full term. Postnatal decrease in plasma glucose concentration in preterm infants is much greater

S.U. Devaskar is supported by grants from the National Institutes of Health (HD33997 and HD25024).

* Corresponding author.
E-mail address: sdevaskar@mednet.ucla.edu (S.U. Devaskar).

0095-5108/06/$ - see front matter © 2006 Elsevier Inc. All rights reserved.
doi:10.1016/j.clp.2006.10.001

than in term infants, suggesting poor postnatal adaptation [5]. The incidence of hypoglycemia in preterm infants is three times greater than in full-term newborn infants, and nearly two-thirds of these infants require intravenous dextrose infusions [4]. Further, the compensatory mechanisms responsible for protecting the brain from hypoglycemic injury are not entirely in place, posing a greater risk to this subpopulation of late preterm infants. Association of hypoglycemia with neurodevelopmental abnormalities has prompted increased recognition, anticipation, diagnosis, and therapy of neonatal hypoglycemia [6–9]. Severe hypoglycemia is recognized to cause neuronal cell death and subsequent adverse neurodevelopment [7,10]; however, the level at which hypoglycemia becomes clinically important, warranting intervention, is not well-defined [11,12]. Although current methods for assessing effects of hypoglycemia are imperfect, the injury to central nervous system depends on the degree of prematurity, presence of intrauterine growth restriction (IUGR), intrauterine compromise, genotype, blood flow, metabolic rate, and availability of other substrates. Therefore, early recognition of glucose metabolic abnormalities pertaining to late preterm infants is essential to provide appropriate and timely interventions in the newborn nursery. Although many of the investigations have targeted full-term infants, premature infants inclusive of the extremely low birth weight infants and the intrauterine growth-restricted infants, adequately powered studies restricted to only the late preterm infants are required and need future consideration.

Incidence

At birth, the glucose concentration is approximately 80% of maternal glucose, but it falls to its lowest nadir between 30 and 90 minutes after birth and stabilizes between 40 to 100 mg/dL. During this transition in the first 2 to 4 hours of life, 8% of babies develop hypoglycemia that requires intervention. How many of these babies belong to the late preterm subpopulation is unknown. The incidence of scheduled cesarean section versus cesarean section following labor or vaginal delivery contributing toward the development of hypoglycemia has not been investigated specifically. The presence of labor may prove to be essential for some of the hormonal and enzymatic adaptations that are necessary to preserve circulating glucose concentrations.

Pathophysiology

Fetus

Eighty percent of the fetal energy consumption is provided by glucose. The fetus is solely dependent on maternal glucose that is supplied transplacentally by a process of facilitative diffusion. This passive diffusion process is mediated primarily by a saturable, stereo-specific, carrier-mediated system consisting of a family of closely related membrane-spanning glycoproteins termed the facilitative glucose transporters (GLUT1). Isoform GLUT1 (Michaelis-Menten constant aka Michaelis constant or Km 1 to 2 mmol) is the predominant transporter in the human placenta, with the isoform GLUT3 (Km 0.8 mM) found during early gestation and in fetal vasculature [13]. These two isoforms provide the basis for transplacental transport of glucose. The fetal glucose concentration generally is maintained at two thirds that of the mother to provide the gradient necessary for passive transport of glucose from mother to fetus. Under normal conditions, the fetus is incapable of producing endogenous glucose. Under conditions of limited transplacental glucose supply, however, the fetus has the ability to produce glucose by glycogenolysis and gluconeogenesis.

Transition at birth

Once the cord is clamped, the newborn has to adapt swiftly to a life of independence and learn to produce endogenous glucose to meet the energy (ATP) demands of cellular oxidation. During this transition, the newborn infant's circulating glucose concentration decreases to one third of the maternal concentration (40 to 60 mg/dL) by 2 to 4 hours of age. In the late premature infant, this concentration may be lower at 30 to 40 mg/dL [11,12,14]. The maintenance of euglycemia depends on postnatal induction of hepatic glycogenolysis and gluconeogenesis in response to postnatal changes in plasma catecholamines, glucagon, insulin, and corticosteroids that are conducive to glucose production. The increase in plasma concentrations of catecholamines (epinephrine, norepinephrine and dopamine) is preserved in preterm and late preterm newborns with an accentuated epinephrine response compared with term newborns [15]. This change is accompanied by a decline in circulating insulin concentrations and a subsequent surge in glucagon concentrations. Glucose-regulated insulin secretion by the pancreatic β–islets is immature, resulting in unregulated insulin production during hypoglycemia [16]. Nevertheless, disturbances in glucose homeostasis are common, because metabolic reserves including glycogen are low in late preterm infants, similar to IUGR infants. The risk of hypoglycemia increases further when energy demands increase because of coexisting conditions of sepsis, birth asphyxia, or cold stress [11,17,18]. The blood glucose level stabilizes at a normal value of 60 to 80 mg/dL within 12 to 24 hours after birth. The neonatal glucose requirement is 6 to 8 mg/kg/min as measured by stable isotope tracer technology, a value higher than that observed in adults (3 mg/kg/min) [19]. Hepatic glucose production by glycogenolysis and gluconeogenesis is essential for maintaining euglycemia. Other gluconeogenic substrates, consisting of increased concentrations of circulating glycerol and fatty acids, are encountered because of the dramatic postnatal increase in fat oxidation secondary to catecholamine-induced lipolysis [5,20]. Available amino acids also are converted to glucose. Further, other substrates such as ketones and lactate are used as alternate fuels by the brain in the presence of hypoglycemia. Late preterm and IUGR infants face the challenge of maintaining euglycemia secondary to developmentally immature hepatic enzyme systems (eg, PEPCK) for gluconeogenesis [21] and lower accumulation of hepatic glycogen reserves that are depleted quickly after birth. The immaturity of the gluconeogenic enzymatic pathways was determined when the administration of alanine failed to improve gluconeogenesis in preterm infants [22].

Definition

Although it is recognized that low circulating glucose concentrations have detrimental effects, the actual level at which such effects occur remains unknown, making it difficult to come up with a clinically useful definition of hypoglycemia. During earlier times, statistical definitions were relied upon for clinical decision making, based on values that represented two standard deviations below the mean glucose value of a given population. This definition determined the incidence in a particular population, but it did not define hypoglycemia adequately. A physiological definition subsequently was rendered at less than 45 mg/dL based on abnormal electroencephalographic or increased latency of auditory brainstem-evoked responses (ABR) [23]. The latter observation was made in 10 out of 11 children with a blood glucose of less than 47 mg/dL [24]. At a glucose concentration less than 18 mg/dL, the electroencephalogram (EEG) was isoelectric, demonstrating the critical nature of such low values. More recently, 340 term newborn infants were examined, and higher numbers of rhythmic EEG patterns of less than 10s with asymmetry were observed in infants who had hypoglycemia [25]. Examination of 20 term newborn infants compared with 20 controls revealed frontal sharp transients in hypoglycemic infants with bilateral asynchrony along with coarser theta waves and the appearance of delta waves [26]. Further in the low birth weight infants, persistent hypoglycemia for 5 days was associated with a poor neurological outcome [27]. Although this physiological definition may herald immediate neurological dysfunction in term babies, the impact of these EEG and ABR changes on long-term outcome is unknown. Meta analysis of different investigations suggested that plasma glucose of less than 25 mg/dL for several hours increased the relative risk for adverse neurological outcome with a 21% (confidence interval [CI] from 14% to 27%) incidence of significant neurological sequelae [28]. This study, however, did not rule out adverse neurological outcomes at other glucose values. Hence the search for a functional definition that impacts long term neurological outcome in the late preterm infants is ongoing. More importantly, a quest for a cut-off value continues toward developing bedside management guidelines for these infants. Although the definitions of asymptomatic versus symptomatic hypoglycemia have assisted toward the need for immediate intervention, given that some of the symptoms are nonspecific, the recognition of symptomatic hypoglycemia may not be that easy. Signs and symptoms of hypoglycemia include:

- Changes in level of consciousness: irritability, excessive crying, lethargy, or stupor
- Apnea episodes, cyanosis
- Feeding poorly
- Tachypnea, tachycardia, grunting
- Hypothermia
- Hypotonia-limpness
- Tremor-seizures, jitteriness

Even if the health care team is astute at detecting hypoglycemia-related symptoms that usually are caused by either counter-regulation or the absence of alternate substrates to fuel brain oxidative metabolism, the cause for lack of symptoms remains evasive. The asymptomatic state may relate to a lack of the compensatory counter-regulatory hormonal response similar to the unaware-ness state described in older children, which may be ominous, or the presence of adequate alternate substrates protecting the brain's energy requirement. Most investigations in asymptomatic hypoglycemic term infants have re-vealed a neurologically intact outcome, supporting the latter [29]. Similar studies do not exist specifically in the subpopulation of late preterm infants.

The more challenging task is to come up with a cut-off circulating glucose threshold value that dictates intervention in the late preterm infant. The rea-son this is difficult is because circulating glucose concentrations are merely the tip of an iceberg, reflecting the net effect of glucose production, use, and clear-ance. Although glucose concentrations less than 45 mg/dL are acceptable during the transition phase of life, glucose concentrations less than 50 to 60 mg/dL following the transition are considered abnormal. The ideal parameter to assess is not the glucose concentration but rather the glucose delivery to tissues. This is calculated by the Fick's principle: (a-v) glucose concentration × cardiac output. This demonstrates that tissue glucose delivery depends, not only on the arterio–venous difference in circulating glucose concentration, but also on the cardiac output/tissue blood flow. Thus, the glucose concentra-tion that predetermines a detrimental effect may vary depending on the car-diac output, being higher in situations of hypotension and shock and lower when normotensive. Thus the threshold varies depending on the clinical pre-sentation. This concept is helpful and can be derived when caring for ill neo-nates, but most often one needs to decipher the significance of a glucose value obtained by a bedside screening test followed by a laboratory assessed value. The American Academy of Pediatrics guidelines suggest glucose screening to be undertaken at the bedside. This is now routine in most nurseries, and the bedside test should be reliable yet easy to perform on a large scale. In addi-tion, the site of sampling, the hematocrit of blood at the time of sampling, presence of alcohol or heparin in a collected sample, and the timeliness of per-forming the test after blood collection all influence the ultimate result.

"Prolonged hypoglycemia should be avoided by close bedside monitoring of vulnerable infants whilst avoiding excessively invasive management in populations of neonates, which may jeopardize the successful establishment of breast feeding" [30].

This statement applies to late preterm infants, because establishment of breast feeding is a challenge in this subpopulation setting them up for hypoglycemia. Because most of the bedside monitoring devices involve a blood draw and are fraught with inaccuracies (ranging from 10% to 15%), a need for developing a noninvasive continuous glucose monitoring sensor exists. To this end, 96 measurements were performed in 16 very low birth weight infants at 23 to 30 weeks who were 584 to 1387 g in body weight [31]. Researchers used disposable glucose oxidase-based platinum electrode sensor that catalyzes interstitial glucose oxidation, generating an electrical current every 10 seconds using a Minimed sensor (Medtronic, Northridge, California) that can last for 7 days of monitoring. The R^2 obtained was 0.87, with $P<.001$ at less than 10 mM. The glucose values obtained from Minimed at <10 mM glucose concentration were 0.06 mM lower than the values obtained by the Yellow Springs Instrument (Yellow Springs, Ohio; YSI) and correlated significantly ($r^2 = 0.87$, $P<.001$. However at >10 mM glucose concentration the difference was -0.106 mM when compared to the YSI laboratory measurements with a lower correlation ($r^2 = 0.69$ at $P<.001$).

Hyperinsulinism

It is important to address the state of hyperinsulinism that frequently is encountered in infants of diabetic mothers and those born to obese insulin-resistant mothers. Given the incredible increase in overweight and obese individuals in the United States, the incidence of gestational diabetes is increasing, resulting in macrosomic infants [32,33]. These infants usually are delivered by cesarean section because of cephalo–pelvic disproportion or shoulder dystocia. Thus these infants run the risk of becoming late preterm infants with hyperinsulinism (Box 1). In the presence of uteroplacental insufficiency, these infants may be growth restricted yet appropriate for gestational age. These infants are at high risk for developing hypoglycemia that may require aggressive intervention. In addition, persistent hyperinsulinemic hypoglycemia of infancy (PHHI) syndromes also can present in the late preterm infant, requiring aggressive and timely intervention to prevent neurological impairment [34,35]. It is clear from animal and human studies that the hyperinsulinemic hypoglycemia is worse than the low glycogen reserve-related hypoglycemia of the late preterm infant. Thus if a late preterm infant presents with a PHHI syndrome, the neurological outcome is worse. This is related to extremely low ketone concentrations secondary to the high insulin concentrations [36]. Thus, the alternate substrate also is lacking, making the brain highly vulnerable to injury. In the infant of a diabetic mother, the increase in free iron in brain incites oxidant injury to the detriment of the infant [37,38].

Box 1. Causes of hypoglycemia in the late preterm infant

Transient hypoglycemia in the late preterm infant
Maternal conditions
- Glucose infusion in the mother
- Preeclampsia
- Drugs: tocolytic therapy, sympathomimetics
- Infant of diabetic mother

Neonatal conditions
- Prematurity
- Respiratory distress syndrome
- Twin gestation
- Neonatal sepsis
- Perinatal hypoxia-ischemia
- Temperature instability: hypothermia
- Polycythemia
- Specific glucose transporter deficiency
- Isoimmune thrombocytopenia, Rh incompatibility

Persistent hypoglycemia in the late preterm infant
Hyperinsulinism
- Nesidioblastosis, beta cell hyperplasia, sulfonylurea receptor defect
- Beckwith-Wiedemann syndrome
- Infant of diabetic mother

Endocrine disorders
- Pituitary insufficiency
- Cortisol deficiency
- Congenital glucagon deficiency

Inborn errors of metabolism
- Carbohydrate metabolism: glycogen storage disease, galactosemia, fructose-1-6-diphoshatase deficiency
- Amino acid metabolism: maple syrup urine disease, propionic acidemia, methylmalonic acidemia hereditary tyrosinemia
- Fatty acid metabolism: acyl-coenzyme dehydrogenase defect, defects in carnitine metabolism, beta-oxidation defects

Defective glucose transport

Protective mechanisms in brain

The higher glucose requirement in neonates reflects the glucose uptake by brain, which accounts for ~80% of total glucose produced. Glucose is transported across the blood–brain barrier into neurons and glia (astrocytes) by two major glucose transporter isoforms, GLUT1 found mainly in the blood–brain barrier and astrocytes and GLUT3 in neurons. The astrocytes are the local power houses of glycogen stores serving as an immediate source of glucose. In addition to glucose, other substrates, particularly ketones and lactate, are transported across the blood–brain barrier and into astrocytes by the monocarboxylate transporter (MCT) isoform 1 and into neurons by MCT2 [39]. The lactate shuttle, recently described as an alternate protective mechanism in the presence of hypoglycemia, consists of lactate being produced in astrocytes that then is transported as fuel to meet the energy requirements of neurons in the presence of limited glucose supply [40,41]. Whether the astrocytic glycogen stores are replete in the late preterm infant remains unknown. What is known is that alternate fuels such as lactate, pyruvate, amino acids, free fatty acids, ketone bodies, and glycerol are used by the brain during hypoglycemia. Unlike term infants, however, late preterm infants and IUGR infants are incapable of mounting an adequate mature peripheral counter-regulatory ketogenic response [5] to hypoglycemia. This is because of inadequate lipolysis in these infants who do not have the necessary adipose tissue stores and fail to demonstrate adequate milk intake. In lieu of these protective responses, these infants are vulnerable to adverse long-term neurodevelopmental outcome [27,42,43]. Another built-in protective mechanism is that cerebral glucose use is low at birth (18 μmol/min/100 g), increasing to 60 μmol/min/100 g only at 50 weeks postconceptional age, which reflects the value at six years of age [44]. The late preterm infant is also able to increase brain blood flow by recruiting underperfused capillaries in response to hypoglycemia as determined by near infrared spectroscopy (NIRS) [45]. Despite this response, the lack of an adequate ketogenic response with limited glycogen reserves that build up only in late gestation enhances vulnerability to neurological injury [46]. This is of particular importance, because the cerebral extraction coefficient for ketone bodies is highest only when expressed as a fraction of cerebral coefficient for oxygen, which is low in the newborn [30,47].

Clinical neurological presentation

Perinatal hypoxia–ischemia may decrease availability of ketone bodies further; therefore hypoglycemia after hypoxic–ischemic events may cause further damage in late preterm or IUGR infants. Initial hypoglycemia with severe fetal acidemia was observed to cause brain injury in term infants. Retrospective examination of 185 term infants with an umbilical arterial pH of less than 7.00 and an initial blood glucose within 30 minutes of birth [48] demonstrated that 27 (14.5%) infants had an initial blood glucose of less than 40 mg/dL. Fifteen (56%) of these 27 infants with a blood glucose of less than 40 mg/dL versus 26 (16%) of the 158 infants with a blood glucose of greater than 40 mg/dL had an abnormal neurological outcome. Although no difference in the requirement for cardiopulmonary resuscitation or a 5-minute Apgar score of less than 5 was observed between the groups, an increased incidence of abnormal fetal heart rate tracing and meconium staining in hypoglycemic infants was noted. This study suggests that asphyxial injury is associated with a higher incidence of hypoglycemia and sets the stage for subsequent development of neurodevelopmental compromise.

Another multi-center trial that was not targeted at hypoglycemia specifically identified 668 infants with hypoglycemia (blood glucose of less than 40 mg/dL); 433 infants had moderate hypoglycemia, and 104 infants presented with persistent hypoglycemia between 3 and 30 days of life. When hypoglycemia was recorded on 5 or more separate days, the adjusted mental and motor developmental scores at 18 months (corrected age) were reduced by 13 to 14 points, and the incidence of developmental delay was increased by a factor of 3.5 [49]. A longer follow-up study involving 85 small for gestational age (SGA) preterm neonates determined the incidence of hypoglycemia to be 73%. Infants with repeated episodes of hypoglycemia presented with a reduced head circumference and lower scores on psychometric testing at 3.5 and 5 years of age [27]. A retrospective study of children with occipital epilepsy at 12 years of age demonstrated that all these children were hypoglycemic at birth and developed epilepsy as early as 5 months of age [50]. Eighteen infants (six infants who were SGA, two infants of diabetic mothers, and 10 normal infants born between 36 and 42 weeks gestational age) were examined in a separate study. These infants had at least one episode of hypoglycemia (less than 45 mg/dL) after 6 hours of age to exclude transient hypoglycemia, and were symptomatic. Symptoms included tremors, apathy, tachypnea, irritability, hypotonia, and feeding difficulties, which all disappeared when treated. The control group consisted of 10 healthy infants with no hypoglycemia. Ultrasound and MRI at birth, and at 2 months of age, were performed. Thirty nine percent of abnormalities, consisting of patchy hyperintense lesions in the occipital periventricular white matter and thalamus, were observed. These injuries may be related to processes of axonal migration and synaptogenesis that occur in the occipital region during the neonatal period. On developmental follow-up, most of the abnormalities recovered to baseline at 2 months of age; however, no longer-term follow-up was reported [51]. Another small cohort of 8-year-old children born to diabetic mothers and who suffered neonatal hypoglycemia presented with neurological dysfunction related to the attention deficit disorder, including hyperactivity, impulsiveness, and easy distractibility, in addition to deficits in motor control and perception [52].

Detection of brain injury

Although EEG changes have been defined, proton spectroscopy has determined the presence of increased lactate during hypoglycemia [53]. In contrast, phosphorus spectroscopy can detect decreased ATP levels when alternate fuels are exhausted [53]. Ultrasound changes have not been found to be sensitive enough, and CT has limited usefulness. MRI, however, particularly the diffusion-weighted T1 and T2 images, has revealed occipital white matter and thalamus changes caused by acute insult, while chronic changes have presented as periventricular leukomalacia. Positron emission tomography has been useful in determining 2-deoxyglucose and lactate uptake by the brain in infants. More recently, investigations have focused on functional MRI in an attempt to pinpoint the affliction in response to visual and auditory stimuli and in response to specific tasks.

Neuronal injury

Neonatal hypoglycemia can cause seizures, permanent neuronal injury, and death. Hypoglycemia is associated with gray and white matter injuries in the immature brain, and the specific mechanisms responsible for hypoglycemic brain injury have formed the subject of many investigations. Many animal studies have demonstrated that longer periods of hypoglycemia are required than that of hypoxic–ischemia to produce the same degree of brain injury [54]. Hypoglycemia superimposed on hypoxic–ischemia causes more severe injury [55]. Hypoglycemia leads to excitotoxicity with accumulating aspartate and glutamate in brain [53]. The superficial cerebral cortex, the dentate gyrus, hippocampus, and caudate nucleus are vulnerable areas to hypoglycemic injury [10].

The neonatal brain, and especially the cerebral white matter, have relatively low oxygen consumption. Therefore glucose supply is essential to meet the metabolic demands [56]. The major source of brain glucose to meet the metabolic requirements is from an adequate blood flow in addition to plasma glucose concentration (a-v glucose concentration × brain blood flow). Hypoglycemic conditions result in a compensatory increase in cerebral blood flow, and this response is shown to be preserved in preterm infants [6,45,57]. When hypoglycemia is prolonged and the alternate substrate use is exhausted, biochemical effects of brain metabolism develop (Fig. 1). The activities of glutamate receptor/channel complexes are enhanced in the immature brain to promote activity-dependent plasticity. Excitotoxicity is an important mechanism involved in perinatal brain injury. Excitatory synaptic transmission in the mammalian brain is mediated primarily by means of α-amino-3-hydroxy-5-methyl-4-isoxazolpropionic acid (AMPA) and N-methyl-D-aspartate (NMDA)-type receptors [58] (Fig. 2). Glutamate is the major excitatory neurotransmitter, and most neurons, oligodendrocytes, and astrocytes possess receptors for glutamate. Perinatal insults such as hypoxia–ischemia,

BRAIN INJURY

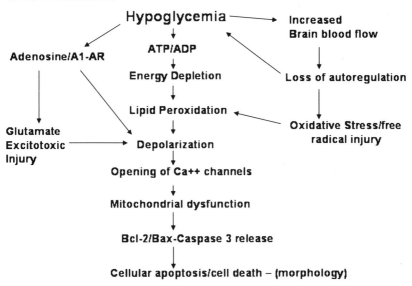

Fig. 1. Intracellular consequences of hypoglycemia.

Brain Neurochemical Changes

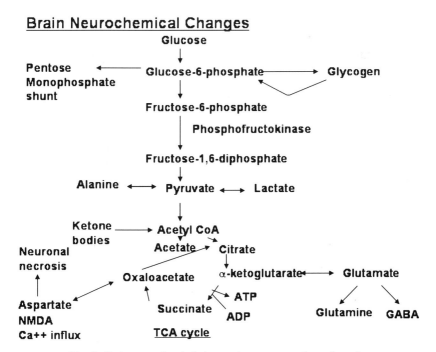

Fig. 2. Brain neurochemical changes in response to hypoglycemia.

stroke, hypoglycemia, and kernicterus, can disrupt synaptic function, leading to accumulation of extracellular glutamate and excessive stimulation of these receptors [10]. Excessive stimulation of glutamate receptor/ion channel complexes trigger calcium influx that stimulates a cascade of intracellular events, resulting in apoptosis or necrosis (see Fig. 1). Reactive oxygen species (ROS) also play a role in brain injury caused by neonatal hypoglycemia [59]. The ability of mitochondria to produce ROS is increased after hypoglycemia in the immature brain. This, in turn, can alter brain structure and function because of oxidant injury sustained by mitochondrial proteins, DNA, or signal transduction pathways in brain [59]. In addition, hypoglycemia is known to release adenosine, which in turn results in neuronal death (see Fig. 1). Hence adenosine receptor subtype antagonists have been observed to reverse hypoglycemia-induced neuronal injury [60]. This is of importance, given that caffeine is an adenosine receptor A1 and A2a receptor antagonist and known to reduce the sensitivity to hypoglycemia [61]. The effect of maternal consumption of caffeine on the infant's response to hypoglycemia is unknown.

Transient anoxia/hypoglycemia is associated with a marked increase of excitatory neurotransmission, which shares similarities with the mechanisms underlying long-term potentiation (LPS), and increases synthesis of excitatory receptor subunits [58]. Both hypoxia and hypoglycemia increase the Ca^{++} influx, which can control the activation of proteolytic enzymes, apoptotic genes, and production of reactive oxygen species directly [62], thus mediating the ultimate neurological insult encountered.

Immature brain also may be more sensitive to limitations of substrate availability because of the presence of minimal cerebral reserves of high-energy phosphates [63]. Thus, there may be enhanced vulnerability of the fetus and newborn to excitotoxic brain injury during hypoglycemia. Acute insulin-induced hypoglycemia leads to specific changes in the cerebral NMDA receptor-associated ion channel in the newborn piglet [64].

In animal studies, many hypoglycemia-induced biochemical alterations in neonatal brain are similar to adults, yet the neurological function and electrical activity are preserved in the neonatal brain at lower plasma glucose concentrations [65]. Although the biochemical changes causing CNS injury in hypoglycemia and hypoxic–ischemic injury are the same, MRI findings suggest that hypoglycemia induces cerebral damage by a mechanism separate from the effects of cerebral hypoxia–ischemia (HIE) [10,66,67]. Severe perinatal hypoglycemia illustrates diffuse cortical and subcortical white matter damage, with the parietal and occipital lobes being affected most severely [42,68] (Fig. 3). This specific pattern of injury correlates with the pathological reports of neonatal hypoglycemia, suggesting that the pattern of damage results from regional hypoperfusion and excitotoxicity with cell type-specific injury [10]. The MRI changes from HIE typically involve parasagittal lesions involving the parieto–occipital cortex that is not limited to the posterior pole of the brain. Occipital brain injury associated with neonatal hypoglycemia can result in long-term disability, epilepsy, and visual

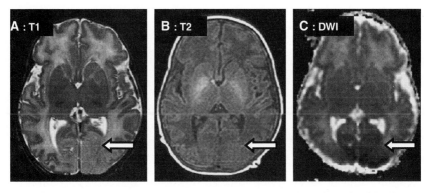

Fig. 3. MRI of brain in neonatal hypoglycemia. Severe neonatal hypoglycemia with seizures 5 days after birth. (*A*) T2-W image. (*B*) T1-W image. (*C*) DWI. On both the T2-W and T1-W images, the occipital cortex of both hemispheres shows increased and decreased signal intensity, which may be confused with subcortical white matter (*arrows*). On the DWI, a clear diffusion restriction is demonstrated. (*Adapted from* Triulzi F, Parazzini C, Righini A. Patterns of damage in the mature neonatal brain. Pediatr Radiol 2006;36(7):608–20; with permission.)

impairment. MRI brain imaging can delineate the extent of brain injury and help prognosticate the long-term outcome of these infants. Transient neonatal hypoglycemia in some full-term infants is reported to be associated with patchy hyperechogenic white matter abnormalities in the frontal and parieto–occipital lobes on cranial ultrasound and cerebral MRI [42,51], the functional significance of which needs to be ascertained. Pathological studies document superficial cerebral cortex, dentate gyrus, hippocampus, and caudate nucleus being most affected [51]. Clinical relevance of these findings, however, is not defined by long-term neurodevelopmental examinations in these full-term infants. Similar studies are nonexistent in late preterm infants, providing a fertile ground for future investigations.

Interventions targeted at hypoglycemia

There are no definitive clinical or laboratory indicators of injury specific to glucose deficiency. Therefore, clinicians must maintain a high index of suspicion to the risk of hypoglycemia in late preterm infants and have a low threshold for investigating and diagnosing hypoglycemia, with frequent monitoring of plasma/blood glucose concentration toward maintaining safe glucose concentrations. Additionally, there is no absolute cut-off value or duration of hypoglycemia that dictates neurological injury. Further, when low blood glucose values are detected, the exact duration of the detected low value cannot be surmised with accuracy unless a normal value was obtained previously at a given time. During the period of transition, late preterm and term infants are treated for blood glucose values less than 45 mg/dL or in the presence of symptoms. Hypoglycemia therapy includes:

- Early feeds-formula
- Glucose infusion (200 mg/kg bolus plus 6 to 8 mg/kg/min)
- Hydrocortisone (intravenous dose: 1–5 mg/kg/day divided every 12–24 hours; not recommended for hyperinsulinemia)
- Glucagon (300 μg/kg, maximum dose 1 mg)
- Epinephrine (0.1 to 1 μg/kg/min)
- Diazoxide (5 to 15 mg/kg/d in two to three doses)
- Octreotide (IV 1–10 μg/kg/d in one to two doses, can be increased gradually to a maximum of 40 μg/kg/d divided in 3 to 6 doses.)

Early feeds are the best intervention; however, in infants being breast fed, the establishment of adequate milk let down and ingestion may take 1–2 days. In these cases, introduction of formula may create some controversy with respect to the success in subsequently establishing breast feeding. This has led to introduction of oral glucose solution (10 to 20 mL/kg) in late preterm and term infants. The risk of rebound hypoglycemia, however, is a possibility and needs close monitoring. Intravenous therapy should be initiated if this intervention does not succeed. This should consist of 200 mg/kg of dextrose bolus followed by a rate of 6 to 8 mg/kg/min dextrose [69,70]. Poor feeding in the presence of low glucose may constitute a symptom leading to introduction of intravenous fluids sooner. Treatment also includes treating the underlying conditions and providing a neutral thermal environment. Glucose levels are monitored every 20 to 30 minutes until stable. The bolus may be repeated if hypoglycemia persists, followed by increasing glucose delivery by 2 mg/kg/min to a maximum of 12 to 15 mg/kg/min. Blood sugar monitoring is continued for the first 24 to 48 hours or until stabilized, especially when any of the risk factors for hypoglycemia are present. Once the glucose level is stabilized, the intravenous infusion should be withdrawn, monitoring blood glucose concentration closely. Hypoglycemia secondary to maternal conditions usually resolves within 48 to 72 hours. Most infants with neonatal conditions that increase the risk for persistent hypoglycemia are symptomatic of the primary disorder. Thus, if the blood glucose fails to respond to adequate intravenous glucose delivery, other causes of persistent hypoglycemia must be entertained and the treatment tailored accordingly.

Prevention of neurological impairment

In late preterm infants with limited ketogenic capability, there is evidence that prolonged hypoglycemia is associated with neurological impairment. Although the entire health care system is not geared toward managing these infants as a separate category from term infants in the well baby nursery and the infants in NICUs, it is imperative that a separate structure be provided to support adequate monitoring and intervention in these infants toward preventing irreversible neurological sequelae. Early discharge of the late preterm infants can result in rehospitalizations and increased morbidity. The associated risk of permanent brain damage leaves the physician vulnerable to litigation.

Future investigations

The recent awareness of the increasing trend in late preterm births and the poor transition faced by these infants should galvanize increasing investigations targeted at their outcomes. In particular, most of the investigations related to hypoglycemia undertaken so far have involved all infants with mixed diagnosis. Some have been retrospective with inadequate controls, or have involved small numbers with inadequate power to test the stated hypothesis. Given the advances in brain imaging and the development of noninvasive glucose monitoring devices, the time is ripe to conduct a well-controlled, adequately powered prospective study on late preterm infants who present with hypoglycemia during transition and follow them closely along with adequate brain imaging techniques and a battery of neurological and developmental testing to determine the long-term outcome of this subpopulation of infants. Timely interventions targeted toward amelioration of neonatal hypoglycemia need to be considered in the study design and analysis. Subsequent investigations targeted at preventing or reversing hypoglycemia-induced brain injury can be contemplated. Until then, anticipation preempting prompt diagnosis and timely intervention are the only ways to prevent adverse long-term neurological outcomes in late preterm infants who are discharged home, sometimes before they have established adequate milk intake during breast feeding.

References

[1] Davidoff MJ, Dias T, Damus K, et al. Changes in the gestational age distribution among US singleton births: impact on rates of late preterm birth, 1992 to 2002. Semin Perinatol 2006; 30(1):8–15.

[2] Engle WA. A recommendation for the definition of late preterm (near-term) and the birth weight–gestational age classification system. Semin Perinatol 2006;30(1):2–7.

[3] Raju TN, Higgins RD, Stark AR, et al. Optimizing care and outcome for late-preterm (near-term) infants: a summary of the workshop sponsored by the National Institute of Child Health and Human Development. Pediatrics 2006;118(3):1207–14.

[4] Wang ML, Dorer DJ, Fleming MP, et al. Clinical outcomes of near-term infants. Pediatrics 2004;114(2):372–6.

[5] Hawdon JM, Ward Platt MP, Aynsley-Green A. Patterns of metabolic adaptation for preterm and term infants in the first neonatal week. Arch Dis Child 1992;67:357–65.

[6] Cornblath M, Ichord R. Hypoglycemia in the neonate. Semin Perinatol 2000;24(2):136–49.

[7] Vannucci RC, Vannucci SJ. Hypoglycemic brain injury. Semin Neonatol 2001;6(2):147–55.

[8] Cornblath M, Hawdon JM, Williams AF, et al. Controversies regarding definition of neonatal hypoglycemia: suggested operational thresholds. Pediatrics 2000;105(5):1141–5.

[9] Rozance PJ, Hay WW. Hypoglycemia in newborn infants: features associated with adverse outcomes. Biol Neonate 2006;90(2):74–86.

[10] Barkovich AJ, Ali FA, Rowley HA, et al. Imaging patterns of neonatal hypoglycemia. AJNR Am J Neuroradiol 1998;19(3):523–8.

[11] Halamek LP, Benaron DA, Stevenson DK. Neonatal hypoglycemia, part I: background and definition. Clin Pediatr (Phila) 1997;36(12):675–80.

[12] Halamek LP, Benaron DA, Stevenson DK. The value of neurophysiologic approaches in the anticipation and evaluation of neonatal hypoglycemia. Acta Paediatr Jpn 1997;39(Suppl 1): S33–43.

[13] Zamudio S, Baumann MU, Illsley NP. Effects of chronic hypoxia in vivo on the expression of human placental glucose transporters. Placenta 2006;27(1):49–55.

[14] Ward Platt M, Deshpande S. Metabolic adaptation at birth. Semin Fetal Neonatal Med 2005;10(4):341–50.

[15] Mehandru PL, Assel BG, Nuamah IF, et al. Catecholamine response at birth in preterm newborns. Biol Neonate 1993;64(2–3):82–8.

[16] Hughes SJ. The role of reduced glucose transporter content and glucose metabolism in the immature secretory responses of fetal rat pancreatic islets. Diabetologia 1994;37(2):134–40.

[17] Halamek LP, Stevenson DK. Neonatal hypoglycemia, part II: pathophysiology and therapy. Clin Pediatr (Phila) 1998;37(1):11–6.

[18] Greisen G, Pryds O. Neonatal hypoglycaemia. Lancet 1989;1(8650):1332–3.

[19] Bier DM, Leake RD, Haymond MW, et al. Measurement of true glucose production rates in infancy and childhood with 6,6-dideuteroglucose. Diabetes 1977;26(11):1016–23.

[20] Hawdon JM. Neonatal metabolic adaptation after preterm delivery or intrauterine growth retardation. Biochem Soc Trans 1998;26(2):123–5.

[21] Hume R, Burchell A. Abnormal expression of glucose-6-phosphatase in preterm infants. Arch Dis Child 1993;68(2):202–4.

[22] van Kempen AA, Romijn JA, Ruiter AF, et al. Alanine administration does not stimulate gluconeogenesis in preterm infants. Metabolism 2003;52(8):945–9.

[23] Koh TH, Aynsley-Green A, Tarbit M, et al. Neural dysfunction during hypoglycaemia. Arch Dis Child 1988;63(11):1353–8.

[24] Koh TH, Eyre JA, Aynsley-Green A. Neonatal hypoglycaemia—the controversy regarding definition. Arch Dis Child 1988;63(11):1386–8.

[25] Oliveira AJ, Nunes ML, Haertel LM, et al. Duration of rhythmic EEG patterns in neonates: new evidence for clinical and prognostic significance of brief rhythmic discharges. Clin Neurophysiol 2000;111(9):1646–53.

[26] Nunes ML, Penela MM, da Costa JC. Differences in the dynamics of frontal sharp transients in normal and hypoglycemic newborns. Clin Neurophysiol 2000;111(2):305–10.

[27] Duvanel CB, Fawer CL, Cotting J, et al. Long-term effects of neonatal hypoglycemia on brain growth and psychomotor development in small-for-gestational-age preterm infants. J Pediatr 1999;134(4):492–8.

[28] Alkalay AL, Sarnat HB, Flores-Sarnat L, et al. Population meta-analysis of low plasma glucose thresholds in full-term normal newborns. Am J Perinatol 2006;23(2):115–9.

[29] Brand PL, Molenaar NL, Kaaijk C, et al. Neurodevelopmental outcome of hypoglycaemia in healthy, large for gestational age, term newborns. Arch Dis Child 2005;90(1): 78–81.

[30] Hawdon JM. Hypoglycaemia and the neonatal brain. Eur J Pediatr 1999;158(Suppl 1):S9–12.

[31] Beardsall K, Ogilvy-Stuart AL, Ahluwalia J, et al. The continuous glucose monitoring sensor in neonatal intensive care. Arch Dis Child Fetal Neonatal Ed 2005;90(4):F307–10.

[32] King JC. Maternal obesity, metabolism, and pregnancy outcomes. Annu Rev Nutr 2006;26: 271–91.

[33] Heiskanen N, Raatikainen K, Heinonen S. Fetal macrosomia—a continuing obstetric challenge. Biol Neonate 2006;90(2):98–103.

[34] Menni F, de Lonlay P, Sevin C, et al. Neurologic outcomes of 90 neonates and infants with persistent hyperinsulinemic hypoglycemia. Pediatrics 2001;107(3):476–9.

[35] Ismail D, Werther G. Persistent hyperinsulinaemic hypoglycaemia of infancy: 15 years' experience at the Royal Children's Hospital (RCH), Melbourne. J Pediatr Endocrinol Metab 2005;18(11):1103–9.

[36] Hussain K, Aynsley-Green A. Hyperinsulinism in infancy: understanding the pathophysiology. Int J Biochem Cell Biol 2003;35(9):1312–7.

[37] de Deungria M, Rao R, Wobken JD, et al. Perinatal iron deficiency decreases cytochrome c oxidase (CytOx) activity in selected regions of neonatal rat brain. Pediatr Res 2000;48(2): 169–76.

[38] Petry CD, Eaton MA, Wobken JD, et al. Iron deficiency of liver, heart, and brain in newborn infants of diabetic mothers. J Pediatr 1992;121(1):109–14.

[39] Fung C, Devaskar SU. Nutrient regulation in brain development: glucose and alternate fuels. In: Thureen P, Hay W Jr, editors. Neonatal nutrition and metabolism. 2nd edition. New York: Cambridge University Press; 2006. p. 91–103.

[40] Tsacopoulos M, Magistretti PJ. Metabolic coupling between glia and neurons. J Neurosci 1996;16(3):877–85.

[41] Pellerin L, Magistretti PJ. Glutamate uptake into astrocytes stimulates aerobic glycolysis: a mechanism coupling neuronal activity to glucose utilization. Proc Natl Acad Sci U S A 1994;91(22):10625–9.

[42] Filan PM, Inder TE, Cameron FJ, et al. Neonatal hypoglycemia and occipital cerebral injury. J Pediatr 2006;148(4):552–5.

[43] Alkalay AL, Flores-Sarnat L, Sarnat HB, et al. Brain imaging findings in neonatal hypoglycemia: case report and review of 23 cases. Clin Pediatr (Phila) 2005;44(9):783–90.

[44] Chugani HT. A critical period of brain development: studies of cerebral glucose utilization with PET. Prev Med 1998;27(2):184–8.

[45] Skov L, Pryds O. Capillary recruitment for preservation of cerebral glucose influx in hypoglycemic, preterm newborns: evidence for a glucose sensor? Pediatrics 1992;90:193–5.

[46] Ogata ES. Carbohydrate metabolism in the fetus and neonate and altered neonatal glucoregulation. Pediatr Clin North Am 1986;33(1):25–45.

[47] Kraus H, Schlenker S, Schwedesky D. Developmental changes of cerebral ketone body utilization in human infants. Hoppe Seylers Z Physiol Chem 1974;355(2):164–70.

[48] Salhab WA, Wyckoff MH, Laptook AR, et al. Initial hypoglycemia and neonatal brain injury in term infants with severe fetal acidemia. Pediatrics 2004;114(2):361–6.

[49] Lucas A, Morley R, Cole TJ. Adverse neurodevelopmental outcome of moderate neonatal hypoglycaemia. BMJ 1988;297(6659):1304–8.

[50] Caraballo RH, Sakr D, Mozzi M, et al. Symptomatic occipital lobe epilepsy following neonatal hypoglycemia. Pediatr Neurol 2004;31(1):24–9.

[51] Kinnala A, Rikalainen H, Lapinleimu H, et al. Cerebral magnetic resonance imaging and ultrasonography findings after neonatal hypoglycemia. Pediatrics 1999;103:724–9.

[52] Stenninger E, Flink R, Eriksson B, et al. Long-term neurological dysfunction and neonatal hypoglycaemia after diabetic pregnancy. Arch Dis Child Fetal Neonatal Ed 1998;79(3):F174–9.

[53] Petroff OA, Young RS, Cowan BE, et al. 1H nuclear magnetic resonance spectroscopy study of neonatal hypoglycemia. Pediatr Neurol 1988;4(1):31–4.

[54] Agardh CD, Kalimo H, Olsson Y, et al. Hypoglycemic brain injury: metabolic and structural findings in rat cerebellar cortex during profound insulin-induced hypoglycemia and in the recovery period following glucose administration. J Cereb Blood Flow Metab 1981;1(1): 71–84.

[55] Cavaliere F, Dinkel K, Reymann K. The subventricular zone releases factors which can be protective in oxygen/glucose deprivation-induced cortical damage: an organotypic study. Exp Neurol 2006;201(1):66–74.

[56] Takahashi T, Shirane R, Sato S, et al. Developmental changes of cerebral blood flow and oxygen metabolism in children. AJNR Am J Neuroradiol 1999;20(5):917–22.

[57] Pryds O, Christensen NJ, Friis-Hansen B. Increased cerebral blood flow and plasma epinephrine in hypoglycemic, preterm neonates. Pediatrics 1990;85(2):172–6.

[58] Quintana P, Alberi S, Hakkoum D, et al. Glutamate receptor changes associated with transient anoxia/hypoglycaemia in hippocampal slice cultures. Eur J Neurosci 2006;23(4): 975–83.

[59] McGowan JE, Chen L, Gao D, et al. Increased mitochondrial reactive oxygen species production in newborn brain during hypoglycemia. Neurosci Lett 2006;399(1–2):111–4.

[60] Kim M, Yu ZX, Fredholm BB, et al. Susceptibility of the developing brain to acute hypoglycemia involving A1 adenosine receptor activation. Am J Physiol Endocrinol Metab 2005; 289(4):E562–9.

[61] Ciruela F, Casado V, Rodrigues RJ, et al. Presynaptic control of striatal glutamatergic neurotransmission by adenosine A1–A2A receptor heteromers. J Neurosci 2006;26(7):2080–7.

[62] Ruscher K, Isaev N, Trendelenburg G, et al. Induction of hypoxia inducible factor 1 by oxygen glucose deprivation is attenuated by hypoxic preconditioning in rat cultured neurons. Neurosci Lett 1998;254(2):117–20.

[63] Aynsley-Green A, Hawdon JM, Deshpande S, et al. Neonatal insulin secretion: implications for the programming of metabolic homeostasis. Acta Paediatr Jpn 1997;39(Suppl 1):S21–5.

[64] McGowan JE, Zanelli SA, Haynes-Laing AG, et al. Modification of glutamate binding sites in newborn brain during hypoglycemia. Brain Res 2002;927(1):80–6.

[65] Auer RN, Siesjo BK. Hypoglycaemia: brain neurochemistry and neuropathology. Baillieres Clin Endocrinol Metab 1993;7(3):611–25.

[66] Barkovich AJ. MR and CT evaluation of profound neonatal and infantile asphyxia. AJNR Am J Neuroradiol 1992;13(3):959–72 [discussion 973–955].

[67] Miller SP, Ramaswamy V, Michelson D, et al. Patterns of brain injury in term neonatal encephalopathy. J Pediatr 2005;146(4):453–60.

[68] Triulzi F, Parazzini C, Righini A. Patterns of damage in the mature neonatal brain. Pediatr Radiol 2006;(May):18.

[69] Lilien LD, Pildes RS, Srinivasan G, et al. Treatment of neonatal hypoglycemia with minibolus and intravenous glucose infusion. J Pediatr 1980;97(2):295–8.

[70] Hawdon JM, Ward Platt MP, Aynsley-Green A. Prevention and management of neonatal hypoglycaemia. Arch Dis Child Fetal Neonatal Ed 1994;70(1):F60–4 [discussion F65].

ELSEVIER
SAUNDERS

CLINICS IN
PERINATOLOGY

Clin Perinatol 33 (2006) 871–882

Infection in Late Preterm Infants

Daniel K. Benjamin Jr, MD, PhD, MPH[a,*], Barbara J. Stoll, MD[b,c]

[a]*Department of Pediatrics, Duke Clinical Research Institute, Duke University, P.O. Box 17969, Durham, NC 27705, USA*
[b]*Department of Pediatrics, Emory University, Atlanta, GA, USA*
[c]*Children's Healthcare of Atlanta, Atlanta, GA, USA*

Late preterm neonates have unique susceptibilities to infection. The closed setting of the neonatal ICU (NICU) and the immunologic immaturity of premature infants set the stage for the development of nosocomial infections. Timing of presentation is one of the crucial factors in determining the cause, evaluation, and appropriate early treatment of neonatal infections. Timing of presentation can be divided broadly into three categories:

- Congenital infections: generally acquired before delivery
- Early onset: usually acquired during delivery and presenting within the first 72 hours of life
- Late onset: often acquired in the hospital and presenting after 72 hours of life

The overall neonatal mortality rate is low for late preterm infants. The tragedy of neonatal infections among these infants is that infection increases risk of neonatal complications, prolongs hospital stay, and increases mortality.

Epidemiology

Congenital and perinatal infections

These infections are acquired before delivery or during the intrapartum period. They result most commonly from *Toxoplasma gondii*, rubella virus, cytomegalovirus, herpes virus, HIV, parvovirus B19 and *Treponema*

Dr. Benjamin received support from NICHD HD-044799-01.

* Corresponding author.

E-mail address: danny.benjamin@duke.edu (D.K. Benjamin Jr).

0095-5108/06/$ - see front matter © 2006 Elsevier Inc. All rights reserved.
doi:10.1016/j.clp.2006.09.005

pallidum. Risk of transmission varies depending on trimester of pregnancy during which maternal infection occurs. *Toxoplasma* transmission rates range from less than 5% during the first trimester to approximately 60% in the third trimester [1]. Severity of the infection also depends on the stage of pregnancy at which the maternal infection occurred. Congenital toxoplasmosis and rubella acquired during the first trimester often result in stillbirth or severe anomalies. Transmission of cytomegalovirus is dependent on whether the maternal infection is a primary infection or a recurrence. Nearly 40% of neonates born to mothers experiencing a primary cytomegalovirus infection during the pregnancy are affected, while only 1% of neonates are affected in pregnancies with recurrent cytomegalovirus infections [2]. Although both HIV and human herpes virus infections can occur in utero during pregnancy, these infections most often are acquired intrapartum; thus timing of rupture of membranes and modes of delivery influence risk. Similar to cytomegalovirus, maternal–infant transmission of herpes is more frequent if a mother has a primary infection with herpes at the time of delivery. Risk of HIV transmission is influenced by maternal viral load.

Early-onset sepsis

This almost always is caused by perinatally acquired infections. The neonate initially is colonized by exposure to various organisms present in the maternal genital tract, including nonpathogenic organisms such as *Lactobacillus*, *Peptostreptococcus*, and *Saccharomyces*. The neonate, however, also is exposed to potential pathogens such as group B *Streptococcus* (GBS), *Escherichia coli*, and *Candida*. Risk factors for development of sepsis such as preterm delivery, prolonged rupture of membranes (greater than 18 hours), maternal fever, and chorioamnionitis often are present in neonates developing early-onset sepsis [3]. Although GBS remains the most common cause of early-onset sepsis, the widespread use of intrapartum prophylaxis in women with known GBS colonization or with risk factors for disease has decreased the incidence of this organism as a cause of early-onset disease. Rates have declined by 70% [4]. In very low birth weight infants, some studies have suggested an increase in early-onset sepsis caused by gram-negative organisms that parallels the decline in early-onset GBS disease [5]. It is unclear whether there has been a shift in pathogen distribution among late preterm infants.

Late-onset sepsis

Late-onset sepsis may be caused by perinatally or postnatally acquired organisms, but it usually is a consequence of nosocomial transmission. Pathogens associated with late-onset infections in the late preterm infant include, *Staphylococcus aureus*, *Candida* species, or gram-negative rods [6,7]. GBS remains an important pathogen, because intrapartum prophylaxis has shown little effect on the rates of late-onset disease [3].

The organisms responsible for late-onset sepsis present a challenging management approach. Treatment is complicated because of the rapid emergence of antimicrobial resistance. Methicillin-resistant strains of *S aureus* are common isolates. *Enterococcus faecalis* and *Enterococcus faecium* are important causes of invasive infection because of the potential for vancomycin resistance [8,9].

Most studies of the epidemiology of late-onset sepsis have been conducted among hospitalized very low birth weight infants. There are limited recent multi-center data for the late preterm infant. But data from the very low birth weight population suggest that gram-negative bacilli are important causes of neonatal hospital-acquired infections. The dominant gram-negative pathogens differ among hospitals, and their importance in a given NICU varies over time. The most commonly isolated gram negative rod (GNR) organisms, in approximately equal distribution [10,11], are *E coli, Klebsiella, Enterobacter, Serratia,* and *Pseudomonas.* Because many pathogens are resistant to commonly employed antimicrobial agents, the importance of recognizing the occurrence and antimicrobial susceptibility pattern of strains indigenous in a given nursery setting cannot be overemphasized. Routine use of third-generation cephalosporin agents as empirical therapy should be avoided, because their use promotes expression of chromosomal β-lactamases associated with resistance of *Enterobacter.* Additionally, their use has led to outbreaks of extended spectrum β-lactamase producing organisms [12]. *Candida* species are important causes of disseminated infection in the very low birth weight infant, and they may occur in the late preterm infant who has other risk factors, such as recent surgery or otherwise complicated inpatient clinical course. Extended use of broad-spectrum antibiotics, day of life (less than 30 days), and birth weight are the key factors enhancing the risk for invasive candidiasis [13–15]. *Candida albicans* and *Candida parapsilosis* are the most common species isolated from the infected neonate.

Community-acquired viruses, such as respiratory syncytial virus, influenza virus, parainfluenza virus, rotavirus, and varicella virus, can be transmitted nosocomially, especially in neonates not afforded the protection of maternally derived protective antibodies.

Clinical presentation

Congenital and perinatal infections

Although caused by various organisms, congenital and perinatal infections may present with similar clinical findings. Infections that are acquired before delivery (eg, cytomegalovirus, rubella, toxoplasmosis, and syphilis) often present with a combination of findings including intrauterine growth restriction, jaundice, rash, intracranial calcifications, microcephaly, chorioretinitis, and thrombocytopenia. Hepatosplenomegaly, although a nonspecific finding, should encourage thorough evaluation for congenital infection in the newborn. Many of the sequelae of congenitally acquired infections are present at birth; others (hearing loss, visual impairment/blindness, and developmental delay) may not manifest for months or years.

Early-onset sepsis

This is often nonfocal and fulminant in onset in contrast to late-onset disease, which may present focally as meningitis, urinary tract infections, septic arthritis, or pneumonia. Over 90% of neonates with early-onset sepsis present in the first 24 hours. Signs of perinatally and nosocomially acquired sepsis are often nonspecific and subtle, but sepsis is uncommon in the asymptomatic neonate [16,17]. Signs of neonatal sepsis include: temperature instability, lethargy, irritability, apnea, respiratory distress, hypotension, bradycardia, tachycardia, cyanosis, abdominal distension, hyperglycemia, jaundice, and feeding intolerance [18]. These signs overlap with a myriad of other disease processes presenting in the neonatal period, including: anemia, intestinal obstruction, congenital heart disease, respiratory distress syndrome, and metabolic disorders.

Late onset infection

Late-onset infection presents more frequently with signs of focal infection than early-onset disease; however, nonfocal and fulminant presentations remain common. Key risk factors for late-onset sepsis include increased risk with younger postconception age and prolonged NICU stay. Other risk factors include central vascular access, invasive procedures, and use of broad-spectrum antibiotics such as third-generation cephalosporins.

Laboratory evaluation

Congenital infections

High pretest probability for congenital infections may be achieved through clinical presentation and a review of the maternal history; history and physical examination often provide guidance as to which laboratory tests should be obtained. Diagnostic methods for congenital infections have advanced substantively in the polymerase chain reaction (PCR) era [19–23]. HIV should be diagnosed by means of DNA PCR. Herpes virus can be diagnosed by DNA PCR of cerebrospinal fluid (CSF) or culture of skin lesions, mouth, nasopharynx, and eyes. Varicella can be diagnosed by IgM antibody or DNA PCR. Likewise, parvovirus B19 can be diagnosed by IgM antibody or DNA PCR. Cytomegalovirus can be diagnosed by shell vial assay, culture of virus from urine, or DNA PCR, and *Toxoplasma* can be diagnosed by IgM or IgA antibody, blood or urine culture, or DNA PCR. Treponema diagnosis and early empirical or presumptive therapy for neonatal syphilis are based on guidelines that have been outlined by the American Academy of Pediatrics [24].

Early- and late-onset infections

Screening tests, including white blood cell counts and acute phase reactants, such a C-reactive protein (CRP), have poor positive predictive values in septic neonates: 40% in symptomatic neonates and as low as 1% to 2% in asymptomatic neonates at risk for GBS [16,25]. The development of effective screening tests continues to be an unmet medical need in neonatal infections.

For bacterial and fungal infections, culture of normally sterile body fluids remains the standard for diagnosis; however the performance of the blood culture is extremely variable. There is no consensus as to the recommended number of blood cultures or volume of blood to culture. Obtaining blood cultures from multiple sites, however, increases the ability to distinguish between cultures contaminated with skin flora and those representing true infection [27]. Although a blood culture inoculum of 0.5 mL is used commonly in preterm infants and is thought to have good sensitivity in neonates for bacteria, some studies have shown that 0.5 mL of blood may not detect low-level bacteremia [28,29]. The performance of the blood culture likely is compromised further by maternal intrapartum antibiotic administration or empirical antibiotics administered to the neonate. Positive blood cultures for pathogenic bacteria are evident by 48 hours of incubation in most cases [26]; however, blood cultures are often negative for *Candida*.

The incidence of bacterial meningitis is higher in the first month of life than at any other time and complicates up to one third of the cases of bacterial sepsis in this population [30]. Diagnosis of meningitis and identification of the offending organisms requires examination of CSF. Unless neurologic signs are present at the time of the sepsis evaluation, clinicians often defer the lumbar puncture until the blood cultures are positive for a pathogenic organism or the neonate is more stable [31]. Studies of otherwise asymptomatic neonates with respiratory distress syndrome found evidence of meningitis in less than 1% of cases on admission to the NICU [31]. Blood cultures, however, were noted to be negative in 28% (12/43) of neonates with culture-proven bacterial meningitis diagnosed in the first 72 hours of life in a series of nearly 170,000 neonates [32]. Investigators of the National Institute of Child Health and Human Development (NICHD)-sponsored Neonatal Research Network found that blood cultures were negative in 34% (45/134) of very low birth weight neonates with culture-proven meningitis [33]. Frequent blood culture-CSF culture discordance also was reported by investigators from the Pediatrix Group and Duke University [7]. The culture discordance observed in the Pediatrix dataset was supported by CSF parameters (white cell, red cell, protein, and glucose) and included late preterm neonates.

The similar findings from different nurseries, reported by different investigators across time, lend strength to the advice that clinicians should include the lumbar puncture as part of the neonatal sepsis evaluation provided that the infant is sufficiently stable to tolerate the procedure.

Urine cultures should be obtained as part of the sepsis evaluation in neonates after day of life 3, but they are of low yield before this point [34]. Urine cultures should be obtained by suprapubic tap or catheterization. Bag specimens are difficult to evaluate because of contamination and may lead to unnecessary antibiotic administration and radiological studies.

Antimicrobial therapy

Therapy may be considered broadly as definitive, presumptive, empirical, and prophylaxis. Definitive treatment is the administration of antimicrobial agents for documented disease (eg, administration of ampicillin and gentamicin for 10 days because GBS has been isolated from the blood). Presumptive therapy is administered when the clinician strongly suspects disease, but the documentation is incomplete. For example, an infant has a positive blood culture for GBS; due to clinical instability, a lumbar puncture is deferred initially. After the blood culture results are known, the lumbar puncture is obtained and reveals 330 white blood cells, 0 red cells, protein 120, and glucose 20, but the CSF culture is negative. Even though the CSF culture is negative, the infant is presumed to have meningitis caused by GBS because of the extremely high likelihood of disease as documented by the CSF white cell count. Empirical therapy is given when disease is suspected for brief preselected time frame (eg, 48 hours) while culture results are pending. Prophylaxis is given to a group of patients who are at risk of acquiring disease independent of culture results.

Note that as clinical management moves from definitive to presumptive to empirical therapy to prophylaxis, the proportion of infants with disease decreases. Thus, the number of infants without disease who are exposed to the antimicrobial agent increases. As clinical management moves from definitive therapy to prophylaxis, the proportion of infants who potentially benefit from therapy drops, and the proportion of infants who are potentially harmed by needless therapy rises. In the settings of empirical therapy and prophylaxis, because so many more infants potentially are harmed by therapy and so few will receive benefit, the conduct of prospective multicenter trials that document the safety, long-term outcomes, and rare adverse events is crucial to public health.

Empirical therapy and definitive treatment

Congenital infections

If congenital nonbacterial infection is suspected, it is often prudent to seek the advice of infectious disease specialists. Treatment for possible exposure to several agents (HIV, herpes virus, toxoplasmosis, and *Treponema pallidum)* often is indicated. Transmission of HIV has been reduced from almost a third to less than 2% through a series of interventions including maternal antenatal and intrapartum and neonatal antiretroviral therapy and delivery by cesarean section. Recent cohort data have emerged regarding the safety of long-term treatment of toxoplasmosis with pyrimethamine and sulfadiazine [41]. Close follow-up is essential for infants with possible intrapartum exposure to ensure proper management (eg, parental acyclovir is given to all infants with suspected herpes virus infections). Active neonatal syphilis can occur in newborns who are asymptomatic at birth and in those with multi-organ involvement. Thus, no infant should be discharged from the hospital without confirmation of evaluation of mother's serologic status for syphilis. Infants born to seropositive mothers need further evaluation and close follow-up.

Early- and late-onset infections

For newborns with suspected bacterial infections, ampicillin and an aminoglycoside are considered standard empirical therapy. Ampicillin provides coverage for gram-positive infections (GBS). Gentamicin provides gram-negative coverage (*E coli* and other *Enterobactericeae*) and also provides synergy with ampicillin against GBS. Cefotaxime, a third-generation cephalosporin with superior CSF penetration compared with gentamicin, may be considered in cases of documented gram-negative meningitis. Vancomycin, or nafcillin, sometimes is substituted for ampicillin for suspected nosocomial infections [35]. Duration of antibiotic therapy is generally 10 days for confirmed bacteremia, 14 days for meningitis caused by gram-positive organisms, and 21 days for gram-negative meningitis.

Empirical therapy for *Candida* can be considered in symptomatic late preterm neonates who have risk factors for fungal infections (thrombocytopenia, history of invasive surgical procedures, or exposure to broad-spectrum antibiotics). The safety and efficacy of this approach are unproven, however, and treatment should not be employed casually. Amphotericin B deoxycholate has a wide spectrum of activity, and it generally is tolerated well in neonates compared with adults; it should therefore be considered first line treatment of *Candida* infections in this population. Fluconazole is an alternative drug when treating an isolate known to be sensitive.

Isolation of *Candida* from the bloodstream warrants prompt removal or replacement of central vascular catheters. Removal has been defined as taking out the catheter at the time of positive blood culture and use of no vascular access or peripheral vascular access. Replacement has been defined as removal of the catheter that is in situ at the time of the acquisition of positive blood culture and placement of a new catheter at a different anatomic location [36,37]. Prompt replacement or removal following candidemia has been associated with more rapid clearance of organism, improved survival, and improved neurodevelopmental outcomes. Prompt removal or replacement following bacteremia with *S aureus*, *Enterococcus*, and gram-negative organisms is probably ideal, but the data are not as consistent as those with candidiasis [37,38]. Following one positive culture, blood cultures should be performed daily to ensure sterility. Persistent bacteremia is an indication for catheter removal or replacement and suggests the possibility of accompanying infection in an intravascular thrombus or endocarditis.

Prevention

Congenital infections

Prevention of HIV infection in the exposed neonate has been a remarkable achievement. The neonatologist can help to ensure prevention of maternal–infant transmission by advocating for routine testing of pregnant women and follow-up of infected pregnant women, timely and appropriate therapy with antiretroviral drugs, collaboration with obstetrical and infectious disease colleagues for mothers in labor and infants in the peripartum period, and follow-up for the infant after discharge from the nursery. Syphilis can be prevented with thorough screening by means of antibody testing of the mother, documentation of administration of three doses of penicillin to the infected mother, and documentation of a fourfold decrease in maternal antibodies.

Early-onset infections

Early infection caused by GBS has been reduced with the use of intrapartum chemoprophylaxis. Using a strategy of universal prenatal cultures [24] at 35 to 37 weeks, intrapartum antimicrobial prophylaxis is indicated if:

- If the mother has had a previous infant with invasive GBS disease
- If GBS bacteriuria is present in the current pregnancy
- If there is a positive GBS screening culture during the current pregnancy (unless a planned cesarean delivery is performed in the absence of labor or membrane rupture),
- If GBS status is unknown and any if any of the following are present: delivery at less than 37 weeks' gestation, membranes have been ruptured for at least 18 hours, intrapartum fever

Intravenous penicillin G to the mother is the drug of choice for GBS prophylaxis because of efficacy and narrow spectrum of activity. Alternatively, intravenous ampicillin may be provided. Detailed algorithms for the management of infants at risk of GBS infection are presented in Fig. 1.

Late-onset

Hand hygiene remains a key component of infection control in the nursery. So too are adequate staffing, avoiding overcrowding, nursery design,

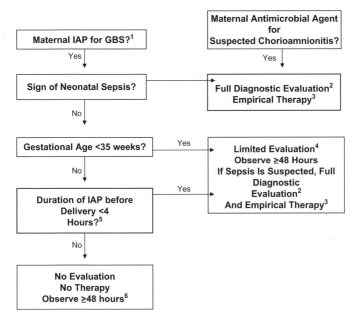

Fig. 1. Empirical therapy following intrapartum antimicrobial prophylaxis (IAP) for Prevention of Group B streptococcal disease [24].

[1] If no maternal IAP for group B *Streptococcus* was administered despite an indication being present, data are insufficient to recommend a single management strategy.

[2] Includes complete blood cell (CBC) count with differential and blood culture. Check radiograph if respiratory abnormalities are present. When signs of sepsis are present, a lumbar puncture, if feasible, should be preformed.

[3] Duration of therapy varies depending on results of blood culture, cerebrospinal fluid findings (if obtained), and the clinical course of the infant. If laboratory results and clinical course do not indicate bacterial infection, duration may be as short as 48 hours.

[4] CBC including white blood cell count with differential and blood culture.

[5] Applies only to penicillin, ampicillin, or cefazolin and assumes recommended dosing regimens.

[6] A healthy-appearing infant who was at least 38 weeks' gestation at delivery and whose mother received at least 4 hours of IAP before delivery may be discharged home after 24 hours if other discharge criteria have been met and a person able to comply fully with instructions for home observation will be present. If any one of these conditions is not met, the infant should be observed in the hospital for at least 48 hours and until criteria for discharge are achieved.

workload capacity, appropriate staff-to-infant ratios, and catheter management teams [39,40]. Advantages of good infection control practices in the NICU include the avoidance of the pressing need for antimicrobial prophylaxis measures and subsequent medication-associated adverse events, drug dosing errors, and antimicrobial resistance.

Two products have been approved for prevention of severe respiratory syncytial virus disease in children younger than 24 months who have bronchopulmonary dysplasia or a history of premature birth. Of the two,

Palivizumab, a humanized monoclonal antibody that is given intramuscularly, is administered more commonly to at risk infants [24].

Summary

Evaluation of the infant with possible infection should include careful review of the maternal and perinatal history and an assessment of the symptoms of infection exhibited by the neonate. A diagnostic evaluation for congenital infections should be considered in neonates who have intrauterine growth restriction and multi-organ involvement. Evaluation for potential sepsis in neonates should include blood and CSF cultures and urine cultures in neonates older than 72 hours of age. Prompt empirical antibiotic therapy is necessary if bacterial sepsis is suspected, and this should cover the organisms to which the neonate is at highest risk. Good infection control practices remain the standard for prevention of invasive disease.

References

[1] Dunn D, Wallon M, Peyron F, et al. Mother-to-child transmission of toxoplasmosis: risk estimates for clinical counseling. Lancet 1999;353:1829–33.
[2] Raynor BD. Cytomegalovirus infection in pregnancy. Semin Perinatol 1993;17:394–402.
[3] Centers for Disease Control and Prevention. Prevention of perinatal group B streptococcal disease. MMWR Morb Mortal Wkly Rep 2002:1–18.
[4] Centers for Disease Control and Prevention. Prevention of perinatal group B streptococcal disease. Revised guidelines from CDC. MMWR Recomm Rep 2002;52(RR-11):1–22.
[5] Stoll BJ, Hansen N, Fanaroff AA, et al. Changes in pathogens causing early-onset sepsis in very-low-birth-weight infants. N Engl J Med 2002;347:240–7.
[6] Bizzarro MJ, Raskind C, Baltimore RS, et al. Seventy-five years of neonatal sepsis at Yale: 1928–2003. Pediatrics 2005;116:595–602.
[7] Garges HP, Moody MA, Cotten CM, et al. Neonatal meningitis: what is the correlation between cerebrospinal fluid cultures, blood cultures, and CSF parameters? Pediatrics 2006;117:1094–100.
[8] Luginbuhl LM, Rotbart HA, Facklam RR. Neonatal enterococcal sepsis: case–control study and description of an outbreak. Pediatr Infect Dis J 1987;6:1022.
[9] Harvey BS, Baker CJ, Edwards MS. Contributions of complement and immunoglobulin to neutrophil-mediated killing of enterococci. Infect Immun 1992;60:3635.
[10] Benjamin DK Jr, DeLong ER, Cotten MC, et al. Mortality following blood culture in premature infants: increased with gram-negative bacteremia and candidemia, but not gram-positive bacteremia. J Perinatol 2004;24:175–80.
[11] Stoll BJ, Hansen N, Fanaroff AA, et al. Late-onset sepsis in very low birth weight neonates: the experience of the NICHD Neonatal Research Network. Pediatrics 2002;110:285–91.
[12] Sohn AH, Garrett DO, Sinkowitz-Cochran RL, et al. Prevalence of nosocomial infections in neonatal intensive care unit patients: results from the first national point-prevalence survey. J Pediatr 2001;139:821.
[13] Benjamin DK Jr, DeLong ER, Steinbach WJ, et al. Empirical therapy for neonatal candidemia in very low birth weight infants. Pediatrics 2003;112:543–7.
[14] Benjamin DK Jr, Ross K, Benjamin DK, et al. When to suspect fungal infections in neonates: a clinical comparison of Candida albicans and Candida parapsilosis fungemia with coagulase-negative staphylococcal bacteremia. Pediatrics 2000;106:712–8.

[15] Roilides E, Farmaki E, Evdoridou J, et al. Neonatal candidiasis: analysis of epidemiology, drug susceptibility, and molecular typing of causative isolates. Eur J Clin Microbiol Infect Dis 2004;23:745–50.

[16] Ottolini MC, Lundgren K, Mirkinson LJ, et al. Utility of complete blood count and blood culture screening to diagnose neonatal sepsis in the asymptomatic at risk newborn. Pediatr Infect Dis J 2003;22:430–4.

[17] Bonadio WA, Hennes H, Smith D, et al. Reliability of observation variables in distinguishing infectious outcome of febrile young infants. Pediatr Infect Dis J 1993;12:111–4.

[18] Fanaroff AA, Korones SB, Wright LL, et al. Incidence, presenting features, risk factors and significance of late-onset septicemia in very low birth weight infants. The National Institute of Child Health and Human Development Neonatal Research Network. Pediatr Infect Dis J 1998;17:593–8.

[19] Kailasam C, Brennand J, Cameron AD. Congenital parvovirus B19 infection: experience of a recent epidemic. Fetal Diagn Ther 2001;16:18–22.

[20] Kravetz JD, Federman DG. Toxoplasmosis in pregnancy. Am J Med 2005;118:212–6.

[21] Banatvala JE, Brown DW. Rubella. Lancet 2004;363:1127–37.

[22] Best JM. Laboratory diagnosis of intrauterine and perinatal virus infections. Clin Diagn Virol 1996;5:121–9.

[23] Cuthbertson G, Weiner CP, Giller RH, et al. Prenatal diagnosis of second-trimester congenital varicella syndrome by virus-specific immunoglobulin M. J Pediatr 1987;111:592–5.

[24] American Academy of Pediatrics. Red book. Report of the Committee on Infectious Diseases. 27th edition. Elk Grove Village (IL): American Academy of Pediatrics; 2006.

[25] Gerdes JS. Clinicopathologic approach to the diagnosis of neonatal sepsis. Clin Perinatol 1991;18:361–81.

[26] Kurlat I, Stoll BJ, McGowan JE Jr. Time to positivity for detection of bacteremia in neonates. J Clin Microbiol 1989;27:1068–71.

[27] Wiswell TE, Hachey WE. Multiple site blood cultures in the initial evaluation for neonatal sepsis during the first week of life. Pediatr Infect Dis J 1991;10:365–9.

[28] Jawaheer G, Neal TJ, Shaw NJ. Blood culture volume and detection of coagulase negative staphylococcal septicaemia in neonates. Arch Dis Child Fetal Neonatal Ed 1997;76: F57–8.

[29] Schelonka RL, Chai MK, Yoder BA, et al. Volume of blood required to detect common neonatal pathogens. J Pediatr 1996;129:275–8.

[30] Feigin RD, McCracken GH Jr, Klein JO. Diagnosis and management of meningitis. Pediatr Infect Dis J 1992;11:785–814.

[31] Weiss MG, Ionides SP, Anderson CL. Meningitis in premature infants with respiratory distress: role of admission lumbar puncture. J Pediatr 1991;119:973–5.

[32] Wiswell TE, Baumgart S, Gannon CM, et al. No lumbar puncture in the evaluation for early neonatal sepsis: will meningitis be missed? Pediatrics 1995;95:803–6.

[33] Stoll BJ, Hansen N, Fanaroff AA, et al. To tap or not to tap: high likelihood of meningitis without sepsis among very low birth weight infants. Pediatrics 2004;113:1181–6.

[34] Visser VE, Hall RT. Urine culture in the evaluation of suspected neonatal sepsis. J Pediatr 1979;94:635–8.

[35] O'Grady NP, Alexander M, Dellinger EP, et al. Guidelines for the prevention of intravascular catheter-related infections. The Hospital Infection Control Practices Advisory Committee, Centers for Disease Control and Prevention. Pediatrics 2002;110:e51.

[36] Benjamin DK Jr, Miller W, Garges H, et al. Bacteremia, central catheters and neonates: when to pull the line. Pediatrics 2001;107:1272–6.

[37] Benjamin DK Jr, Stoll BJ, Fanaroff AA, et al. Neonatal candidiasis among extremely low birth weight infants: risk factors, mortality, and neurodevelopmental outcomes at 18–22 months. Pediatrics 2006;117:84–92.

[38] Nazemi KJ, Buescher ES, Kelly RE Jr, et al. Central venous catheter removal versus in situ treatment in neonates with Enterobacteriaceae bacteremia. Pediatrics 2003;111:e269–74.

[39] Moisiuk SE, Robson D, Klass L, et al. Outbreak of parainfluenza virus type 3 in an intermediate care neonatal nursery. Pediatr Infect Dis J 1998;17:49.

[40] Harbarth S, Sudre P, Dharan S, et al. Outbreak of *Enterobacter cloacae* related to understaffing, overcrowding, and poor hygiene practices. Infect Control Hosp Epidemiol 1999;20:598.

[41] McLeod R, Boyer K, Karrison T, et al. Outcome of treatment for congenital toxoplasmosis, 1981–2004: the National Collaborative Chicago-Based Congenital Toxoplasmosis Study. Clin Infect Dis 2006;42:1383–94.

ELSEVIER
SAUNDERS

CLINICS IN
PERINATOLOGY

Clin Perinatol 33 (2006) 883–914

The Late Preterm Infant and the Control of Breathing, Sleep, and Brainstem Development: A Review

Robert A. Darnall, MD[a],[*], Ronald L. Ariagno, MD[b],
Hannah C. Kinney, MD[c]

[a]*Department of Physiology, Dartmouth-Hitchcock Medical Center,
1 Medical Center Drive, Lebanon, NH 03756, USA*
[b]*Department of Pediatrics, Division of Neonatal-Perinatal Medicine, Stanford University
School of Medicine, 750 Welch Road, Suite 315, Stanford, CA 94304, USA*
[c]*Department of Pathology, Children's Hospital Boston, 300 Longwood Avenue,
Boston, MA 02115, USA*

Late preterm infants born between 34 and 37 weeks' gestation might appropriately be termed "great imposters" [1] because they often appear to be as old as term infants. Indeed in many hospitals they are treated much like term infants. In reality, however, they are premature and have many problems common to smaller and more immature infants, including increased risk for temperature instability, hypoglycemia, jaundice, respiratory distress, feeding issues, and apnea. Brainstem development and neural control of respiration are less mature than those in a full-term infant. Unfortunately, there is a paucity of clinical, physiologic, neuroanatomic, and neurochemical data in this specific group of infants. What little information we have indicates that the maturation of the brainstem and related rostral brain elements involved in respiratory and state control have variable and nonlinear development profiles with respect to neuronal origin and proliferation, migration pathways, morphologic and neurochemical differentiation, neurotransmitter receptors, transporters, and enzymes, dendritic arborization, spine formation, synaptogenesis, axonal outgrowth, and myelination. Nevertheless, the physiologic maturity of various respiratory reflexes in this late preterm group of infants appears to lie on a continuum that extends from more immature infants to some time beyond term. This article focuses on

---
* Corresponding author.
E-mail address: robert.a.darnall@hitchcock.org (R.A. Darnall).

0095-5108/06/$ - see front matter © 2006 Elsevier Inc. All rights reserved.
doi:10.1016/j.clp.2006.10.004   *perinatology.theclinics.com*

issues related to brainstem development, cardiorespiratory control and apnea, sleep, and their interactions in the late preterm infant.

Brainstem development

This review of human brainstem development provides a neuroanatomic guide to understanding the neurophysiology of respiratory control, sleep, and arousal in the human fetus, as well as addresses the issue of potential critical periods in brainstem development in the late preterm period. Vital functions, however, are not "governed" by the brainstem alone, but rather, involve a complex interplay between the brainstem and structures rostral to it, primarily located in the limbic system [2]. Consequently, brainstem and forebrain development must be considered relative to one another. At 34 gestational weeks, the total brain weight is 65% of that at term [3]. The question arises, what is the timetable of the development of the brainstem relative to the forebrain in the human fetus? While the precise maturational sequences of individual gray matter regions are uncertain, the overall sequential order is defined by the embryonic (and phylogenic) pattern of structural development (ie, with caudal to rostral progression and rhomboencephalic before diencephalic before telencephalic development, and neocortical primary before association area development). These patterns are indicated by regional sequences of myelination [4], with the underlying premise that myelination follows neuronal maturation and is a marker of "completed" neuronal/axonal maturation. Myelination sequences progress in a hierarchical order that putatively determines the neurodevelopment of the fetus (eg, "primitive" brainstem functions developing before "advanced" cortical cognitive functions). Indeed, this caudal-to-rostral pattern mimics that of McLean's "triune brain" in which the brain's functional organization is based upon three structures layered over one another across the evolutionary scale: 1) the early primitive brain (archipallidum), which is comprised of the brainstem and cerebellum and is involved in vital functions (eg, respiration, blood pressure), self-preservation (homeostasis), and movement; 2) the intermediate, limbic brain (palleopallidum), which is involved in hunger, instincts, emotions, fight/flight reactions, memory, sensory input, and sexual behavior; and 3) the evolutionary most "advanced" component, the cerebral cortex (neopallidum), which is involved in reason, perception, and motor control [5].

The brainstem is at its greatest (measurable) weight relative to the forebrain at the end of the first trimester, at which time it accounts for 8.3% of total brain weight compared with 88.6% of the forebrain (and 3.1% cerebellum) (Fig. 1) [6]. The greatest change in relative forebrain-brainstem weights occurs between 12 and 24 gestational weeks, with a decrease of 4.8% in brainstem weight and an increase of 4.5% in forebrain weight (see Fig. 1) [6]. The change over the last part of gestation, spanning the

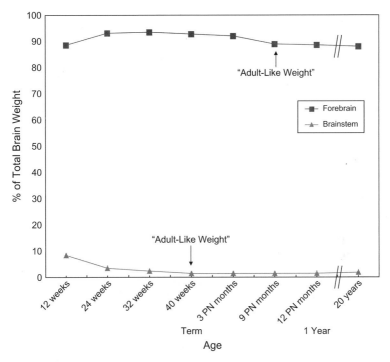

Fig. 1. The greatest change in relative forebrain-brainstem weights occurs between 12 and 24 gestational weeks, with a decrease of 4.8% in brainstem weight and an increase of 4.5% in forebrain weight [6]. The change over the last part of gestation, spanning the late preterm period, however, is small (ie, less than 1% of either structure, with "adult" relative proportions reached by the end of the first postnatal year) [6].

late preterm period, however, is small (ie, less than 1% of either structure, with "adult" relative proportions reached by the end of the first postnatal year) (see Fig. 1) [6]. In parallel to the emergence of forebrain dominance (by weight), the brainstem increases significantly in length and volume, as demonstrated in comparable cross-sections of the human medulla from the end of the first trimester through the first year of postnatal life (infancy) (Fig. 2). Again, the most dramatic changes occur during the first half of gestation, with more incremental changes occurring over the second half of gestation, including the late preterm period (see Fig. 2). Of note, the brainstem is not fully mature even at term, as indicated by the incomplete myelination of the central tegmental tract, comprised of interconnections of the brainstem reticular formation and rostral projections of the ascending arousal systems, and the tract of the nucleus of the solitary tract, comprised of visceral sensory input [4]. This protracted maturation is not surprising, considering the ongoing changes in the neurodevelopment of autonomic and respiratory control and sleep–wake cycling in infants and children (see later discussion).

Mid-Medulla

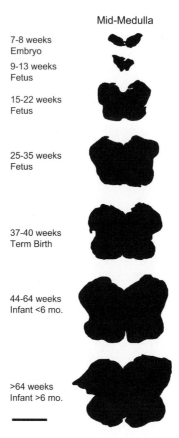

7-8 weeks
Embryo

9-13 weeks
Fetus

15-22 weeks
Fetus

25-35 weeks
Fetus

37-40 weeks
Term Birth

44-64 weeks
Infant <6 mo.

>64 weeks
Infant >6 mo.

Fig. 2. During the fetal period, the brainstem increases significantly in length and volume, as demonstrated in comparable cross-sections of the human medulla from the end of the first trimester through the first year of postnatal life (infancy). The changes are dramatic during the first half of gestation but appear incremental thereafter until the end of infancy.

Yet, the brainstem is a heterogeneous structure with a complex organization, and its development cannot be regarded as merely a "sum of its parts." With the DiI method for tract-tracing in the postmortem human fetal brainstem, the authors found that the basic circuitry of respiratory control in the medulla is established by midgestation [7,8]. Thereafter, dramatic changes involving up and down regulation of molecular, cellular, and neurochemical elements occur across nuclei in an increasingly integrated and synchronized manner, as judged by increasing clinical stability in respiratory functions and sleep–wake patterns (see later discussion). Nevertheless, changes occur in a nonlinear fashion with the development of different elements beginning and ending at different times progressing at different rates. This principal is well-illustrated by the interplay of increasing, decreasing, and unchanging receptor binding levels for six different neurotransmitter systems in the inferior olive (cerebellar-relay) in the human fetus and infant [9]. Respiratory-related regions with similar complex and nonlinear development include: the raphé complex, nucleus of the solitary tract, paragigantocellularis lateralis, the putative homolog of the pre-bötzinger complex in animals, with regard to respiratory control; nucleus ambiguus and nucleus of the solitary tract with regard to laryngeal reflexes; hypoglossal nucleus in regards to swallowing and upper airway control; medullary raphé complex with regard to thermoregulation; lateral dorsal tegmental nucleus and pedunculopontine nucleus with regard to REM sleep; and locus coeruleus, rostral raphé complex, and mesopontine reticular formation with regard to arousal. Variable developmental profiles are observed in neuronal origin and proliferation, migration pathways, morphologic and neurochemical differentiation, neurotransmitter receptors, transporters, and enzymes, dendritic arborization, spine formation, synaptogenesis, axonal outgrowth, and myelination [10–12]. Also, changes of seemingly small magnitude in one nucleus correlate with substantial changes in others even in the same developmental parameter. This point is well-illustrated by changes in serotonergic (5-HT) receptor binding in three regions of the medulla that are part of the medullary 5-HT system involved in homeostatic modulation and integration [3,13,14]. In the medullary 5-HT system, more than 50% reductions occur in receptor binding in the raphé (raphé obscurus) and extra-raphé (paragigantocellularis lateralis) sites, and substantially less than 50% reductions occur in the arcuate nucleus, the putative human homolog of respiratory central chemoreceptor areas along the ventral medullary surface in experimental animals [3,14,15]. In addition, dramatic changes occurr in the different neurotransmitter systems across different brain regions in parallel, as illustrated in the differential patterns of 5-HT and nicotinic receptor binding in the human medulla between midgestation and term birth (Fig. 3).

The dynamic maturation of the fetal brainstem during the second half of gestation reflects a masterful synchrony and integration of multiple transcription, growth, and other factors. This point is illustrated by findings in our laboratory demonstrating rapid and dramatic changes occurring in receptor binding across brainstem regions during this period for opioid, glutamatergic, muscarinic, nicotinic, and serotonergic receptors [9,13,14,16–20]. Little is known about the development of the GABAergic system within or rostral to the brainstem during early human life. The 5-HT system in the medulla, for example, begins to develop in the embryonic period as early as 7 weeks and results from the mediation of several signaling factors (eg, sonic hedgehog, PET-1, Lmx1b, GATA-3) that interact with one another in a cascade-like fashion, leading to the specification, differentiation, and survival of 5-HT precursor neurons into mature neurons [21]. Serotonin subsequently acts as a growth factor in neuronal proliferation, differentiation, and synaptogenesis [22]. In developmental studies, we found that the "crude" topographic configuration of the medullary 5-HT system is in place at 13 to 15 gestational weeks, and appears "adult-like" at birth. Serotonin receptor binding is likewise

³H-LSD   ³H-Nicotine

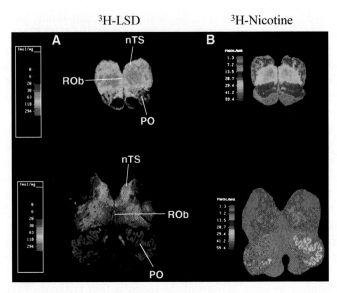

Fig. 3. The binding patterns to 5-HT receptors (*A*) and nicotinic receptors (*B*) changes differentially relative to one other in the medulla, with binding reductions in the tegmental nuclei and reticular formation occurring in both instances from the fetal to infant period. Tissue receptor autoradiography with ³H-LSD radioligand to the 5-HT$_{1A-D}$ and 5-HT$_2$ receptors [13], and with ³H-nicotine to multiple nicotinic receptor subtypes [18].

present at midgestation, and is already differentially distributed across the medullary nuclei [13]. Over the last half of gestation, however, binding to the broad radioligand ³H-LSD decreases dramatically in virtually all medullary nuclei (Fig. 4) [13,14], changes that may reflect regressive changes ("pruning") of receptor number, binding affinity, spine number, dendritic number, or axonal collateralization. By birth, the differential distribution of 5-HT receptor binding is the same as in the neonatal period but quantitative changes occur into infancy for different receptor subtypes (eg, 5-HT$_{1A}$ receptor binding in the hypoglossal nucleus) [14]. In light of the general understanding of the development of neural circuitry, these postnatal changes may, at least in part, be considered as refinements in the system that are potentially driven by activity. Imagine, then, the sequence of 5-HT development in the context of the development of over 100 other neurotransmitters alone in the brainstem, and the bewildering complexity and astounding integration of brainstem development becomes apparent.

Can developmental changes in brainstem neuroanatomy and neurochemistry be correlated with functional changes in the late preterm infant? Clearly, specific functions are regulated by the integration by more than one neurotransmitter system or region, and such correlations are likely to be overly simplistic. Yet, we are beginning to understand the underlying biologic substrate of physiologic maturation in the human brainstem, as exemplified for the ventilatory response to carbon dioxide between the fetal

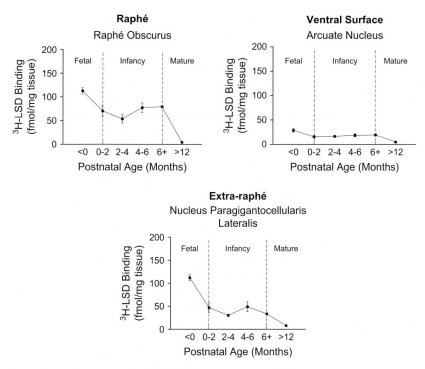

Fig. 4. Serotonin receptor binding is likewise present at midgestation, and is already differentially distributed across the medullary nuclei (Fig. 3). Over the last half of gestation, binding to the broad radioligand ^{3}H-LSD decreases dramatically in virtually all nuclei with different rates of reduction, as illustrated in three nuclei, which contain 5-HT cell bodies (ie, nucleus raphé obscurus, arcuate nucleus, and paragigantocellularis lateralis). The measurements in the fetal cases were taken at midgestation (approximately 20 weeks) such that the downward trajectory of changes across the late preterm period can only be assumed. By birth, the differential distribution of 5-HT receptor binding is the same as in the infancy with minor subtle changes with this particular radioligand.

periods and early infancy. We have found dramatic changes in 5-HT receptor binding in the human arcuate nucleus and the medullary raphé complex from the midgestation to birth [13,14] of relevance because of the homology of 5-HT neurons in these regions to those at the ventral medullary surface and in the midline (raphé) that have been shown to be chemosensitive in experimental models [15,23,24].

We know little about the specific developmental changes in the late preterm brainstem because this period has not been dissected apart from early and mid preterm periods nor from term itself, and thus critical periods (defined by rapid and dramatic changes) in any one parameter have not been reported. In the authors' studies to date, the developmental trajectory is suggested by assessment of midgestation compared with term or post-term periods that span the late preterm period (see Figs. 3 and 4). Linearity in the trajectory cannot be assumed in the development of every brainstem circuit and its interconnections with forebrain sites, even though clinical observations suggest a continuous and upward progression in the stability of cardiorespiratory function, sleep, and arousal (see later discussion). Information about the baseline development of the human brainstem in the fetal and infant periods, including close to term, is an essential step toward deciphering the cause(s) and pathogenesis of central respiratory disorders during this timeframe, including apnea of prematurity, apnea of infancy, congenital central hypoventilation syndrome, and sudden infant death syndrome [3,25]. Such information is also valuable in the determination of brainstem maturation relative to pre- and postnatal insults. The transient overexpression of nicotinic receptors in the mesopontine reticular formation and locus coeruleus, for example, suggest a site of interaction for exogeneous nicotine in maternal cigarette smoke that crosses the placenta and in turn adversely influences the maturation of the fetal cholinergic system in these regions, thereby potentially resulting in postnatal deficits in cholinergic-mediated arousal (see Fig. 3) [12,18]. In addition, the transient expression of kainate receptors that bind to glutamate in the brainstem reticular formation in the fetus suggest that this region is vulnerable to hypoxicischemic (excitotoxic) injury at this early age, in contrast to its relative vulnerability postnatally when such receptors are virtually negligible [26].

Cardiorespiratory control

Although the maturation of the neural control of breathing, heart rate, and blood pressure appears to be on a continuum extending from fetal life until sometime after birth, this is not simply the result of a linear course of growth and development for all of the responsible neural elements and their interactions.The control of lung volume, laryngeal reflexes, upper airways, chemoreceptor activity, coordination of sucking, swallowing, breathing, the incidence of apnea and periodic breathing, and the control of heart rate are still developing during late gestation, regardless of the trajectory of development. In addition, all of these reflexes are influenced by sleep and arousal state, the neurobiologic substrate that is also undergoing maturation. There are little data about the control of breathing from the group of infants born between 33 and 38 weeks' gestation. Early studies in preterm infants that often included infants in this gestational age range indicate that ventilatory responses to CO_2 and hypoxia as well as autonomic control of heart rate are not yet mature, even at 36 weeks postmenstrual age (PMA). Clinically, late preterm infants have more apnea and periodic breathing than term infants. Immature coordination of sucking, swallowing, and breathing is an important clinical issue in this group of infants, often delaying their ability to feed without accompanying bradycardia, decreases in oxyhemoglobin saturation, and even apnea. This section focuses on the maturation of respiratory control, and the coordination of sucking, swallowing, and breathing.

Neurophysiology of the respiratory control system

A full review of the neurophysiology of respiratory control is beyond the scope of this article, however the reader is referred to recent excellent summaries [27–29]. Normal respiration results from the rhythmic discharge of networks of neurons that drive the respiratory muscles including the diaphragm, the external intercostal muscles, and the upper airway (Fig. 5). In contrast, the elastic recoil forces accumulated during inspiration largely accomplish expiration. Although voluntary control of breathing in the newborn may originate in the cerebral cortex, activities that can affect breathing, such as arm and leg movement, crying, and sucking, originate largely in the brainstem or spinal cord. In contrast, the involuntary component of the control system originates almost entirely in the medulla and pons. Neurons in

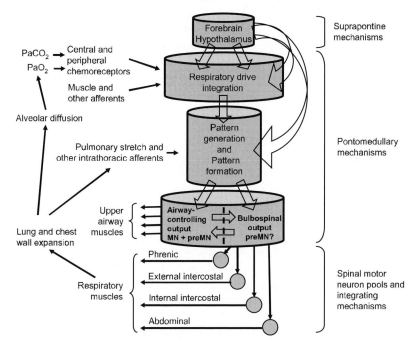

Fig. 5. Organization of the respiratory control system. Emphasis is placed on the mechanisms for respiratory drive integration, respiratory pattern generation and formation, and their influences on the two main output systems that control the upper airway and respiratory muscles. The behavioral component of the control system with direct connections between the cerebral cortex and the lower motor neurons is not shown (*Adapted from* Euler CV. Breathing and behavior. In: Euler CV, Lagercrantz H, editors. Neurobiology of the control of breathing: Proceedings of the 10th Nobel Conference of the Karolinska Institute. Philadelphia: Lippincott, Williams & Wilkins; 1987. p. 4; with permission.)

"the pre-bötzinger complex" located in the medulla appear to be essential components of the neural networks responsible for rhythmogenesis [30]. Many of these neurons exhibit bursting pacemaker properties and are believed to be necessary for respiratory rhythm generation [31]. However, much of the information about the functions of various neuronal networks has been derived from reduced preparations, each of which has its own particular characteristics. Thus major questions remain about the relative contribution of these regions to rhythmic breathing. For example, uncertainties exist as to whether bursting neurons in ventrolateral medulla are most important for "eupnia" or normal respiration, or "gasping", a type of discharge that occurs during extreme hypoxia [30,32,33]. Other regions close to the facial nucleus have also been implicated in primary rhythm generation [34]. Moreover, pontine mechanisms may be necessary for normal respiration [35]. Excitatory and inhibitory neurons of many neurochemical phenotypes, including glutamate, GABA, acetylcholine, endorphins, prostaglandins and serotonin comprise these networks, which are in turn influenced by excitatory and inhibitory inputs from chemoreceptors, mechanoreceptors, and more rostral areas of the brain, including the amygdala, hippocampus, and hypothalamus. As reviewed, important neurotransmitter systems, including serotonin, glutamate, GABA, and acetylcholine are undergoing rapid and varying changes during late gestation resulting in continuing instability in the control systems involved in breathing.

Control of lung volume and mechanoreflexes

The respiratory system in the newborn, especially the premature newborn, is characterized by a high compliance of the chest wall [36,37]. Inward distortion of the anterior chest wall is commonly observed in preterm infants, even in those without respiratory disease. This is also accentuated during REM sleep, which comprises approximately 60% of total sleep time in the late preterm infant [38]. End-expiratory volume is higher than passively determined functional residual capacity during quiet sleep, but is considerably lower during REM sleep [39] and is maintained by actively interrupting expiration and initiating inspiration before passive deflation is complete coupled with active laryngeal narrowing during expiration [36]. With maturation, chest wall compliance decreases and the mechanical advantage improves enhancing the mechanical stability of the respiratory system.

During lung inflation, slowly adapting pulmonary stretch receptors innervated by the vagus nerve are stimulated and help to terminate inspiration. This phenomenon is known as the Hering-Breuer inflation inhibition reflex and was first demonstrated in human newborn infants by Cross and colleagues [40]. The reflex is an important respiratory control mechanism in premature infants whereas in older children and adults, it may not operate in the tidal volume range. There are also rapidly adapting pulmonary receptors, such as irritant receptors, that can be stimulated both chemically (smoke, noxious gases) and mechanically (particulate matter or changes in airflow). These receptors are located mostly in the larger airways and appear to be poorly developed in premature infants. Another important reflex in the newborn is the "paradoxical" reflex of Head [41]. When the lungs are rapidly inflated, there is a paradoxical further inspiration, rather than inhibition. This reflex is commonly observed in neonates in the form of a sigh. Sighs are common in premature infants, are more frequent during REM sleep than during quiet sleep, and are also more common during periodic breathing. It is believed that the high incidence of sighs in premature infants reflects a greater need for lung recruitment at this age [42]. Between 33 and 38 weeks' gestation there continues to be important changes in dynamic lung compliance, the diaphragmatic work of breathing, and the volume displacement of the diaphragm (Fig. 6) [37].

Airway control during breathing

The airway of the newborn is more compliant than in the adult, and the anatomic arrangement of the upper airway favors obstruction, particularly when the neck is flexed. Thus the maintenance of an open upper airway during inspiration becomes particularly important (Fig. 7). During extreme flexion, the airway can collapse even under conditions of positive pressure [43–45]. The protection of the upper airway is maintained by several reflex mechanisms, including inhibition of diaphragm muscle activity during periods of obstruction, the timing of the onset of upper airway muscle with respect to diaphragm muscle activity, and the differential effects of ventilatory drive on diaphragm and upper airway muscles [36]. Even in full-term infants, unlike the coordinated activity observed in adults, the posterior crico-arytenoid, a muscle that pulls the vocal cords open, contracts simultaneously with or after the diaphragm in approximately 21% of breaths [46]. The percentage of such "lag" breaths is even greater in the premature infant, including those born after 33 weeks' gestation [46,47]. Many upper airway reflexes are more immature in preterm infants who have apnea compared with those who do not have apnea. For example, in infants who have apnea, there is less recruitment of the genioglossus muscle [48] and obstruction of the upper airway after nasal occlusion occurs more commonly [49,50].

Laryngeal reflexes

The larynx contains mechanoreceptors and chemoreceptors that respond to various stimuli, including pressure and airflow, hyperosmolar solutions, milk, water, and CO_2 [51,52]. In older infants and adults, a typical response to the introduction of certain liquids into the larynx includes cough, expiratory efforts, and swallowing [53]. In newborns, however, the response can include apnea and bradycardia followed by swallowing [54]. This response pattern is most marked in premature infants (Fig. 8) [53]. Although there

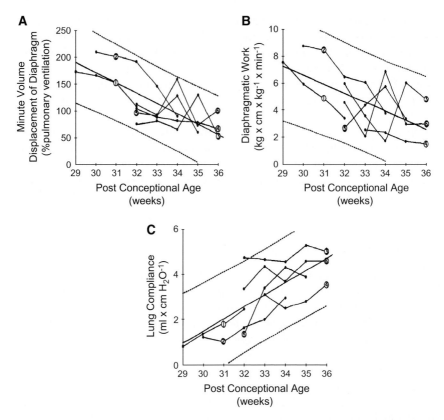

Fig. 6. (*A*) Changes in average minute volume displacement of the diaphragm expressed as % of pulmonary ventilation in 6 infants. There was a significant decrease ($P < .005$) with maturation. (*B*) Average diaphragmatic work for each weekly study in 6 infants. There was a - significant decrease ($P < .005$) with maturation. (*C*) Dynamic lung compliance for each infant versus postmenstrual age. There was a significant increase ($P < .01$) with maturation. For each figure is a line fit to group data by linear regression with 95% confidence limits. (*From* Heldt GP. Development of stability of the respiratory system in preterm infants. J Appl Physiol 1988;65(1):443; with permission.)

is no statistically significant relationship between gastroesophageal reflux and apnea of prematurity [55], severe gastroesophageal reflux can stimulate laryngeal receptors inducing prolonged apnea and bradycardia.

Chemical regulation of breathing

Respiratory rate and tidal volume are regulated by feedback mechanisms involving chemoreceptors that sense Pao_2 and $Paco_2$, which in turn trigger changes in minute ventilation to maintain normal concentrations of oxygen, CO_2, and pH. An increase in $Paco_2$ or a decrease in Pao_2 increases excitatory input to central respiratory neural networks, increasing respiratory muscle activity, augmenting the exchange of CO_2 and O_2. Under normoxic

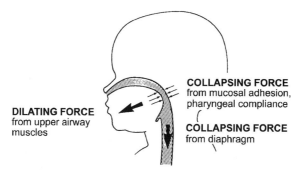

Fig. 7. Collapsing and dilating forces acting on the upper airway. This sagittal section of the upper airway demonstrates various forces operating either to collapse the pharynx or to maintain its patency during normal respiration. (*Adapted from* Miller MJ, Martin RJ. Pathophysiology of apnea of prematurity. In: Polin RA, Fox WW, editors: Fetal and neonatal physiology, Philadelphia: WB Saunders 1992. p. 877; with permission.)

conditions, $Paco_2$ largely determines minute ventilation. Respiratory responses to inhaled CO_2 or hypoxic gas mixtures are commonly used to assess chemoreceptor activity.

Response to hypercapnia

Neurons (and possibly glia) sensitive to changes in local CO_2 or H^+ concentrations are largely responsible for sensing changes in CO_2. These

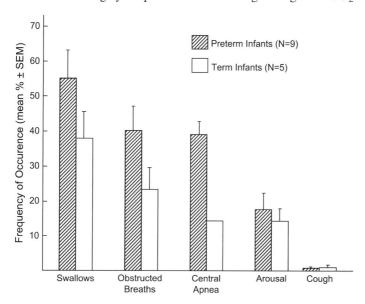

Fig. 8. The percent occurrence of swallows, obstructed breaths, central apnea, arousals, and coughs in response to a saline bolus stimuli of 0.4 mL or less for 2 groups of infants. (*From* Pickens DL, Schefft GL, Thach BT. Pharyngeal fluid clearance and aspiration preventive mechanisms in sleeping infants. J Appl Physiol 1989;66(3):1167; with permission.)

neurons are located predominantly on the ventral surface of the medulla, but also in many other widespread locations [56]. One homologous area at the ventral medullary surface in the human fetus and infant may be the arcuate nucleus (see former discussion). Stimulation of neuronal structures sensitive to CO_2 results in an increase in minute ventilation. In the newborn infant, the response to CO_2 is usually assessed by measuring respiratory variables after increasing the inspired CO_2 to a steady state concentration of 3% to 5%. It should be noted, however, that approximately 20% to 50% of the total ventilatory response originates from peripheral chemoreceptors located mainly within the carotid body [57] which become increasingly sensitive to advancing postnatal age [58]. Although at term, the slope of the ventilatory response curve (sensitivity) is equivalent to that of an adult [59], the position of the curve is shifted to the left by about 4 mm Hg [60]. Thus, for any given $PaCO_2$, minute ventilation is greater in the term infant compared with the adult, which may reflect the greater metabolic rate (greater production of CO_2) during infancy [28]. In preterm infants sensitivity of the response is related to both gestational and chronologic age [61]. This increase is likely secondary to a combination of the maturation of central mechanisms and to improved lung mechanics. Studies that have included late preterm infants suggest that infants born between 33 and 38 weeks' gestation have ventilatory responses that are greater than more immature infants and less than infants born at term, depending on the chronologic age at the time of study [62]. Most of these studies, however, were not controlled for sleep state. From 34 to 37 weeks' gestational age, the percentage of NON-REM sleep increases from 20% to 40%, whereas the percentage of REM stays rather constant at approximately 60% [38]. By term, newborn infants spend approximately 50% of their sleep time in REM. A few studies in human newborns have shown blunted ventilatory responses to hypercapnia during REM [63]. It has also been reported that the ventilatory response to hypercapnia is also decreased in premature infants who have apnea of prematurity compared with those who do not have apnea [64,65]. A cause-and-effect relationship, however, has not been clearly established. Thus the late preterm infant continues to have a slightly blunted ventilatory response to CO_2, spends more than 50% of sleep time in REM, and continues to have apnea and periodic breathing, with a prevalence of 10% compared with 60% in infants born at less than 1500 g [66].

Response to hypoxia

In the fetus, breathing movements are decreased or abolished during hypoxia [67]. Very immature preterm infants also have little if any increase in ventilation in response to 15% oxygen breathing [68]. In the later preterm and full-term newborn infant, a decrease in PaO_2 causes an initial increase in minute ventilation, followed by a more sustained decrease, often to baseline levels, or even apnea [61]. In the adult, the response tends to be more sustained [69], although a secondary decrease in ventilation has been described during steady state hypoxia [70]. Thus, differences in the ventilatory responses of the fetus, newborn, and adult to hypoxia appear to represent a developmental continuum in which similar mechanisms may be involved, but the balance and timing of the excitatory and depressive components of the response may change with development. Fig. 9 shows a typical newborn and adult response to sustained hypoxia [69]. The maturation of this response appears to be related more to PMA than to chronologic age. Thus premature infants of varying gestational and chronologic ages continue to have a biphasic response when studied between 33 and 38 weeks postmenstrual age [71].

In the biphasic ventilatory response to hypoxia and initial increase in minute ventilation results from stimulation of peripheral chemoreceptors located primarily in carotid bodies. During the secondary decrease in ventilation, the excitatory input from the carotid bodies to the brainstem appears to be sustained [72]. It is likely that the late decrease in minute ventilation originates centrally and ultimately overrides the excitatory inputs, resulting in a net decrease in ventilation. The mechanisms responsible for the central "depression" of ventilation have not been completely elucidated but probably include changes in metabolism, local perfusion, and the production of inhibitory neuromodulators, including adenosine [73–76] and GABA [77]. There is recent evidence suggesting that certain areas in the midbrain or rostral pons may also contribute to the decrease in ventilation produced by hypoxia in the fetus and neonate [67]. Moreover, certain neurons may

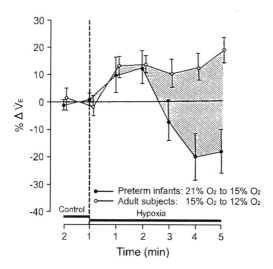

Fig. 9. Ventilatory response to hypoxia in premature infants and adults. Percent change in ventilation when 15% oxygen was substituted for 21% oxygen in preterm infants (*closed circles*) and when 12% oxygen was substituted for 15% oxygen in adult subjects (*open circles*). The initial increase in ventilation is sustained in adults but not in preterm infants. (*Adapted from* Rigatto H. Maturation of breathing. Clin Perinatol 1992;4:750; with permission.)

function as "oxygen sensors" that, when activated, inhibit brain stem respiratory neurons [78]. Late preterm infants continue to have immature ventilatory responses to hypoxia. In a series of studies, infants born at 37 weeks' gestation had biphasic responses of the same magnitude as those born at 32 weeks' gestation [79]. In addition, preterm infants with an average postmenstrual age of 36 weeks exhibited a blunted excitatory component of the ventilatory response to hypoxia during REM sleep compared with both NON-REM sleep and wakefulness [80].

Coordination of sucking, swallowing, and breathing

Feeding-related bradycardia and desaturation are common among premature infants, including those born between 33 and 38 weeks' gestation. Problems with coordination of sucking, swallowing, and breathing stem from anatomic and neurodevelopmental issues: 1) the upper airway is the common conduit of both the respiratory and digestive tracts (the basis for commonly occurring pulmonary aspiration syndromes) [81]; 2) feeding and breathing have conflicting priorities; 3) oral feeding involves sucking and swallowing that need to be integrated with breathing; 4) several upper airway muscles are involved, and 5) aspiration can occur if the airway is unprotected [82]. The physiologic organization of sucking becomes almost fully organized by 36 weeks PMA [83], whereas swallow rhythm is established by 32 weeks PMA [83,84]. The timed activation of several upper airway muscles is critical for suck–swallow coordination, but unlike sucking, swallowing interrupts breathing [85,86], thus protecting the airway, decreasing the risk for aspiration. Overall, minute ventilation decreases during nipple feeding and this is more pronounced in the preterm infant (Fig. 10) [87].

Coordination of breathing and swallowing is also important during nonnutritive swallowing, an important mechanism for clearing oral and nasal secretions. The laryngeal chemoreflex is apparently responsible for initiating nonnutritive swallowing, stimulated by increasing fluid volumes in the piriform fossae. Unlike the adult, nonnutritive swallowing can be initiated at any time during the respiratory cycle in the newborn and when it occurs during inspiration, the diaphragm continues to contract [88,89]. Thus, a small prolongation of inspiration or expiration is produced, resulting in only minimal "coordination" [86].

The number of swallows associated with respiratory pauses during feeding becomes less frequent as the infant matures in parallel with maturation of the auditory evoked response [90] and maturation of the laryngeal chemoreflex [91]. As the infant matures the sequence of breathing and swallowing becomes more consistent: inspiration→ swallow → expiration, with no pauses in breathing (Fig. 11) [92]. It is likely that the frequent feeding issues encountered by the late preterm infant have their origin largely in the immaturity of the coordination of sucking, swallowing, and breathing.

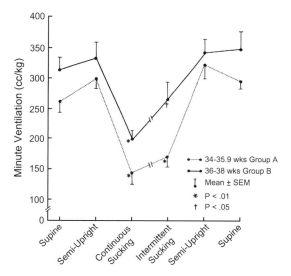

Fig. 10. Minute ventilation during feeding in two groups of premature infants. Ventilation during the continuous sucking phase is significantly lower than control in both groups. Note that greater reduction in ventilation occurs in the more immature group. (*From* Shivpuri CR, Martin RJ, Carlo WA, Fanaroff AA. Decreased ventilation in preterm infants during oral feeding. J Pediatr 1983;103(2):285–9; with permission.)

Apnea of prematurity

Apnea of prematurity is the most frequently encountered clinical problem of respiratory control in the neonatal intensive care nursery. The pathogenesis of apnea is multifactorial with immature lung volume and upper airway control, ventilatory responses to hypoxia and CO_2, and feeding, as well as physiologic and iatrogenic anemia, all contributing to the pathogenesis. Some of these factors have their origin in immature brainstem neuronal circuitry; others are related to the anatomy of the upper airway and chest wall. Importantly, late preterm infants born between 33 and 38 weeks' gestation continue to have apnea and are at risk for the resulting periods of bradycardia and hypoxia [66].

Periodic breathing

Periodic breathing, or alternating periods of hyperpnea and apnea, is a common breathing pattern in premature infants. Clinically important apnea of prematurity is almost always associated with periodic breathing [93]. Although this immature pattern of breathing occurs mostly during REM sleep, as the infant matures, and non-REM (or quiet) sleep can be better defined, periodic breathing can be identified in both sleep states. The difference is that during REM sleep, the periodicity is accompanied by irregular breathing, whereas during quiet sleep the periodic breathing is regular,

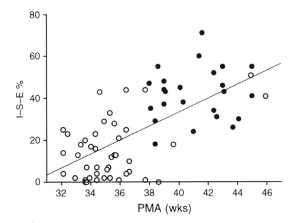

Fig. 11. The percentage of swallows in an inspiration-swallow-expiration (I-S-E) phase relation. I-S-E is the predominant swallow-breath pattern in term infants (*closed circles*) and is significantly higher compared with preterm infants (*open circles*). I-S-E is directly correlated with increasing PMA ($r^2 = 0.456$; $P < 0.001$) (*From* Gewolb IH, Vice FL. Maturational changes in the rhythms, patterning, and coordination of respiration and swallow during feeding in preterm and term infants. Dev Med Child Neurol 2006;48:593; with permission.)

with breathing and apneic intervals of similar duration [93]. Although the mechanisms have not been fully elucidated, it is likely that the periods of hyperpnea or hyperventilation may decrease Pa_{CO_2} and reduce the stimulus to breathe, resulting in apnea. The transition from regular to periodic breathing, however, does not usually occur abruptly. In premature infants, the depth of breathing tends to oscillate in relatively slow cycles. True periodic breathing or apnea emerges when the segments of the cycle with the lowest depth of breathing actually become pauses [94].

Thermoregulation, metabolism, and the control of breathing

Metabolic rate increases after birth to meet the demands for growth and heat production. The increased oxygen demand and CO_2 production in turn increase respiratory drive. Temperature-related stimulation of respiratory drive may be particularly important for sustained breathing after birth [95]. The relatively narrow thermoneutral range of the neonate may also affect respiratory control. Under steady-state conditions, ventilation is closely matched to metabolic rate [96]. Fig. 12 illustrates the general relationships between ambient and body temperature, metabolism, and ventilation. In the newborn infant, heat production is largely accomplished by the oxidative metabolism of brown fat producing nonshivering thermogenesis, an oxidative process that requires normal development of the sympathetic nervous system. In particular, 5-HT and glutamatergic neurons located in the medullary raphé are important for the activation of nonshivering thermogenesis and peripheral vasoconstriction, the major mechanisms for

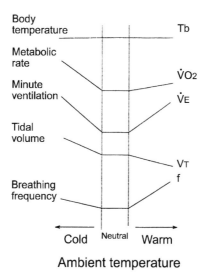

Fig. 12. Thermoregulation and breathing. Relationship between ambient temperature and body temperature (Tb), metabolic rate (VO$_2$), minute ventilation (VE), tidal volume (VT), and breathing frequency (f). For modest drops or increases in ambient temperature (as assumed here), Tb does not change. VO$_2$ and VE have minimal values at thermoneutrality, and VT increases and decreases, respectively, below and above thermoneutrality; f increases slightly with low ambient temperature and markedly above thermoneutrality. (*Adapted from* Mortola JP, Gautier H. Interaction between metabolism and ventilation: Effects of respiratory gases and temperature. In: Dempsey JA, Pack AI, editors: Regulation of Breathing. New York: Marcel Dekker; 1995. p. 1034; with permission. © Copyright 1995. Reproduced by permission of Routledge/Taylor & Francis Group, LLC.)

heat production and heat loss reduction, respectively [97,98]. Infants who are hypoxic, therefore, cannot respond normally to cold stress. In addition, in many species, the metabolic response to cooling is blunted during REM sleep [99], but this is less apparent in the newborn human [100]. It is not clear why human infants are different from other mammalian species, however, it might offer an advantage to the human newborn, who spends 50% to 60% of sleep time in REM. Over the first few weeks of life, the activation of nonshivering thermogenesis declines and is replaced by shivering thermogenesis. In animals and possibly in human neonates, increasing environmental temperature reduces the gain of respiratory responses. This, combined with the reduced metabolic respiratory drive at warmer temperatures, may predispose an infant to develop apnea. Heating can prolong the laryngeal chemoreflex [101] in animals and cause fictive apnea in reduced preparations [102]. In a clinical setting clusters of apnea are often observed after a rapid rise in incubator air temperature. Infants who are weaned from their incubators too quickly can also be at increased risk for apnea. In this case a large energy expenditure is necessary to maintain body temperature, which in extreme cases can lead to decreased ability to defend against hypoxia with increasing ventilation, resulting in more apnea and periodic breathing. Late preterm infants are often treated more like term infants. In some cases attendance to some of the basic principles of thermoregulation may be overlooked resulting in large variations in environmental temperature that could result in both cold stress (baths) and overheating (bundling).

Data from the Collaborative Home Infant Monitoring Evaluation study

The multicenter Collaborative Home Infant Monitoring Evaluation (CHIME) study performed during the 1990s included late preterm infants comprising approximately 19% of all enrolled infants 37 weeks gestation or less. In this study, 443 infants 34 weeks gestation or less were classified as either having (symptomatic) or not having (asymptomatic) apnea within 5 days of discharge. Of the symptomatic preterm infants, 2.6% were born at 34 weeks' gestation, and of the asymptomatic preterm infants, 4.9% were born at 34 weeks' gestation. The majority of late preterm infants were enrolled after having experienced an acute life-threatening event (ALTE), or as siblings of infants who died of sudden infant death syndrome (SIBS). In contrast to the asymptomatic and symptomatic preterm groups, prematurity was defined as being born 37 weeks or less gestation in the ALTE and SIBS infants. Of the 45 ALTE preterm infants 86.7% were late preterms. Similarly, of the 50 preterm SIBS, 86.0% were late preterms. Table 1 shows the distribution of late preterm infants by CHIME classification.

In late preterm infants the incidence of conventional (apnea duration >20 seconds, heart rate (HR) <60 for ≥5 seconds or ≤80 for ≥15 seconds if <44 weeks PMA; HR <50 for ≥5 seconds or <60 for ≥15 seconds if

Table 1
Late preterm infants included in the Collaborative Home Infant Monitoring Evaluation study

Gestational age	Number of infants	Percent
Symptomatic preterm ≤34 wk	76	
34 wk	2	2.6
Asymptomatic preterm ≤34 wk	367	
34 wk	18	4.9
ALTE ≤37 wk	45	
34 wk	3	6.7
35 wk	10	22.2
36 wk	10	22.2
37 wk	16	35.6
34-37 wk	*39*	*86.7*
SIBS ≤37 wk	50	
34 wk	3	6.0
35 wk	10	20.0
36 wk	9	18.0
37 wk	19	38.0
34–37 wk	*43*	*86.0*
Total ≤37 wk	538	
Total 34–37 wk	102	19.0

≥44 weeks PMA) and extreme (apnea duration >30 seconds, HR <60 for ≥10 seconds if <44 weeks PMA; HR <50 for ≥10 seconds if ≥44 weeks PMA) events was intermediate between preterm infants born 34 weeks or less gestation and full-term infants [66]. Fifty-four percent of all conventional events and 37% of all extreme events in the SIBS and ALTE groups occurred in the late preterm infants. The relative risk for at least one extreme event in late preterm infants in the ALTE or sibling group was increased (5.6 and 7.6, respectively, $P < .008$) compared with the reference term infants [66]. The chance of having at least one extreme event remained higher in late preterm infants compared with full-term infants until 43 weeks PMA (Fig. 13) [66,103]. The incidence of SIDS in preterm infants born at 33 to 36 weeks is 1.37 out of 1000 live births compared with 0.69 out of 1000 in term infants [104]. Affected late preterm infants also die at an older mean

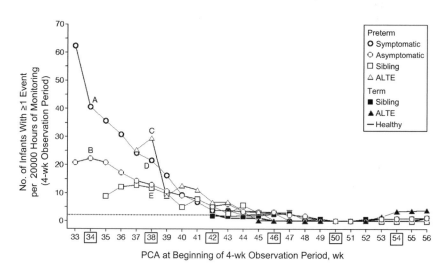

Fig. 13. Rate of infants with one or more events exceeding the extreme threshold during 4-week postconceptional age periods: Each point indicates the number of infants in a given study group who experienced at least one event exceeding the extreme threshold, per 20,000 hours of monitor use during a 4-week observation period beginning at the specified postconceptional age week. Poisson analyses were used to calculate relative rates for nonoverlapping 4-week periods (beginning at the postconceptional age weeks enclosed in a box) compared with the reference group of healthy term infants observed from 42 to 45 weeks. Significantly higher relative rates were observed in (A) preterm symptomatic group at 34 to 37 weeks (relative rate, 19.7; 95% CI, 4.1–94.0; $P<.001$); (B) preterm asymptomatic group at 34 to 37 weeks (relative rate, 10.5; 95% CI, 2.4–47.0; $P = .002$); (C) ALTE preterm group at 38 to 41 weeks (relative rate, 14.3; 95% CI, 2.6–80.1; $P = .002$); (D) preterm symptomatic group at 38 to 41 weeks (relative rate, 10.2; 95% CI, 2.2–47.8; $P = .003$); (E) preterm asymptomatic group at 38 to 41 weeks (relative rate, 6.0; 95% CI, 1.4–26.5; $P = .02$); and SIBS preterm group at 38 to 41 weeks (relative rate, 5.7; 95% CI, 1.0–31.1; $P = .05$). (From Ramanathan R, Corwin MJ, Hunt CE, et al. Cardiorespiratory events recorded on home monitors-comparison of healthy infants with those at increased risk for SIDS. JAMA 2001;285:2206; with permission.)

PMA compared with less mature infants (48 and 46 weeks, respectively), but die at a younger PMA than full-term infants (53 weeks, $P < 0.05$) [105].

Resolution of apnea as an indicator of the maturation
of respiratory control

The resolution of recurrent apnea involves the maturation of the multiple interacting neurophysiologic and mechanical factors that influence respiratory control and remains poorly understood [36]. It is therefore not surprising that chronologic age at the resolution of recurrent apnea is inversely proportional to gestational age at birth. However, there is an aspect of maturity that is not simply related to time. Several lines of evidence indicate that infants born at term are "more mature" than infants born earlier who reach term PMA [106]. Thus, infants less than 28 weeks' gestation often do not resolve their recurrent apnea until well after the average resolution time of 37 weeks PMA (Figs. 14 and 15) [107,108]. The time of resolution of apnea might be considered one measure of the maturation of brain structures involved in respiratory control. However, because the upper airway and other mechanical factors also contribute to the etiology of apnea, its resolution may reflect the maturation of other factors as well. In addition, even these data are confounded by the differing definitions of apnea used clinically and those incorporated into many studies.

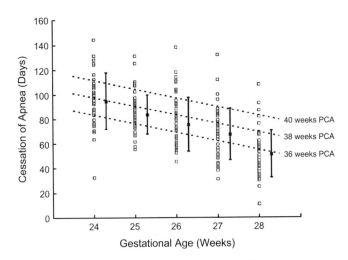

Fig. 14. Individual (*open squares*) and mean (*closed squares*) ($\pm$ SD) values for the last postnatal day with a documented apnea or bradycardia event of any type for each gestational group. Dotted lines indicate when infants in each gestational age group reach 36, 38, and 40 weeks PMA. (*From* Eichenwald EC, Aina A, Stark AR. Apnea frequently persists beyond term gestation in infants delivered at 24 to 28 weeks. Pediatr 1997;100(3 Pt 1):356; with permission.)

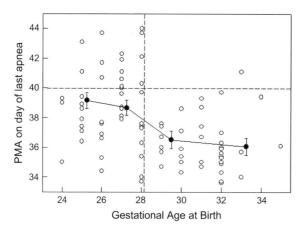

Fig. 15. Relationship between the gestational age at birth and the PMA on the day of the last apnea. Each open circle represents 1 infant. The closed circles are the least-square means of the same data compressed into quartiles (means ± SEM). Reference lines have been included at 40 weeks PMA and at 28 weeks' gestational age to illustrate the distribution of infants who experience their last clinically significant apnea at 40 weeks PMA or greater. Nearly all such infants were born at 28 weeks' gestation or less. (*From* Darnall RA, Kattwinkel J, Nattie C, Robinson M. Margin of safety for discharge after apnea in preterm infants. Pediatr 1997;100(5):798; with permission.)

Sleep and circadian rhythms

Sleep maturation and brain development

The development of behavioral states is one of the most significant aspects of brain maturation in the fetal and infant periods [109]. Behavioral states, classified as quiet (NREM) sleep, active (REM) sleep, and wakefulness are characterized by a number of state specific criteria defined by behavioral, cardiorespiratory, and electroencephalography (EEG) criteria, which emerge over time. By 32 weeks PMA, active sleep and quiet sleep can be differentiated, although a large proportion of the time, which cannot be classified as active sleep or quiet sleep is spent in indeterminant sleep [110,111]. Between 32 and 40 weeks' gestation there are significant increases in quiet sleep and a decrease in indeterminant sleep, whereas the amount of active sleep remains relatively constant [110,112,113]. Longitudinal observations in preterm infants indicate that quiet sleep significantly increases, indeterminant sleep decreases, and active sleep remains relatively constant from 32 to 38 weeks PMA [114] (Fig. 16), and are consistent with cross-sectional studies looking at groups of infants at increasing PMA [112,113,115]. It appears, therefore, that the time course of sleep development is not affected by preterm birth and can be used as another measure of brain development.

Perhaps one of the most fascinating sleep-related phenomenon in human brain development is the transition from the dominance of REM sleep by non-REM sleep that begins around the time of birth [116]. REM sleep

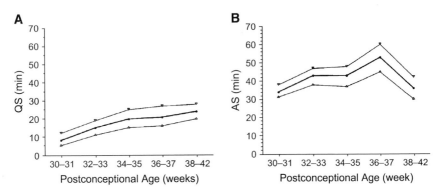

Fig. 16. (*A*) Development of quiet sleep (QS) as a function of postconceptional age in preterm infants born at less than 30 weeks' gestational age. Data is presented as the mean and 95% confidence interval of 2 h longitudinal recordings of 96 infants. (*B*) Development of active sleep (AS) in preterm infants as in (*A*). (*From* Mirmiran M, Mass YG, Ariagno RL. Development of fetal and neonatal sleep and circadian rhythms. Sleep Med Rev 2003;7(4):323; with permission.)

predominates the sleep time in the last trimester [117], comprises approximately 60% at 36 weeks' gestation, and about 50% at term [38]. The time spent in REM decreases steadily after birth, reaching a plateau of 25% to 30% by 9 months of age [116]. Of note, the peak period of the development of REM occurs in the human between 30 and 40 weeks' gestation [118,119]. The high level of endogenous neuronal activation during REM may be critical for promoting brain development during a period in which environmental (external) experiences are limited in the intrauterine environment [117]. REM sleep also appears to be important for brain plasticity as evidenced by experiments in which REM-deprived rats fail to respond to environmental enrichment with increase in the size of the cerebral cortex, increased number of synapses, and problem solving ability [120]. In the visual system, the abundance of REM during early development may be a source of symmetrical stimulation to all lateral geniculate body relay cells, irrespective of eye innervation and promote symmetrically appropriate brain development [121–123].

Development of circadian rhythms

In nonhuman primates, a fetal biologic clock, which is responsive to maternal entraining signals, is functional in the last trimester of pregnancy [124–126]. In the human fetus, a light–dark heart rate rhythm is synchronized with maternal rest–activity cycles, heart rate, cortisol and melatonin levels, and body temperature [127,128]. Early studies in the human infant found little or no evidence of circadian rhythms at the time of birth; however, a nocturnal nadir in body temperature, which is an indicator of human circadian rhythms, can be found by 6 to 12 weeks [129]. Longitudinal studies of preterm infants (mean gestational age, 30 weeks) report circadian rhythms of body temperature could be evident as early as 36 weeks PMA. The magnitude of the temperature rhythms is greater at 35 to 37 weeks than at 32 to 34 weeks PMA. Late preterm infants from 33 to 36 weeks' gestation secrete melatonin during the first week of life [130,131]. Term infants can establish a cortisol circadian rhythm by 8 to 12 weeks of life [131] and many preterm infants born at 31 to 34 weeks' gestation have cortisol rhythms by 2 to 8 weeks of life [132]. There are many environmental and other factors, however, that affect the development of circadian rhythms during infancy, including feeding patterns, use of maternal breast milk, environmental lighting, regular versus irregular light–dark cycles, and chronologic and PMA [133,134]. Indeed, the inherent fetal biologic clock continues oscillating after birth if not disturbed by interfering environmental factors such as fixed feeding schedules and nighttime bright light [135–138]. Preterm infants are particularly vulnerable to the effects of continuous or unpredictable lighting cycles and the lack of maternal entrainment factors. Late preterm infants are often exposed to unpredictable lighting and decreased maternal entrainment and are at risk for delays in developing normal circadian rhythms.

Interaction of sleep and arousal with cardiorespiratory control

A striking feature of the resting breathing pattern of the premature newborn is its irregularity; a large degree of breath-to-breath variability accompanied by long stretches of periodic breathing with apnea is characteristic [93,139]. The resting breathing pattern of the neonate is greatly modulated by sleep. The preterm infant sleeps the majority of time, and 60% to 90% of that time is REM sleep. Quiet or NREM sleep is difficult to define before 32 weeks' gestation. Sleep generally depresses ventilatory and arousal responses and many respiratory reflexes. During sleep in the preterm newborn, brief periods of regular breathing alternate with longer periods of irregular breathing. In both the newborn and the adult, it is likely that sleep removes excitatory inputs from brainstem and other ascending arousal systems mediating wakefulness. During REM sleep, breathing is irregular, with marked variability in its rate and depth. In addition, there is loss of muscle activity in intercostal and airway-maintaining musculature. In the newborn, the loss of phasic inspiratory activity in upper airway muscles contributes to a greater risk of upper airway obstruction. The inhibition of respiratory muscle activity, especially those muscles contributing to expiratory braking mechanisms, in combination with the generally compliant chest wall, puts the infant at a mechanical disadvantage, increasing the potential for reduced end-expiratory lung volume contributing to apnea.

Arousal from sleep is an important component of the protective responses to physiologic challenges, helping to protect the infant from potentially dangerous situations. Arousals occur spontaneously or may be elicited by stimuli such as hypercapnia, hypoxia, laryngeal stimulation, changes in blood pressure, sound, or touch. There are several "levels" of arousal including subcortical (spinal and brainstem) and cortical (EEG) arousals. Subcortical arousals associated with changes in breathing, blood pressure, heart rate, and heart rate variability may be particularly important in infants. Infant sleeping position also affects both elicited and spontaneous arousals. Thresholds for elicited arousals are significantly higher in both REM and NREM sleep when preterm infants sleep prone at 36 to 38 weeks PMA and at 2 to 3 months postterm [140]. Also, late preterm infants born at 34 ± 2 weeks' gestation, studied at 1 and 3 months corrected age have fewer spontaneous arousals during active sleep and quiet sleep when prone compared with supine [141]. It has been postulated that less frequent arousals during prone sleeping may contribute to the association of prone sleeping and sudden infant death.

Summary

The brainstem development of infants born between 33 and 38 weeks' gestation is less mature than that of a full-term infant. During late gestation, there are dramatic and nonlinear developmental changes in the brainstem with respect to neuronal origin and proliferation, migration pathways, morphologic and neurochemical differentiation, neurotransmitter receptors, transporters, and enzymes, dendritic arborization, spine formation, synaptogenesis, axonal outgrowth, and myelination. This translates into immaturity of upper airway and lung volume control, laryngeal reflexes, chemical control of breathing, and sleep mechanisms. Ten percent of late preterm infants have significant apnea of prematurity and they frequently have delays in establishing coordination of feeding and breathing. Eighty six percent of the 45 preterm infants who were enrolled in the CHIME study after experiencing an ALTE were between 34 and 37 weeks' gestation. Clearly these infants are at risk for respiratory-related problems compared with infants born at term. Unfortunately, there is a paucity of clinical, physiologic, neuroanatomic, and neurochemical data in this specific group of infants. Research focused on this group of infants will not only further our understanding of brainstem maturation during this high-risk period, but will help develop focused plans for their management.

References

[1] Buss Frank M. The great imposter. Adv Neonatal Care 2005;5(5):233–6.
[2] Krimsky WR, Leiter JC. Physiology of breathing and respiratory control during sleep. Semin Respir Crit Care Med 2005;26(1):5–12.
[3] Kinney HC. The near-term (late preterm) human brain and risk for periventricular leukomalacia: a review. Semin Perinatol 2006;30(2):81–8.
[4] Kinney HC, Brody BA, Kloman AS, et al. Sequence of central nervous system myelination in human infancy. II. Patterns of myelination in autopsied infants. J Neuropathol Exp Neurol 1988;47(3):217–34.

[5] Ploog DW. The place of the triune brain in psychiatry. Physiol Behav 2003;79(3):487–93.

[6] Blinkov SM, Glezer II. The human brain in figures and tables: a quantitative handbook. New York: Plenum Press; 1968.

[7] Zec N, Kinney HC. Anatomic relationships of the human nucleus paragigantocellularis lateralis: a DiI labeling study. Auton Neurosci 2001;89(1–2):110–24.

[8] Zec N, Kinney HC. Anatomic relationships of the human nucleus of the solitary tract in the medulla oblongata: a DiI labeling study. Auton Neurosci 2003;105(2):131–44.

[9] Armstrong DD, Assmann S, Kinney HC. Early developmental changes in the chemoarchitecture of the human inferior olive: a review. J Neuropathol Exp Neurol 1999;58(1):1–11.

[10] Blanchi B, Sieweke MH. Mutations of brainstem transcription factors and central respiratory disorders. Trends Mol Med 2005;11(1):23–30.

[11] Landsberg RL, Awatramani RB, Hunter NL, et al. Hindbrain rhombic lip is comprised of discrete progenitor cell populations allocated by Pax6. Neuron 2005;48(6):933–47.

[12] Kinney HC, Rava LA, Benowitz LI. Anatomic distribution of the growth-associated protein GAP-43 in the developing human brainstem. J Neuropathol Exp Neurol 1993;52(1):39–54.

[13] Zec N, Filiano JJ, Panigrahy A, et al. Developmental changes in [3H]lysergic acid diethylamide ([3H]LSD) binding to serotonin receptors in the human brainstem. J Neuropathol Exp Neurol 1996;55(1):114–26.

[14] Paterson DS, Belliveau RA, Trachtenberg F, et al. Differential development of 5-HT receptor and the serotonin transporter binding in the human infant medulla. J Comp Neurol 2004;472(2):221–31.

[15] Paterson DS, Thompson EG, Kinney HC. Serotonergic and glutamatergic neurons at the ventral medullary surface of the human infant: observations relevant to central chemosensitivity in early human life. Auton Neurosci 2006;124(1–2):112–24.

[16] Kinney HC, Panigrahy A, Rava LA, et al. Three-dimensional distribution of [3H]quinuclidinyl benzilate binding to muscarinic cholinergic receptors in the developing human brainstem. J Comp Neurol 1995;362(3):350–67.

[17] Kinney HC, Ottoson CK, White WF. Three-dimensional distribution of 3H-naloxone binding to opiate receptors in the human fetal and infant brainstem. J Comp Neurol 1990;291(1):55–78.

[18] Kinney HC, O'Donnell TJ, Kriger P, et al. Early developmental changes in [3H]nicotine binding in the human brainstem. Neuroscience 1993;55(4):1127–38.

[19] Panigrahy A, Rosenberg PA, Assmann S, et al. Differential expression of glutamate receptor subtypes in human brainstem sites involved in perinatal hypoxia-ischemia. J Comp Neurol 2000;427(2):196–208.

[20] Mansouri J, Panigrahy A, Assmann SF, et al. Distribution of alpha 2-adrenergic receptor binding in the developing human brain stem. Pediatr Dev Pathol 2001;4(3):222–36.

[21] Cordes SP. Molecular genetics of the early development of hindbrain serotonergic neurons. Clin Genet 2005;68(6):487–94.

[22] Whitaker-Azmitia PM, Druse M, Walker P, et al. Serotonin as a developmental signal. Behav Brain Res 1996;73(1–2):19–29.

[23] Richerson GB, Wang W, Hodges MR, et al. Homing in on the specific phenotype(s) of central respiratory chemoreceptors. Exp Physiol 2005;90(3):259–66.

[24] Taylor NC, Li A, Nattie EE. Medullary serotonergic neurones modulate the ventilatory response to hypercapnia, but not hypoxia in conscious rats. J Physiol 2005;566(Pt 2):543–57.

[25] Brazy JE, Kinney HC, Oakes WJ. Central nervous system structural lesions causing apnea at birth. J Pediatr 1987;111(2):163–75.

[26] Panigrahy A, White WF, Rava LA, et al. Developmental changes in [3H]kainate binding in human brainstem sites vulnerable to perinatal hypoxia-ischemia. Neuroscience 1995;67(2):441–54.

[27] Abu-Shaweesh JM. Maturation of respiratory reflex responses in the fetus and neonate. Semin Perinatol 2004;9:169–80.

[28] Cohen G, Katz-Salamon M. Development of chemoreceptor responses in infants. Resp Physiol & Neurobiol 2005;149:233–42.

[29] Haddad GG, Farber JP. Developmental neurobiology of breathing; vol 53. 1st edition. New York: Marcel Dekker; 1991.

[30] Funk GD, Feldman JL. Generation of respiratory rhythm and pattern in mammals: insights from developmental studies. Curr Opin Neurobiol 1995;5:778–85.

[31] Rekling JC, Feldman JL. PreBotzinger complex and pacemaker neurons: hypothesized site and kernel for respiratory rhythm generation. Annu Rev Physiol 1998;60:385–405.

[32] St-John WM. Neurogenesis, control, and functional significance of gasping. J Appl Physiol 1990;68:1305–15.

[33] St-John WM. Gasping and autoresuscitation. In: Mathew OP, editor. Respiratory control and disorders in the newborn. New York: Marcel Dekker; 2003. p. 173:17–38.

[34] Onimaru H, Homma I, Feldman JL, et al. Point: counterpoint: the parafacial respiratory group (pFRG)/pre-Botzinger complex (preBotC) is the primarhy site of respiratory rhythm generation in the mammal. J Appl Physiol 2006;100:2094–8.

[35] St-John WM, Zhou D. Rostral pontine mechanisms regulate durations of expiratory phases. J Appl Physiol 1991;71:2133–7.

[36] Eichenwald EC, Stark AR. Maturation of respiratory control. In: Mathew OP, editor. Respiratory control and disorders in the newborn. New York: Marcel Dekker; 2003. 173:55–372.

[37] Heldt GP. Development of stability of the respiratory system in preterm infants. J Appl Physiol 1988;65(1):441–4.

[38] Lehtonen L, Martin RJ. Ontogeny of sleep and awake states in relation to breathing in preterm infants. Semin Perinatol 2004;9:229–38.

[39] Henderson-Smart DJ, Read JC. Reduced lung volume during behavioral active sleep in the newborn. J Appl Physiol 1979;46(6):1081–5.

[40] Cross KW, Klaus M, Tooley WH, et al. The response of the newborn baby to inflation of the lungs. J Physiol 1960;151:551–65.

[41] Widdicombe J. Henry Head and his paradoxical reflex. J Physiol 2004;559(Pt 1):1–2.

[42] Thach BT, Tauesch HW. Sighing in human newborn infants:role of inflation-augmenting reflex. J Appl Physiol 1976;41:502–7.

[43] Thach BT, Stark AR. Spontaneous neck flexion and airway obstruction during apneic spells in preterm infants. J Pediatr 1979;94(2):275–81.

[44] Mathew OP, Roberts JL, Thach BT. Pharyngeal airway obstruction in preterm infants during mixed and obstructive apnea. J Pediatr 1982;100:964–8.

[45] Mathew OP. Maintenance of upper airway patency. J Pediatr 1985;106:863–9.

[46] Kosch PC, Hutchinson AA, Wozniak JA, et al. Posterior cricoarytenoid and diaphragm activities during tidal breathing in neonates. J Appl Physiol 1988;64:1968–78.

[47] Eichenwald EC, Howell RG, Kosch PC, et al. Developmental changes in sequential activation of laryngeal abductor muscle and diaphragm in infants. J Appl Physiol 1992;73(4): 1425–31.

[48] Gauda EB, Miller MJ, Carlo WA, et al. Genioglossus response to airway occlusion in apneic versus nonapneic infants. Pediatr Res 1987;22(6):683–7.

[49] Cohen G, Henderson-Smart DJ. Upper airway stability and apnea during nasal occlusion in newborn infants. J Appl Physiol 1986;60(5):1511–7.

[50] Cohen G, Henderson-Smart DJ. Upper airway muscle activity during nasal occlusion in newborn babies. J Appl Physiol 1989;66(3):1328–35.

[51] Boggs DF, Bartlett D. Chemical specificity of a laryngeal apneic reflex in puppies. J Appl Physiol 1982;53:455–62.

[52] Anderson JW, Sant'Ambrogio FB, Mathew OP, et al. Water-responsive laryngeal receptors in the dog are not specialized endings. Respir Physiol 1990;79:33–44.

[53] Pickens DL, Schefft GL, Thach BT. Pharyngeal fluid clearance and aspiration preventive mechanisms in sleeping infants. J Appl Physiol 1989;66(3):1164–71.

[54] Davies AM, Koenig JS, Thach BT. Upper airway chemoreflex responses to saline and water in preterm infants. J Appl Physiol 1988;64(4):1412–20.

[55] Poets CF. Gastroesophageal reflux: a critical review of its role in preterm infants. Pediatr 2004;113(2):e128–32.

[56] Nattie EE. Central chemosensitivity, sleep, and wakefulness. Respir Physiol 2001;129(1–2): 257–68.

[57] Rigatto H, Kwiatkowski KA, Hasan SU, et al. The ventilatory response to endogenous CO2 in preterm infants. Am Rev Respir Dis 1991;143(1):101–4.

[58] Carroll JL, Bamford OS, Fitzgerald RS. Postnatal maturation of carotid chemoreceptor responses to O2 and CO2 in the cat. J Appl Physiol 1993;75(6):2383–91.

[59] Avery ME, Chernick V, Dutton RE, et al. Ventilatory response to inspired carbon dioxide in infants and adults. J Appl Physiol 1963;18(5):895–903.

[60] Rigatto H. Control of ventilation in the newborn. Ann Rev Physiol 1984;46:661–74.

[61] Rigatto H, Brady JF, Verduzco RT. Chemoreceptor reflexes in preterm infants: II. The effect of gestational and postnatal age on the ventilatory response to inhaled carbon dioxide. Pediatr 1975;55:614–20.

[62] Frantz ID, Adler SM, Thach BT, et al. Maturational effects on respiratory responses to carbon dioxide in premature infants. J Appl Physiol 1976;41(1):41–5.

[63] Cohen G, Xu C, Henderson-Smart D. Ventilatory response of the sleeping newborn to CO2 during normoxic rebreathing. J Appl Physiol 1991;71:168–74.

[64] Gerhardt T, Bancalari E. Apnea of prematurity I. Lung function and regulation of breathing. Pediatr 1984;74:58–62.

[65] Gerhardt T, Bancalari E. Apnea of prematurity II. Respiratory reflexes. Pediatr 1984;74: 63–6.

[66] Hunt C. Ontogeny of autonomic regulation in late preterm infants born at 34–37 weeks postmenstrual age. Semin Perinatol 2006;30:73–6.

[67] Johnston BM, Gluckman PD. Lateral pontine lesions affect central chemosensitivity in unanesthetized fetal lambs. J Appl Physiol 1989;67:1113–8.

[68] Alvaro R, Alvarez J, Kwiatkowski K, et al. Small preterm infants (less than equal to1500 g) have only a sustained decrease in ventilation in response to hypoxia. Pediatr Res 1992;32:403–6.

[69] Sankaran K, Wiebe H, Seshia MMK, et al. Immediate and late ventilatory response to high and low O₂ in preterm infants and adult subjects. Pediatr Res 1979;13:875–8.

[70] Weiskopf RB, Gabel RA. Depression of ventilation during hypoxia in man. J Appl Physiol 1975;39(6):911–5.

[71] Martin RJ, DiFiore JM, Jana L, et al. Persistence of the biphasic ventilatory response to hypoxia in preterm infants. J Pediatr 1998;132(6):960–4.

[72] Blanco CE, Hanson MA, Johnson P, et al. Breathing pattern of kittens during hypoxia. J Appl Physiol 1984;56(1):12–7.

[73] Darnall RA, Bruce RD. Effects of adenosine and xanthine derivatives on breathing during acute hypoxia in the anesthetized newborn piglet. Pediatr Pulmonol 1987;3(2):110–6.

[74] Darnall RA Jr. Aminophylline reduces hypoxic ventilatory depression: possible role of adenosine. Pediatr Res 1985;19(7):706–10.

[75] Bruce RD, Darnall RA, Althaus JS. Aminophylline reduces hypoxic ventilatory depression without increasing catecholamines. Pediatr Pulmonol 1986;2(4):218–24.

[76] Lagercrantz H, Runold M, Yamamoto Y, et al. Adenosine: a putative mediator of the hypoxic ventilatory response of the neonate. In: Lagercrantz H, editor. Neurobiology of the control of breathing. New York: Raven Press; 1987. p. 133–9.

[77] Hedner J, Hedner T. On the involvement of GABA in the Central respiratory regulation of the adult and newborn. In: Von Euler C, Lagercrantz H, editors. Neurobiology of the control of breathing. New York: Raven Press; 1987. p. 109–17.

[78] St.-John WM, St.-Jacques R, Li A, et al. Modulation of hypoxic depressions of ventilatory activity in the newborn piglet by mesencephalic mechanisms. Brain Res 1998;.

[79] Rigatto H, Brady Jp, Verduzco RT. Chemoreceptor reflexes in preterm infants: I. The effect of gestational and postnatal age on the ventilatory response to inhalation of 100% and 15% oxygen. Pediatr 1975;55:604–13.

[80] Rigatto H, Kalapesi Z, Leahy FN, et al. Ventilatory response to 100% and 15% O2 during wakefulness and sleep in preterm infants. Early Hum Dev 1982;7:1–10.

[81] Thach BT, Menon A. Pulmonary protective mechanisms in human infants. Am Rev Respir Dis 1985;131(5):S55–8.

[82] Mathew OP. Respiratory control during oral feeding. In: mathew OP, editor. Respiratory control and disorders in the newborn, Vol 173. New York: Marcel Dekker; 2003. p. 373–93.

[83] Gewolb IH, Vice FL, Scheiter-Kenney EL, et al. Developmental patterns of rhythmic suck and swallow in preterm infants. Dev Med Child Neurol 2001;43:22–37.

[84] Qureshi MA, Vice FL, Taciak V, et al. Changes in rhythmic suckle feeding in term infants in the first month of life. Dev Med Child Neurol 2002;44:34–9.

[85] Ardran GM, Kemp FH, Lind J. A cineradiographic study of breast feeding. Br J Radiol 1958;31(363):156–62.

[86] Thach BT. Can we breathe and swallow at the same time. J Appl Physiol 2005;99:1633.

[87] Shivpuri CR, Martin RJ, Carlo WA, et al. Decreased ventilation in preterm infants during oral feeding. J Pediatr 1983;103(2):285–9.

[88] Samson N, St-Hilaire M, Nsegbe E, et al. Effect of nasal continuous or intermittent positive airway pressure on nonnutritive swallowing in newborn lamb. J Appl Physiol 2005;99:1636–42.

[89] Wilson SL, Thach BT, Brouillette RT, et al. Coordination of breathing and swallowing in human infants. J Appl Physiol 1981;50:851–8.

[90] Henderson-Smart DJ, Pettigrew AG, Campbell DJ. Clinical apnea and brainstem neural function in preterm infants. N Engl J Med 1983;308:353–7.

[91] Mathew OP, Saint'Ambrogio FB. Laryngeal reflexes. In: Mathew OP, Saint'Ambrogio FB, editors. Respiratory function of the upper airway. New York: Marcel Dekker; 1988. p. 259–302.

[92] Gewolb IH, Vice FL. Maturational changes in the rhythms, patterning, and coordination of respiration and swallow during feeding in preterm and term infants. Dev Med Child Neurol 2006;48:589–94.

[93] Rigatto H. Periodic Breathing. In: Mathew OP, editor. Respiratory control and disorders in the newborn, Vol 173. New York: Marcel Dekker, Inc; 2003. p. 237–72.

[94] Waggener TB, Stark AR, Cohlan BA, Frantz ID. Apnea duration is related to ventilatory oscillation characteristics in newborn infants. J Appl Physiol 1984;57(2):536–44.

[95] Johnson P, Andrews DC. Thermometabolism and cardiorespiratory control during the perinatal period. In: Beckerman RC, editor. Respiratory Control Diseases in Infants and Children. Baltimore (MD): Williams and Wilkins; 1992. p. 76–88.

[96] Mortola JP, Gautier H. Interaction between metabolism and ventilation: effects of respiratory gases and temperature. In: Dempsey JA, Pack AI, editors. Regulation of breathing, Vol 79. New York: Marcel Dekker; 1995. p. 1011–64.

[97] Morrison SF. Central pathways controlling brown adipose tissue thermogenesis. News Physiol Sci 2004;19:67–74.

[98] Ootsuka Y, Blessing WW. Activation of 5–HT1A receptors in rostral medullary raphe inhibits cutaneous vasoconstriction elicited by cold exposure in rabbits. Brain Res 2006; 1073–1074:252–61.

[99] Parmeggiani PL, Rabini D. Shivering and panting during sleep. Brain Res 1967;6:789–91.

[100] Darnall RA, Ariagno RL. The effect of sleep state on active thermoregulation in the premature infant. Pediatr Res 1982;16:512–4.

[101] Curran AK, Xia L, Leiter JC, et al. Elevated body temperature enhances the laryngeal chemoreflex in decerebrate piglets. J Appl Physiol 2005;98:780–6.

[102] Tryba AK, Ramirez JM. Response of the respiratory network of mice to hyperthermia. J Neurophysiol 2003;89(6):2975–83.

[103] Ramanathan R, Corwin MJ, Hunt CE, et al. Cardiorespiratory events recorded on home monitors-comparison of healthy infants with those at increased risk for SIDS. JAMA 2001;285:2199–207.

[104] Malloy M, Freeman DJ. Birth weight- and gestational age-specific sudden infant death syndrome mortality: United States, 1991 versus 1995. Pediatrics 2000;6:1227–31.

[105] Malloy M, Hoffman H. Prematurity, sudden infant death syndrome, and age of death. Pediatrics 1995;3:464–71.

[106] Hüppi PS, Schuknecht B, Boesch C. Structural and neurobehavioral delay in postnatal brain development of preterm infants. Pediatr Res 1996;1996(39):895–901.

[107] Darnall RA, Kattwinkel J, Nattie C, et al. Margin of safety for discharge after apnea in preterm infants. Pediatr 1997;100(5):795–801.

[108] Eichenwald EC, Aina A, Stark AR. Apnea frequently persists beyond term gestation in infants delivered at 24 to 28 weeks. Pediatr 1997;100(3 Pt 1):354–9.

[109] Mirmiran M. The function of fetal/neonatal rapid eye movement sleep. Behav Brain Res 1995;69:13–22.

[110] Mulder EJ, Visser GH, Bekedam DJ, et al. Emergence of behavioral states in fetuses of type-I diabetic women. Early Hum Dev 1987;15:231–51.

[111] Visser GH, Poelmann-Weesjes G, Cohen TMN, et al. Fetal behavior at 30 to 32 weeks of gestation. Pediatr Res 1987;22:655–8.

[112] Curzi-Dascalova L, Figueroa JM, Eiselt M, et al. Sleep state organization in premature infants of less than 35 weeks gestational age. Pediatr Res 1993;34:624–8.

[113] Curzi-Dascalova L, Peirano P, More-Kahn F. Development of sleep states in normal premature and full term infants. Dev Psychobiol 1988;21:431–44.

[114] Mirmiran M, Mass YG, Ariagno RL. Development of fetal and neonatal sleep and circadian rhythms. Sleep Med Rev 2003;7(4):321–34.

[115] Curzi-Dascalova L, Mirmiran M. Manual of methods for recording and analyzing sleep-wakefulness states in preterm and full-term infants. Paris: Les editions INSERM; 1996.

[116] Curzi-Dascalova L, Challamel MJ. Neurophysiological basis of sleep development. In: Loughlin GM, Carroll JL, Marcus CL, editors. Sleep and breathing in children, Vol 147. New York: Marcel Dekker; 2000. p. 3–37.

[117] Roffwarg HP, Muzio JN, Dement WC. Ontogenetic development of the human sleep-dream cycle. Science 1966;152:604–19.

[118] Birnholz JC. The development of human fetal eye movement patterns. Science 1981;213: 679–81.

[119] Inoue M, Koyanagi T, Nakahara H, et al. Functional development of human eye movement in utero assessed quantitatively with real time ultrasound. Am J Obstetr Gynecol 1986;155:170–4.

[120] Mirmiran M, Uylings HB, Corner MA. Pharmacological suppression of REM sleep prior to weaning counteracts the effectiveness of subsequent environmental enrichment on cortical growth in rats. Brain Res 1983;283:102–5.

[121] Frank MG, Issa N, Stryker MP. Sleep enhances plasticity in the developing visual cortex. Neuron 2001;30:275–87.

[122] Oksenberg A, Shaffery JP, Marks JP, et al. Rapid eye movement sleep deprivation in kittens amplifies LGN cell-size disparity induced by monocular deprivation. Dev Brain Res 1996; 97:51–61.

[123] Shaffery JP, Roffwarg HP, Speciale SG, et al. Ponto-geniculo-occipital-wave suppression amplifies lateral geniculate nucleus cell-size changes in monocularly deprived kittens. Dev Brain Res 1999;114:109–19.

[124] Reppert SM, Schwartz WJ. Functional activity of the suprachiasmatic nucleus in the fetal primate. Neurosci Lett 1984;46:145–9.

[125] Rivkees SA, Hofman PL, Fortman J. Newborn primate infants are entrained by low intensity lighting. Proc Natl Acad Sci USA 1997;94:292–7.

[126] Hao HP, Rivkees SA. The circadian clock of very premature primate infants is responsive to light. Proc Natl Acad Sci USA 1999;96:2426–9.

[127] Mirmiran M, Lunshof S. Perinatal development of human circadian rhythms. Prog Brain Res 1996;111:217–26.

[128] Lunshof S, Boer K, Wolf H, et al. Fetal and maternal diurnal rhythms during the third trimester of normal pregnancy: outcomes of computerized analysis of continuous 24-hr fetal heart rate recordings. Am J Obstetr Gynecol 1998;178:247–54.

[129] Petersen SA, Anderson ES, Lodemore M, et al. Sleeping position and rectal temperature. Arch Dis Child 1991;66:976–9.

[130] Mantagos S, Moustogiannis A, Makri M, et al. The effect of light on plasma melatonin levels in premature infants. J Pediatr Endocrinol Metab 1996;9:387–92.

[131] Mantagos S, Moustogiannis A, Vagenakis AG. Diurnal variation of plasma-cortisol levels in infancy. J Pediatr Endocrinol Metab 1998;11:549–53.

[132] Antonini SR, Jorge SM, Moreira AC. The emergence of salivary cortisol circadian rhythm and its relationship to sleep activity in preterm infants. Clin Endocrinol (Oxf) 2000;52: 423–6.

[133] Salzarulo P, Fagioli I, Solomon F, et al. Sleep patterns in infants under continuous feeding from birth. Electroencephalogr Clin Neurophysiol 1980;49:330–6.

[134] Salzarulo P, Fagioli I, Solomon F. Maturation of sleep patterns in infants under continuous nutrition from birth. Acta Chir Scand Suppl 1980;498:78–82.

[135] Mirmiran M, Ariagno R. Influence of light in the NICU on the development of circadian rhythms in preterm infants. Semin Perinatol 2000;24:247–57.

[136] Sadeh A. Sleep and melatonin in infants: a preliminary study. Sleep 1997;20:185–91.

[137] Sitka U, Weinert D, Berle K, et al. Investigations of the rhythmic function of heart rate, blood pressure, and temperature in neonates. Eur J Pediatr 1994;153:117–22.

[138] Lohr B, Siegmund R. Ultradian and circadian rhythms of sleep-wake and food-intake behavior during early infancy. Chronobiol Int 1999;16:129–48.

[139] Weintraub Z, Cates D, Kwiatkowski K, et al. The morphology of periodic breathing in infants and adults. Resp Physiol 2001;127:173–84.

[140] Horne RS, Bandopadhayay P, Vitkovic J, et al. Effects of age and sleeping position on arousal from sleep in preterm infants. Sleep 2002;25(7):746–50.

[141] Ariagno RL, van Liempt S, Mirmiran M. Fewer spontaneous arousals during prone sleep in preterm infants at 1 and 3 months corrected age. J Perinatol 2006;26:306–12.

Is the Late Preterm Infant More Vulnerable to Gray Matter Injury than the Term Infant?

Saraid S. Billiards, PhD[a,b,*],
Christopher R. Pierson, MD, PhD[a,b,c],
Robin L. Haynes, PhD[a,b,d],
Rebecca D. Folkerth, MD[a,b,c],
Hannah C. Kinney, MD[a,b]

[a]Department of Pathology, Enders Building, Room 1109, Children's Hospital Boston,
300 Longwood Avenue, Boston, MA 02115, USA
[b]Harvard Medical School, 300 Longwood Avenue, Boston, MA 02115, USA
[c]Department of Pathology, Brigham and Women's Hospital,
75 Francis Street, Boston, MA 02115 USA
[d]Department of Neurology, Children's Hospital Boston, 300 Longwood Avenue,
Boston, MA 02115, USA

Although long-term neurodevelopmental abnormalities in preterm (<34 gestational weeks) infants are well recognized, mounting evidence suggests that neurologic morbidity is also a considerable problem for near-term (34–36 gestational weeks) infants [1,2]. Attempts to delay delivery have not been considered essential for the near-term infant because the general perception is that the infant is considered "near-normal" [2–4]. The problem of late preterm birth is significant (approximately 320,000 or 7.9% of all live births in 2003) [5], given that there has been an almost 16% increase in the rate of prematurity between 1990 and 2003 (500,000 infants or 12.3% of all births were delivered preterm in 2003) [5], with approximately two thirds of this increase due to an increase in late preterm births [6]. A shift in the

This work was supported by the National Institute of Neurological Disorders and Stroke (PO1-NS38475); the National Institute of Child Health and Development (P30-HD18655); Children's Hospital Boston Developmental Disabilities Center; and the National Multiple Sclerosis Society.

* Corresponding author. Department of Pathology, Enders Building, Room 1109, Children's Hospital Boston, 300 Longwood Avenue Boston, MA 02115.

E-mail address: saraid.billiards@childrens.harvard.edu (S.S. Billiards).

0095-5108/06/$ - see front matter © 2006 Elsevier Inc. All rights reserved.
doi:10.1016/j.clp.2006.10.003

perception of the susceptibility of the late preterm infant to overall morbidity, including feeding difficulties, respiratory disorders, infection, apnea, hypoglycemia, hyperbilirubinemia, kernicterus, and temperature instability [2], is reflected in the very recent recommendation that the phrase "near-term" be changed to "late preterm." The latter term underscores the vulnerabilities of these infants due to the lack of the full growth and development yet to be reached at term. In a prospective study of 869 low birth weight infants, nearly 20% of the cohort born at 34 to 37 weeks had significant behavior problems that persisted to 8 years of age [6]. These recent clinical data underscore the need for understanding the cellular and molecular mechanisms that underlie the vulnerability of the late preterm brain to devise developmentally relevant interventions and therapy.

The challenging question to pediatric neuropathologists by the editors of this monograph was: is the late preterm infant more vulnerable to brain injury than the term infant? Obviously, brain injury in the premature infant at all gestational ages is complex and involves the whole spectrum of disease, including infection (meningitis), inborn errors of metabolism, genetic anomalies, acquired metabolic disorders (kernicterus and hypoglycemia), neoplasia, malformations, and birth trauma [7,8]. This review focuses upon the vulnerability of the brain's neurons to hypoxia-ischemia in the late preterm versus term infant as an initial step toward answering the editors' question. This review complements the authors' recent review of cerebral white matter vulnerability to hypoxia-ischemia and periventricular leukomalacia in the late preterm infant [9]. This discussion summarizes available information on the developing human brain and addresses approaches of which such information can be enhanced by future human postmortem studies. The authors begin with a brief summary of the pathogenesis of perinatal hypoxia-ischemia to gray matter (neurons) injury as a guide to the analysis of the human fetal brain data relevant to vulnerability. Several recent reviews of hypoxic-ischemic damage in the perinatal period are available [10–12].

Perinatal hypoxic-ischemic injury to the gray matter

The critical consequence of hypoxic-ischemic injury is diminished oxygen supply, with hypoxia-ischemia referring to the two mechanisms of oxygen deficiency (ie, diminished oxygen supply in the blood [hypoxia], and diminished amount of blood perfusing the brain tissue [ischemia]) (Fig. 1). Neuronal cell injury and death is primarily caused by deprivation of oxygen and glucose, the two key energy sources for the brain. Because neither oxygen nor glucose is stored in the brain, deprivation of only a few minutes can cause neuronal energy depletion and death [7]. Initially, hypoxia-ischemia depresses adenosine triphosphate synthesis and hence ion-pump failure. It also depresses the mechanisms involved in the energy-dependent uptake of glutamate, the major excitatory amino acid neurotransmitter in the brain,

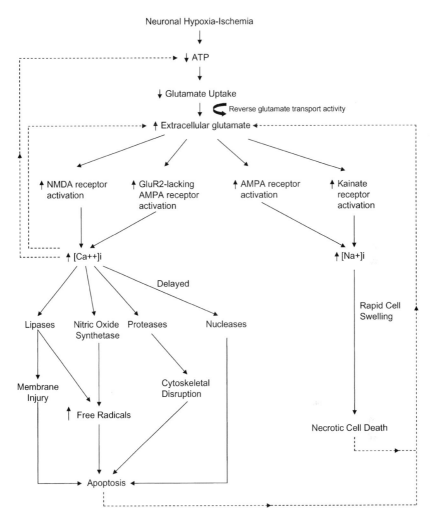

Fig. 1. The cascade of events that ultimately leads to neuronal cell death following hypoxic-ischemic–induced injury is initiated by energy depletion, followed by the accumulation of excitotoxic amino acids (primarily glutamate), excessive glutamate receptor depolarization, increase in intracellular calcium, the generation of free radicals which attack the integrity of the neuron and surrounding tissue, neuronal cell death and dropout, and instigation of the inflammatory response, with reactive astrocytes and activated microglia.

by glutamate transporters in presynaptic nerve terminals and in astrocytes, which, in excessive amounts, leads to neuronal injury and death (excitotoxicity) [10,13–16]. Extracellular glutamate accumulation is followed by excessive glutamate receptor activation and depolarization (see Fig. 1) [14,17–20]. The finding of elevated levels of glutamate in the cerebrospinal fluid of infants who have hypoxic-ischemic brain injury supports a role for excitotoxicity in humans [21].

Increased extracellular glutamate causes prolonged stimulation of the N-methyl-D-aspartate (NMDA) receptors and non-NMDA receptors (kainate and α-amino-3-hydroxy-5-methyl-4-isoxazole [AMPA]), thereby allowing increased calcium or sodium influx into neurons (see Fig. 1) [10,17,22]. Calcium and sodium enter the neuron through the open NMDA channels, whereas sodium enters through the open AMPA and kainate channels (see Fig. 1). The heteromeric AMPA receptor is comprised of four subunits (GluR1, GluR2, GluR3, and GluR4). Of considerable relevance to the pathogenesis of neuronal injury due to hypoxia-ischemia and the key role of calcium cytotoxicity, the lack of the GluR2 subunit renders the channel permeable to calcium [23]. Increases in intracellular sodium and water cause cell swelling and rapid cell death by way of kainate and AMPA receptor-mediated mechanisms. On the other hand, increased intracellular calcium concentrations by way of NMDA and AMPA receptor-mediated mechanisms (in which the GluR2 subunit is lacking) play a major role in delayed cell death with multiple deleterious consequences, including free radical injury (see Fig. 1). Excitotoxicity is complicated by free radical toxicity, which likewise contributes to neuronal injury and death (see Fig. 1). Free radicals are highly reactive compounds that interact with normal cellular components to produce cell injury leading to necrosis or apoptosis, the two principle forms of neuronal death. The majority of free radical sources are directly or indirectly related to increased cytosolic calcium, a major consequence of increased glutamate levels and prolonged glutamate receptor activation (see Fig. 1).

Neuronal necrosis is characterized by cellular swelling, membrane disintegration, and an inflammatory cellular response that, if excessive or prolonged, can damage neighboring cells; it typically occurs after an intense but brief insult. Apoptosis, on the other hand, is a delayed cellular response to prolonged injury that involves gene activation and protein synthesis and mimics the mechanisms of programmed cell death during normal development. In tissue sections of perinatal human brains, the conventional morphologic criteria for apoptosis are: intense, uniform nuclear basophilia; chromatin condensation with nuclear shrinkage (pyknosis) or fragmentation of the nucleus into several rounded and uniformly dense basophilic masses (karyorrhexis); or the formation of apoptotic bodies [24]. Cells are considered necrotic if they have intensely eosinophilic cytoplasm, pyknotic or karyorrhectic nuclei, breakdown of the nuclear and plasma membranes, and cell swelling [8,24]. Immunocytochemical markers for cleaved caspase-3 expression (activation) are considered reliable indicators of cells undergoing apoptosis, particularly when combined with the terminal deoxytransferase-mediated dUTP-biotin nick end labeling (TUNEL) method that identifies dying cells [25,26]. Several factors are likely to influence whether a cell undergoes apoptosis or necrosis after hypoxic-ischemic injury, including the type of initiating insult, the severity and duration of injury, and the stage of cell maturation and cell type [27]. Detection of cleaved caspase-3 in the developing human brain is limited thus far to cases of pontosubicular necrosis [28,29] and has notbeen analyzed specifically in relationship to the late preterm time frame.

Gray matter development in the late preterm brain

The potential for increased vulnerability of the late preterm brain to injury is underscored by recognition of its substantial overall immaturity relative to the term brain, and the immense growth of the gray matter that occurs from 34 weeks to term. At 34 gestational weeks, the total brain weight is 65% of that at term; there is still 35% of brain weight yet to be obtained to reach term (40 weeks) weight over the ensuing 6 weeks [9]. The question arises, what is the timetable of the fetal development of different gray matter regions relative to one another in the human brain? Although the precise maturational sequences of gray matter regions are unknown, the order is defined by the embryonic (and phylogenic) pattern of structural development (ie, with caudal to rostral progression, rhomboencephalon before diencephalon before telencephalon) and primary cortical before association cortical regions. These patterns are indicated by the regional sequences of myelination [30,31] with the underlying concept that myelination follows upon neuronal maturation and is a marker of "completed" neuronal/axonal maturation. The overall concept of central nervous system myelination is that sequences progress in a hierarchical order, which determines the neurodevelopment of the fetus (eg, "primitive" brainstem functions developing before "advanced" cortical cognitive functions). It is known that the brainstem and thalamus (cerebral cortical relay) demonstrate earlier dendritic maturation than the cerebral cortex [7,32,33]. The sequences of neurologic development have begun to be determined in the fetus *in utero* (eg, movement, breathing, arousal, heart rate variability) and postdelivery (eg, muscle tone, sensory perception, reflexes) [34]. Ultimately, the goal is to correlate the biologic sequences of brain development with the clinical sequences of specific neurologic functions and behaviors, to characterize fully the vulnerability to injury at specific time-points.

Perhaps the most information available about neuronal development in the human fetus concerns the cerebral cortex. This body of information serves as a template for the types of information needed for all gray matter regions. Neuroimaging studies of the volume of the cerebral cortex demonstrate that the late preterm infant at 34 postconceptional weeks achieves approximately 55% of the full-term volume, with 45% growth yet to occur [35]. Yet clearly, different gray matter regions develop at different rates. In a neuroimaging study of cerebellar growth in the human fetus, the degree of growth from 28 postconceptional weeks to term is greater (177%) than the increase in total brain volume (107%) (Fig. 2) [36]. Like the cerebral cortex, however, its volume at 34 gestational weeks is approximately 55% of that at term.

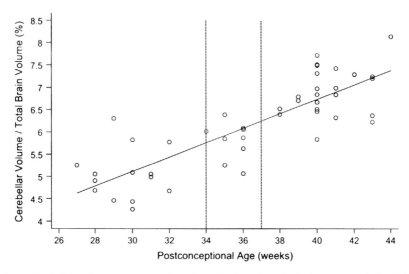

Fig. 2. Cerebellar volume as a proportion of total brain volume in the late preterm infant (*dotted lines*) is approximately 55% that of the term infant. (*Adapted from* Limperopoulos C, Soul JS, Gauvreau K, et al. Late gestation cerebellar growth is rapid and impeded by premature birth. Pediatrics 2005;115(3):688–95; with permission.)

After the cessation of neuronal proliferation and migration to the human cortical plate around midgestation (20–24 weeks), dramatic events occur in the organization of the cerebral cortex to term in synchronized and integrated sequences. These events include: secondary and tertiary gyration; alignment, orientation, and lamination of the migrated cortical neurons; neurotransmitter phenotypic differentiation; dendritic arborization; axonal elongation and collateralization, vascularization, gliogenesis, and even myelination [7,8,30,31,37–39]. The timetable of synaptogenesis in different gray matter regions in the human fetal brain is beginning to be defined with the use of modern immunocytochemical markers for synaptic proteins [8,40–42]. The expression of the growth cone-related phosphoprotein GAP-43, for example, is increasingly expressed over the last half of gestation in the neuropil (ie, the site of synaptic contacts between in-growing axonal terminals and spines) [41] (Fig. 3). The developmental changes in the late preterm brain are not yet established for any cerebral cortical region. Unpublished data from our laboratory about GAP-43 expression determined by quantitative Western blot analysis in the human parietal cortex suggests the that there is a transient elevation in synaptogenesis in the late preterm brain (Fig. 4). Further analysis with larger sample sizes and in different cortical regions for comparison are needed.

A critical component for the correct "wiring" in the development of the cerebral cortex is the subplate neuron. This neuron is the earliest to differentiate in cortical development, emerging from the ventricular zone and migrating to the primitive marginal zone early in the first trimester, before the

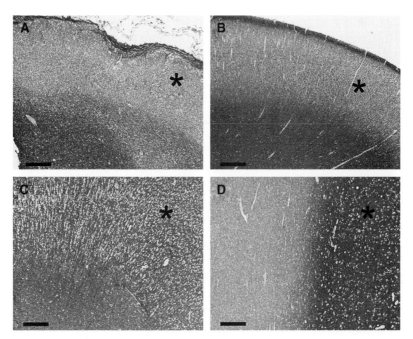

Fig. 3. GAP-43 immunocytochemistry shows differential expression of GAP-43 in the parietal white matter and overlying cortex at the increasing ages of (*A*) 20 postconceptional (PC) weeks; (*B*) 27 PC weeks; (*C*) 37 PC weeks; and (*D*) 144 PC weeks. Note the switch of GAP-43 expression from predominately white matter to cortex (*) around term (*C*). (*From* Haynes RL, Borenstein NS, Desilva TM, et al. Axonal development in the cerebral white matter of the human fetus and infant. J Comp Neurol 2005;484(2):156–67; with permission.)

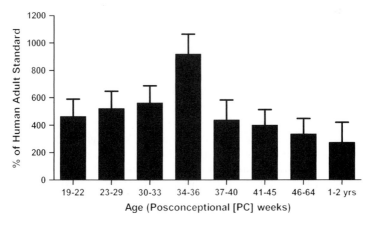

Fig. 4. GAP-43 expression levels in the developing cerebral (parietal) cortex of human infants grouped according to ages (3–5 cases/group) reflecting epochs of brain development (including the late preterm period). Data are expressed as a percent of adult human standard. Of note, during the late preterm period (34–36 weeks), GAP-43 expression in the cerebral cortex remains high, suggesting that axons are still growing ($P = 0.12$) (*Data courtesy of* RL Haynes, PhD, Boston, MA, and Natalia Borenstein, MS, Boston, MA).

generation and migration of neurons to the cortical plate [43–45]. The sub-plate neurons receive synaptic inputs from thalamo-cortical afferents and aids axonal guidance to and from the thalamus [46–48]. Ablation of sub-plate neurons at approximately 70% gestation in a feline model results in an absence of layer IV in the cerebral cortex [47], attributed to an inability of ingrowing thalamocortical axons to reach this layer. Without subplate neurons acting as transient targets, these axons undergo degeneration [7,47]. The human subplate neurons reach their peak density between 22 to 34 weeks of gestation, after which programmed cell death with "pruning back" occurs, until approximately 6 postnatal months [49–51]. Thus, changes in the subplate number and density as well as neurochemical phe-notype are occurring in the late preterm brain, yet the specific details remain to be determined. A small proportion of subplate neurons persist in the ce-rebral white matter into adulthood as "interstitial" neurons [51]. Subplate neurons use glutamate and nitric oxide in neurotransmission with differen-tial expression of glutamate receptors and neuronal nitric oxide synthase across development in animal models [52–54].

Gray matter injury in the late preterm infant

In essence, the pathology of hypoxia-ischemia in the fetal brain reflects cellular and tissue reactions brought about by a complex interplay of the type, timing, and severity of the insult and its changing developmental vul-nerabilities during a period when the brain is at its peak capacity for plas-ticity and repair. Overall brain development is occurring so rapidly that responses to hypoxia-ischemia vary considerably even from midgestation to term, as witnessed by the preferential injury to cerebral white matter in the preterm infant compared with preferential injury to gray matter just a few months later in the postneonatal period. In the human fetal brain, neuronal injury may occur in a widespread distribution or in particular com-binations of sites (eg, thalamus-brainstem pattern). Some patterns of neuro-nal injury (eg, thalamic-brainstem injury, pontosubicular necrosis, and status marmoratus) are seen only in the fetal and term brain, and not in the mature (child or adult) brain. Indeed, the key regions of vulnerability to hypoxia-ischemia in the human adult brain are neurons in the cerebral cortex, hippocampus (Sommer's sector), and cerebellar cortex, with general sparing of brainstem neuronal populations and cerebral white matter [55]. The age at which this mature pattern of vulnerability is reached is uncertain, but based upon our personal clinical experience, it is set around the end of the second year of life, when the brain reaches 80% of adult weight (unpub-lished observations).

A recent survey we conducted of the neuropathology (subacute and chronic injury as indicated by gliosis and neuronal loss) of the premature in-fant in 41 cases revealed that, although cerebral and cerebellar white matter damage was the most common lesion in the preterm brain, it was associated with variable and substantial neuronal injury in multiple gray matter sites [56]. These sites preferentially included the thalamus, basal ganglia, cerebellum, and brainstem cerebellar-relay nuclei (inferior olive and basis pontis), with relative (but not complete) sparing of the cerebral cortex. We also found that the temporospatial profile of gray matter injury varied significantly from midgestation to term: brainstem injury precedes injury in the deep gray nuclei which precedes injury in the cerebral cortex. Parenthetically, this pattern mimics that of the caudal to rostral development of the brain (see earlier discussion). The inferior olive, which provides the sole source of climbing fibers to the cerebellum, appeared to be the most vulnerable site in the preterm brain to injury. In addition, 80% of the cases at birth demonstrated olivary gliosis, suggesting that this lesion arises in utero. Gliosis increased dramatically in the globus pallidus, thalamus, hippocampus, and basis pontis after birth, suggesting that these four gray matter sites are the most vulnerable to postnatal injury in premature infants. Of note, this dataset consisted of extremely ill premature infants who experienced hypoxic-ischemic, infectious/inflammatory, or metabolic insults before death. In recognition of the complex combination of white and gray matter lesion in the brains of premature infants, we termed the spectrum of injury the "encephalopathy of prematurity." Because these autopsied patients had complex clinical problems, we were unable to determine which of the many insults, alone or in combination, were responsible for the neuropathologic findings. Indeed, hypoxia-ischemia, hypoglycemia, and hyperbilirubinemia are all characterized by acute neuronal necrosis, neuronal loss, or gliosis, albeit in different topographic distributions [8], and all share common mechanisms of cell injury, particularly glutamate toxicity [8,57–59]. Thus, the encephalopathy of prematurity is likely secondary to a combination of systemic circulatory insufficiency and impaired cerebrovascular autoregulation in the ventilated premature infant that may be potentiated by inflammatory processes [7,57,60–63] and metabolic derangements [58,59].

Very little is known about the specific pattern of gray matter injury in the late preterm infant because essentially no autopsy (or neuroimaging) studies have focused upon this particular age range in comparison to early preterm or term infants. In our survey of the neuropathology of premature infants, we did not analyze specific age-related patterns of gray matter injury in large part because of the small sample size in each age bin (early, mid, and late preterm) and the lack of term brain analysis for comparison in the same study. The mean gestational age of the infants in our series of premature infants was 31.2 ± 3.9 weeks [56].

One approach to decipher preferential developmental gray matter vulnerability is to analyze the neuropathology by these specific age groups in the fetal and term periods. To demonstrate the principle of such analysis for this review, we performed an exploratory (unpublished) analysis. We compared pathologic variables among the preterm age groups in this series of

41 preterm infants, as well with those in 35 term infants dying in the immediate postnatal period following cardiac surgery of congenital heart disease
that were defined by us in a separate study [64]. We classified the cases according to the following gestational age groups: 23 to 29 weeks (n = 4), 30 to
33 weeks (n = 5), and 34 to 36 weeks (n = 4), thereby incorporating the
early, mid, and late preterm periods, and 37 weeks or greater (n = 35).
All of the preterm cases used in this analysis survived for less than 2 postnatal days, thereby indicating that the injuries sustained occurred in utero
or immediately around birth. We analyzed by site the variable of neuronal
necrosis because we had the most information about it across the second
half of gestation into the neonatal period. We also selected neuronal necrosis as the marker of neuronal injury because it is indicative of acute injury
(within 24 hours of insult) [55], and therefore reflects preferential susceptibility to hypoxia-ischemia around the time of death.

In the cerebral cortex, neuronal necrosis was not identified until 30 to 33
gestational weeks, and appeared to increase with advancing gestational age,
with the incidence of injury relatively comparable between the late preterm
group (75% of cases) and term group (68% of cases) (Fig. 5A) [64]. Different patterns of neuronal necrosis were suggested in different regions: in the
hippocampus, the incidence of neuronal necrosis appeared to increase
steadily with age (Fig. 5B), whereas in the basis pontis, it appeared to
peak in the late preterm period (Fig. 5C). Although these data are obviously
limited because of small sample size, they suggest that neuronal vulnerability
varies substantially by region and age in the human fetal brain. There is no
single pattern of vulnerability in all gray matter regions at one time.

The vulnerability of gray matter regions to hypoxia-ischemia in the late preterm infant

The reasons for selective neuronal vulnerability at different develomental
ages are clearly complex and multifactorial. Circulatory factors play a role
as evidenced by selective neuronal necrosis in vascular border zones of the
middle and anterior cerebral arteries in the term infant [7,57]. Other factors
that have been identified experimentally include developmental differences
in anaerobic glycolytic capacity, energy requirements, lactate accumula-
tions, calcium influx, free radical formation and scavenging capacity, regional distribution of glutamate receptors, and the regional accumulation
of excitotoxic amino acids [7,8,10,11]. In essence, the authors conceptualize
that the basis of a specific topographic pattern of gray matter injury at a particular age of the human fetal brain reflects the balance of protective and
susceptibility factors relevant to glutamate, free radical, and cytokine toxicity. These factors are developmentally regulated and dynamic, in that they
are changing rapidly relative to one another at the precise time in gestation
or at premature delivery when the hypoxic-ischemic insult occurs. Given

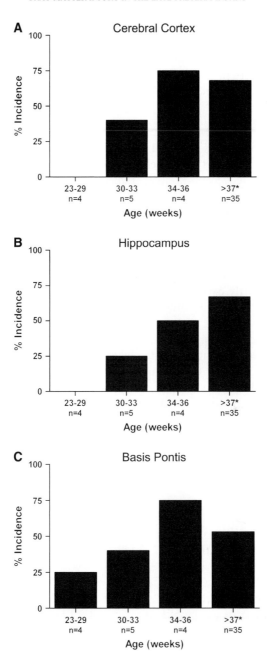

Fig. 5. Neuronal necrosis in the (A) cerebral cortex, (B) hippocampus, and (C) basis pontis of the early, mid, and late preterm, and term human infant. Note the increased incidence of neuronal necrosis during the late preterm period (34–36 weeks) in the cerebral cortex and basis pontis.

that these protective and susceptibility factors follow different temporal profiles in different gray matter sites, it is not unexpected that the pattern of
neuronal injury is complex and variable in the fetal and neonatal brain. Several of these factors in relationship to the vulnerability of the late preterm
brain are summarized below.

Glutamate receptors

Animal data link developmental vulnerability to hypoxia-ischemia in different gray matter regions to age-related transient elevations in pre- or post-
synaptic glutamate receptors [65]. Experimentally, glutamate receptor-
mediated mechanisms are involved in neurite outgrowth, synapse formation
and plasticity, and programmed cell death [66–76]. In developing animals,
NMDA and non-NMDA receptors are differentially distributed throughout
the cerebral cortex, hippocampus, basal ganglia, cerebellum, and brainstem
[65,77–79]. Of note, ontogenetic peaks of glutamate receptor density and
vulnerability to hypoxia-ischemia do not always parallel one another. Dis-
crepancies are partly explained by simultaneous changes in factors, which
contribute to excitotoxicity other than the density of glutamate receptors.
Some immature neurons, for example, may not be able to buffer glutamate-induced increases in intracellular calcium because they have not yet
produced the calcium binding protein calbindin D_{28} [65].

Limited studies of the developmental profile of glutamate receptor subunits are available in perinatal human brains [79–86]. In the human cerebral
cortex, there is a relative increase in GluR2-lacking, calcium-permeable,
AMPA receptor expression with advancing gestation, marked by a transient
peak around term (38–42 postconceptional weeks) (Fig. 6) [79]. These

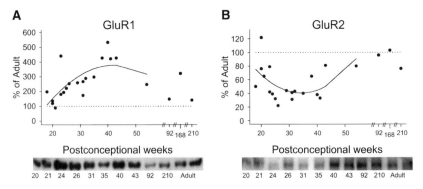

Fig. 6. (*A*) AMPA receptor GluR1 and (*B*) GluR2 expression in the developing human cortex
from midgestation (18 postconceptional weeks) through early infancy (210 postconceptional
weeks). Data are expressed as a percentage of human adult standard (*dotted line*). (*From* Talos
DM, Follett PL, Folkerth RD, et al. Developmental regulation of alpha-amino-3-hydroxy-5-
methyl-4-isoxazole-propionic acid receptor subunit expression in forebrain and relationship
to regional susceptibility to hypoxic/ischemic injury. II. Human cerebral white matter and cortex. J Comp Neurol 2006;497(1):61–77; with permission.)

AMPA receptors are predominantly found on subplate neurons transiently during the preterm period (25–37 weeks) and on pyramidal and nonpyramidal neurons during the term and neonatal periods (38–46 weeks) [79]. Binding levels of glutamate and NMDA receptors in the stratum lucidum of CA3 also follow a bell-shaped curve with peak binding during the early preterm period (18–27 weeks; n = 6) [81]. In the developing human brainstem, there is virtually no NMDA receptor binding at midgestation, but it increases thereafter, with highest values in the inferior olive and hypoglossal nucleus. At term and in early infancy, the binding is 40 fold greater than the levels at midgestation [85]. In contrast, kainate receptor binding is prominent in different nuclei at midgestation, and is transiently expressed during the late preterm and term periods in all areas vulnerable to perinatal: the basis pontis, inferior olive, reticular core, and the inferior colliculus [84,85].

Antioxidant enzymes

To protect against the deleterious effects of oxygen-free radicals, cells possess multiple enzymatic (catalases, peroxidases, and dismutases) and nonenzymatic (glutathione, cholesterol, ascorbic acid, and tocopherol) defenses [87]. Hypoxic-ischemic injury generates free radicals that can overwhelm these endogenous antioxidant systems (see Fig. 1). During hypoxic-ischemic injury, a major source of free radicals is nitric oxide generated from the activation of nitric oxide synthase and from the infiltration of microglia (see Fig. 1). Additional sources of free radicals include increased intracellular calcium and mitochondrial injury, activation of proteases leading to conversion of xanthine dehydrogenase to xanthine oxidase, and activation of phospholipase A_2 leading to increased generation of oxygen free radicals from cyclo-oxygenase and lipoxygenase pathways (see Fig. 1). The fetal gray matter may be particularly susceptible to free radical injury because of a relative developmental deficiency in the antioxidant enzyme systems [7,11,61]. The activity of copper, zinc-superoxide dismutase, for example, that is required for the conversion of oxygen to hydrogen peroxide increases with advancing gestational age in the developing human cerebral cortex, with activity only reaching 50% of adult levels during the neonatal period [88]. Neuronal immunostaining for catalase, required for hydrogen peroxide breakdown, appears around 27 to 28 weeks in the thalamus, basal ganglia, and cerebellum, but not until 35 weeks in the frontal cortex, (ie, during the late-preterm period) [89].

Apoptotic systems

The mechanism by which hypoxia-ischemia induces apoptosis may involve several different and overlapping pathways, including free radical damage and calcium toxicity in which glutamate and nitric oxide are well-known participants [90–92]. Proteins from the caspase family, *Bcl-2* family, and apoptosis protease-activating factor 1 are among the central effectors of these pathways [26,93]. In vitro abnormalities of mitochondrial morphology and function precede caspase-3 activation, indicating a role for mitochondria in the caspase-dependent cell death cascade [92]. The *Bcl-2* family of proto-oncogenes encodes specific proteins, expressed within the mitochondrial matrix, that regulate programmed cell death in different physiologic and pathologic conditions [94]. The ratio of the pro-apoptosis protein BAX and the anti-apoptosis proteins *Bcl-2* and *Bcl-x* is critical in determining cell survival, although the expression ratios following hypoxia-ischemia in the infant rat brain may differ from that in the adult [95]. Caspase-independent modes of programmed cell death are now recognized as well [91].

In the fetal and newborn brain, developmental processes that involve the programmed apoptotic death of redundant cells may be at their peak or near peak, and therefore immature cell types may be particularly vulnerable to apoptotic cell death triggered by hypoxia-ischemia. In the human fetal brain, programmed cell death occurs primarily in the ventricular and subventricular zones beginning at 4.5 gestational weeks, with TUNEL-positive cells appearing in the preplate and ganglionic eminence by 6 to 7 weeks. By 11 to 12 weeks, TUNEL-positive cells are found throughout the telencephalic wall. At midgestation (14–27 weeks), TUNEL-positive cells are detected in the intermediate zone and ganglionic eminence [96,97]. Programmed cell death in the cortical plate is relatively sparse from 4.5 to 27 gestational weeks; however, the apoptotic index (fraction of dying cells as percentage of all cells) is the highest in the two pioneer cortical layers (ie, layer I and subplate) peaking at 17 to 21 weeks [97]. The developmental profile of pro- and anti-apoptotic factors and their functional "balance" with one another in different gray matter regions of the human fetal brain, including in the late preterm period, is an area for future research.

Summary

Here the authors attempt to answer the question: is the late-preterm infant more vulnerable to gray matter injury than the term infant? The short answer seems to be: "it depends." It depends upon the particular balance of susceptibility and protective factors in the particular gray matter region and particular neuronal subtype at that particular age. The basis pontis in the late preterm infant, for example, may be more vulnerable to hypoxic-ischemic injury than in the term infant, but the cerebral cortex may be as vulnerable in the late preterm as term infant. Thus, the late preterm infant may develop a different pattern or degree of neurologic morbidity than the term infant, a direction for future clinical research. In terms of the analysis of the fetal brain itself, considerable information needs to be obtained about the molecular and cellular sequences of different gray matter regions, with a breakdown by the clinically relevant early, mid, and late preterm stages compared with term and beyond. The capability to measure different molecular and cellular factors in the developing human brain at autopsy is greater now than at any other time in neuroscience and human neuropathology, and includes methodologies for genomic and proteonomic analysis. It is incumbent upon neonatologists to request autopsies in their patients to allow such analyses. It is only through combined neurologic and neuropathologic studies that we will be able to answer fully the question: is the late preterm infant more vulnerable to gray matter injury than the term infant?

Acknowledgments

We appreciate the help of Sarah E. Andiman in the preparation of the illustrations and Natalia S. Borenstein for technical assistance with the unpublished GAP-43 western blot data in the developing human cerebral cortex. We thank Dr. Joseph J. Volpe for his critical review of the manuscript.

References

[1] Raju T. Optimizing care and outcomes for late preterm (near-term) infants: part 2. Semin Perinatol 2006;30(2):53.
[2] Amiel-Tison C, Allen MC, Lebrun F, et al. Macropremies: underprivileged newborns. Ment Retard Dev Disabil Res Rev 2002;8(4):281–92.
[3] DePalma RT, Leveno KJ, Kelly MA, et al. Birth weight threshold for postponing preterm birth. Am J Obstet Gynecol 1992;167(4 Pt 1):1145–9.
[4] Hauth JC. Spontaneous preterm labor and premature rupture of membranes at late preterm gestations: to deliver or not to deliver. Semin Perinatol 2006;30(2):98–102.
[5] Martin JA, Kochanek KD, Strobino DM, et al. Annual summary of vital statistics—2003. Pediatrics 2005;115(3):619–34.
[6] Davidoff MJ, Dias T, Damus K, et al. Changes in the gestational age distribution among US singleton births: impact on rates of late preterm birth, 1992 to 2002. Semin Perinatol 2006; 30(1):8–15.
[7] Volpe JJ. Neurology of the newborn. 4th edition. Philadelphia: W.B. Saunders Company; 2001.
[8] Kinney HC, Armstrong D. Perinatal neuropathology. In: Graham DI, Lantos P, editors. Greenfield's neuropathology: erinatal neuropathology vol. 1. London: Arnold; 2002. p. 543–51.
[9] Kinney HC. The near-term (late preterm) human brain and risk for periventricular leukomalacia: a review. Semin Perinatol 2006;30(2):81–8.
[10] Johnston MV. Excitotoxicity in perinatal brain injury. Brain Pathol 2005;15(3):234–40.
[11] Folkerth RD, Kinney HC. Perinatal neuropathology. In: Graham DI, Lantos P, editors. Greenfield's neuropathology, vol. 1. London: Arnold; 2006.
[12] Rees S, Inder T. Fetal and neonatal origins of altered brain development. Early Hum Dev 2005;81(9):753–61.
[13] Choi DW, Rothman SM. The role of glutamate neurotoxicity in hypoxic-ischemic neuronal death. Annu Rev Neurosci 1990;13:171–82.
[14] Silverstein FS, Naik B, Simpson J. Hypoxia-ischemia stimulates hippocampal glutamate efflux in perinatal rat brain: an in vivo microdialysis study. Pediatr Res 1991;30(6):587–90.
[15] Ichord RN, Johnston MV, Traystman RJ. MK801 decreases glutamate release and oxidative metabolism during hypoglycemic coma in piglets. Brain Res Dev Brain Res 2001;128(2): 139–48.

[16] Magistretti PJ, Pellerin L. Astrocytes couple synaptic activity to glucose utilization in the brain. News Physiol Sci 1999;14:177–82.

[17] Choi DW. Excitotoxic cell death. J Neurobiol 1992;23(9):1261–76.

[18] Benveniste H, Drejer J, Schousboe A, et al. Elevation of the extracellular concentrations of glutamate and aspartate in rat hippocampus during transient cerebral ischemia monitored by intracerebral microdialysis. J Neurochem 1984;43(5):1369–74.

[19] Vannucci RC, Brucklacher RM, Vannucci SJ. CSF glutamate during hypoxia-ischemia in the immature rat. Brain Res Dev Brain Res 1999;118(1–2):147–51.

[20] Hagberg H, Gilland E, Diemer NH, et al. Hypoxia-ischemia in the neonatal rat brain: histopathology after post-treatment with NMDA and non-NMDA receptor antagonists. Biol Neonate 1994;66(4):205–13.

[21] Gucuyener K, Atalay Y, Aral YZ, et al. Excitatory amino acids and taurine levels in cerebrospinal fluid of hypoxic ischemic encephalopathy in newborn. Clin Neurol Neurosurg 1999; 101(3):171–4.

[22] Choi DW. Ionic dependence of glutamate neurotoxicity. J Neurosci 1987;7(2):369–79.

[23] Hollmann M, Heinemann S. Cloned glutamate receptors. Annu Rev Neurosci 1994;17: 31–108.

[24] Edwards AD, Yue X, Cox P, et al. Apoptosis in the brains of infants suffering intrauterine cerebral injury. Pediatr Res 1997;42(5):684–9.

[25] Namura S, Zhu J, Fink K, et al. Activation and cleavage of caspase-3 in apoptosis induced by experimental cerebral ischemia. J Neurosci 1998;18(10):3659–68.

[26] Ferrer I, Planas AM. Signaling of cell death and cell survival following focal cerebral ischemia: life and death struggle in the penumbra. J Neuropathol Exp Neurol 2003;62(4): 329–39.

[27] Taylor DL, Edwards AD, Mehmet H. Oxidative metabolism, apoptosis and perinatal brain injury. Brain Pathol 1999;9(1):93–117.

[28] Rossiter JP, Anderson LL, Yang F, et al. Caspase-3 activation and caspase-like proteolytic activity in human perinatal hypoxic-ischemic brain injury. Acta Neuropathol (Berl) 2002; 103(1):66–73.

[29] Takizawa Y, Takashima S, Itoh M. A histopathological study of premature and mature infants with pontosubicular neuron necrosis: neuronal cell death in perinatal brain damage. Brain Res 2006;1095(1):200–6.

[30] Kinney HC, Brody BA, Kloman AS, et al. Sequence of central nervous system myelination in human infancy. II. Patterns of myelination in autopsied infants. J Neuropathol Exp Neurol 1988;47(3):217–34.

[31] Brody BA, Kinney HC, Kloman AS, et al. Sequence of central nervous system myelination in human infancy. I. An autopsy study of myelination. J Neuropathol Exp Neurol 1987;46(3): 283–301.

[32] Mojsilovic J, Zecevic N. Early development of the human thalamus: Golgi and Nissl study. Early Hum Dev 1991;27(1–2):119–44.

[33] Takashima S, Mito T, Becker LE. Neuronal development in the medullary reticular formation in sudden infant death syndrome and premature infants. Neuropediatrics 1985;16(2): 76–9.

[34] Amiel-Tison C. Neurological evaluation of the maturity of newborn infants. Arch Dis Child 1968;43(227):89–93.

[35] Huppi PS, Warfield S, Kikinis R, et al. Quantitative magnetic resonance imaging of brain development in premature and mature newborns. Ann Neurol 1998;43(2):224–35.

[36] Limperopoulos C, Soul JS, Gauvreau K, et al. Late gestation cerebellar growth is rapid and impeded by premature birth. Pediatrics 2005;115(3):688–95.

[37] Chi JG, Dooling EC, Gilles FH. Gyral development of the human brain. Ann Neurol 1977; 1(1):86–93.

[38] Evrard P, Gressens P, Volpe JJ. New concepts to understand the neurological consequences of subcortical lesions in the premature brain. Biol Neonate 1992;61(1):1–3.

[39] Marin-Padilla M. Ontogenesis of the pyramidal cell of the mammalian neocortex and developmental cytoarchitectonics: a unifying theory. J Comp Neurol 1992;321(2): 223–40.

[40] Kinney HC, Rava LA, Benowitz LI. Anatomic distribution of the growth-associated protein GAP-43 in the developing human brainstem. J Neuropathol Exp Neurol 1993;52(1):39–54.

[41] Haynes RL, Borenstein NS, Desilva TM, et al. Axonal development in the cerebral white matter of the human fetus and infant. J Comp Neurol 2005;484(2):156–67.

[42] Sarnat HB, Flores-Sarnat L. Synaptophysin as a marker of synaptogenesis in human fetal brain [abstract 310]. In: XVIth International Congress of Neuropathology. San Francisco (CA): Brain Pathology; 2006. p. S139.

[43] Luskin MB, Shatz CJ. Studies of the earliest generated cells of the cat's visual cortex: cogeneration of subplate and marginal zones. J Neurosci 1985;5(4):1062–75.

[44] McConnell SK, Ghosh A, Shatz CJ. Subplate neurons pioneer the first axon pathway from the cerebral cortex. Science 1989;245(4921):978–82.

[45] Volpe JJ. Subplate neurons—missing link in brain injury of the premature infant? Pediatrics 1996;97(1):112–3.

[46] Ghosh A, Antonini A, McConnell SK, et al. Requirement for subplate neurons in the formation of thalamocortical connections. Nature 1990;347(6289):179–81.

[47] Ghosh A, Shatz CJ. A role for subplate neurons in the patterning of connections from thalamus to neocortex. Development 1993;117(3):1031–47.

[48] Ghosh A. Subplate neurons and the patterning of thalamocortial connections. Ciba Found Symp 1995;193:150–72 [discussion: 192–159].

[49] Mrzljak L, Uylings HB, Kostovic I, et al. Prenatal development of neurons in the human prefrontal cortex: a qualitative Golgi study. J Comp Neurol 1988;271(3):355–86.

[50] Kostovic I, Lukinovic N, Judas M, et al. Structural basis of the developmental plasticity in the human cerebral cortex: the role of the transient subplate zone. Metab Brain Dis 1989; 4(1):17–23.

[51] Kostovic I, Rakic P. Developmental history of the transient subplate zone in the visual and somatosensory cortex of the macaque monkey and human brain. J Comp Neurol 1990; 297(3):441–70.

[52] Wolff JR, Bottcher H, Zetzsche T, et al. Development of GABAergic neurons in rat visual cortex as identified by glutamate decarboxylase-like immunoreactivity. Neurosci Lett 1984;47(3):207–12.

[53] Herrmann K. Differential distribution of AMPA receptors and glutamate during pre- and postnatal development in the visual cortex of ferrets. J Comp Neurol 1996;375(1):1–17.

[54] Judas M, Sestan N, Kostovic I. Nitrinergic neurons in the developing and adult human telencephalon: transient and permanent patterns of expression in comparison to other mammals. Microsc Res Tech 1999;45(6):401–19.

[55] Auer RN, Benveniste H. In: Graham DI, Lantos P, editors. Greenfield's neuropathology: hypoxia and related conditions vol. 1. London: Arnold; 2002. p. 263–314.

[56] Pierson CR, Folkerth RD, Trachtenberg FL, et al. The encephalopathy of prematurity: a neuropathologic study of 41 cases in the modern era of intensive care. Submitted for publication.

[57] Volpe JJ. Neurobiology of periventricular leukomalacia in the premature infant. Pediatr Res 2001;50(5):553–62.

[58] McDonald JW, Shapiro SM, Silverstein FS, et al. Role of glutamate receptor-mediated excitotoxicity in bilirubin-induced brain injury in the Gunn rat model. Exp Neurol 1998;150(1): 21–9.

[59] Suh SW, Aoyama K, Chen Y, et al. Hypoglycemic neuronal death and cognitive impairment are prevented by poly(ADP-ribose) polymerase inhibitors administered after hypoglycemia. J Neurosci 2003;23(33):10681–90.

[60] Volpe JJ. Cerebral white matter injury of the premature infant-more common than you think. Pediatrics 2003;112(1 Pt 1):176–80.

[61] Folkerth RD, Haynes RL, Borenstein NS, et al. Developmental lag in superoxide dismutases relative to other antioxidant enzymes in premyelinated human telencephalic white matter. J Neuropathol Exp Neurol 2004;63(9):990–9.

[62] Greisen G. Effect of cerebral blood flow and cerebrovascular autoregulation on the distribution, type and extent of cerebral injury. Brain Pathol 1992;2(3):223–8.

[63] Haynes RL, Folkerth RD, Keefe RJ, et al. Nitrosative and oxidative injury to premyelinating oligodendrocytes in periventricular leukomalacia. J Neuropathol Exp Neurol 2003;62(5): 441–50.

[64] Kinney HC, Panigrahy A, Newburger JW, et al. Hypoxic-ischemic brain injury in infants with congenital heart disease dying after cardiac surgery. Acta Neuropathol (Berl) 2005; 110(6):563–78.

[65] Barks JD, Silverstein FS. Excitatory amino acids contribute to the pathogenesis of perinatal hypoxic-ischemic brain injury. Brain Pathol 1992;2(3):235–43.

[66] Angelatou F, Mitsacos A, Goulas V, et al. L-aspartate and L-glutamate binding sites in developing normal and 'nervous' mutant mouse cerebellum. Int J Dev Neurosci 1987;5(5–6): 373–81.

[67] Mattson MP, Kater SB. Isolated hippocampal neurons in cryopreserved long-term cultures: development of neuroarchitecture and sensitivity to NMDA. Int J Dev Neurosci 1988;6(5): 439–52.

[68] Parnavelas JG, Cavanagh ME. Transient expression of neurotransmitters in the developing neocortex. Trends Neurosci 1988;11(3):92–3.

[69] McDonald JW, Johnston MV. Physiological and pathophysiological roles of excitatory amino acids during central nervous system development. Brain Res Brain Res Rev 1990; 15(1):41–70.

[70] Johnston MV. Neurotransmitters and vulnerability of the developing brain. Brain Dev 1995; 17(5):301–6.

[71] Ikonomidou C, Bosch F, Miksa M, et al. Blockade of NMDA receptors and apoptotic neurodegeneration in the developing brain. Science 1999;283(5398):70–4.

[72] Ritter LM, Unis AS, Meador-Woodruff JH. Ontogeny of ionotropic glutamate receptor expression in human fetal brain. Brain Res Dev Brain Res 2001;127(2):123–33.

[73] Catsicas M, Allcorn S, Mobbs P. Early activation of Ca(2 +)-permeable AMPA receptors reduces neurite outgrowth in embryonic chick retinal neurons. J Neurobiol 2001;49(3): 200–11.

[74] Haberny KA, Paule MG, Scallet AC, et al. Ontogeny of the N-methyl-D-aspartate (NMDA) receptor system and susceptibility to neurotoxicity. Toxicol Sci 2002;68(1):9–17.

[75] King AE, Chung RS, Vickers JC, et al. Localization of glutamate receptors in developing cortical neurons in culture and relationship to susceptibility to excitotoxicity. J Comp Neurol 2006;498(2):277–94.

[76] Pires RS, Real CC, Hayashi MA, et al. Ontogeny of subunits 2 and 3 of the AMPA-type glutamate receptors in Purkinje cells of the developing chick cerebellum. Brain Res 2006; 1096(1):11–9.

[77] Insel TR, Miller LP, Gelhard RE. The ontogeny of excitatory amino acid receptors in rat forebrain—I. N-methyl-D-aspartate and quisqualate receptors. Neuroscience 1990;35(1): 31–43.

[78] Rao H, Jean A, Kessler JP. Postnatal ontogeny of glutamate receptors in the rat nucleus tractus solitarii and ventrolateral medulla. J Auton Nerv Syst 1997;65(1):25–32.

[79] Talos DM, Follett PL, Folkerth RD, et al. Developmental regulation of alpha-amino-3-hydroxy-5-methyl-4-isoxazole-propionic acid receptor subunit expression in forebrain and relationship to regional susceptibility to hypoxic/ischemic injury. II. Human cerebral white matter and cortex. J Comp Neurol 2006;497(1):61–77.

[80] Greenamyre T, Penney JB, Young AB, et al. Evidence for transient perinatal glutamatergic innervation of globus pallidus. J Neurosci 1987;7(4):1022–30.

[81] Represa A, Tremblay E, Ben-Ari Y. Transient increase of NMDA-binding sites in human hippocampus during development. Neurosci Lett 1989;99(1–2):61–6.

[82] D'Souza SW, McConnell SE, Slater P, et al. Glycine site of the excitatory amino acid N-methyl-D-aspartate receptor in neonatal and adult brain. Arch Dis Child 1993;69(2): 212–5.

[83] Itoh M, Watanabe Y, Watanabe M, et al. Expression of a glutamate transporter subtype, EAAT4, in the developing human cerebellum. Brain Res 1997;767(2):265–71.

[84] Panigrahy A, Filiano JJ, Sleeper LA, et al. Decreased kainate receptor binding in the arcuate nucleus of the sudden infant death syndrome. J Neuropathol Exp Neurol 1997;56(11): 1253–61.

[85] Panigrahy A, Rosenberg PA, Assmann S, et al. Differential expression of glutamate receptor subtypes in human brainstem sites involved in perinatal hypoxia-ischemia. J Comp Neurol 2000;427(2):196–208.

[86] Lee H, Choi BH. Density and distribution of excitatory amino acid receptors in the developing human fetal brain: a quantitative autoradiographic study. Exp Neurol 1992;118(3): 284–90.

[87] Delivoria-Papadopoulos M, Mishra OP. Mechanisms of cerebral injury in perinatal asphyxia and strategies for prevention. J Pediatr 1998;132(3 Pt 2):S30–4.

[88] Nishida A, Misaki Y, Kuruta H, et al. Developmental expression of copper, zinc-superoxide dismutase in human brain by chemiluminescence. Brain Dev 1994;16(1):40–3.

[89] Houdou S, Kuruta H, Hasegawa M, et al. Developmental immunohistochemistry of catalase in the human brain. Brain Res 1991;556(2):267–70.

[90] Edwards AD, Mehmet H. Apoptosis in perinatal hypoxic-ischaemic cerebral damage. Neuropathol Appl Neurobiol 1996;22(6):494–8.

[91] Friedlander RM. Apoptosis and caspases in neurodegenerative diseases. N Engl J Med 2003; 348(14):1365–75.

[92] Hagberg H. Mitochondrial impairment in the developing brain after hypoxia-ischemia. J Bioenerg Biomembr 2004;36(4):369–73.

[93] Cohen GM. Caspases: the executioners of apoptosis. Biochem J 1997;326(Pt 1):1–16.

[94] Bredesen DE. Neural apoptosis. Ann Neurol 1995;38(6):839–51.

[95] Ferrer I, Pozas E, Lopez E, et al. Bcl-2, Bax and Bcl-x expression following hypoxia-ischemia in the infant rat brain. Acta Neuropathol (Berl) 1997;94(6):583–9.

[96] Simonati A, Rosso T, Rizzuto N. DNA fragmentation in normal development of the human central nervous system: a morphological study during corticogenesis. Neuropathol Appl Neurobiol 1997;23(3):203–11.

[97] Rakic S, Zecevic N. Programmed cell death in the developing human telencephalon. Eur J Neurosci 2000;12(8):2721–34.

ELSEVIER
SAUNDERS

CLINICS IN
PERINATOLOGY

Clin Perinatol 33 (2006) 935–945

Emergency Department Visits and Rehospitalizations in Late Preterm Infants

Shabnam Jain, MD[a,b,*], John Cheng, MD[a,b]

[a]Division of Pediatric Emergency Medicine, Emory University, 1645 Tullie Circle Northeast,
Atlanta, GA 30329, USA
[b]Children's Healthcare of Atlanta at Egleston, 1405 Clifton, Road,
NE, Atlanta, GA 30322, USA

There is a rising rate of late preterm babies (8.8% in 2003), up from 7.6% a decade earlier, and the highest since the government starting tracking such births [1,2]. Neonatologists generally recognize that these infants face more problems in the immediate newborn period compared with their full-term counterparts. What is not known completely is how these infants fare after they are discharged from the nursery.

Practitioners outside the nursery are not able to recognize readily the often subtle differences in size and appearance of late preterm infants from more mature infants, and thus, they tend to include them in the same category as full-term infants [3]. This perhaps explains the commonly used phrase near-term infant to describe infants born at 34 to 36 weeks gestational age. Their size and apparent maturity create a false sense of security, delaying the recognition of problems in this vulnerable group.

There is limited literature describing the experience of these late preterm infants after nursery discharge. Wang and colleagues reviewed the clinical outcomes of late preterm infants in the nursery and concluded that these infants had significantly more medical problems at birth, leading to increased hospital costs compared with contemporaneous full-term infants [4]. They recommended that the next steps include closer follow-up of late preterm newborns with particular emphasis on frequency of pediatric visits, hospital readmission, feeding, and growth issues. Shapiro-Mendoza and colleagues studied late preterm birth as a risk factor for neonatal morbidity among singleton newborns discharged early (defined as less than 2 nights' stay in the

---

* Corresponding author.
E-mail address: shabnam.jain@oz.ped.emory.edu (S. Jain).

0095-5108/06/$ - see front matter © 2006 Elsevier Inc. All rights reserved.
doi:10.1016/j.clp.2006.09.007
perinatology.theclinics.com

hospital after vaginal delivery) [5]. As compared with full-term infants, late preterm infants discharged early were at greater risk of neonatal morbidity, with a nearly twofold relative risk of being readmitted to a hospital in the neonatal period. Oddie and colleagues also noted that late preterm infants had the highest rate of readmission to hospital in the first month of life after early discharge [6]. Escobar and colleagues found that late preterm babies with short neonatal ICU (NICU) stays had the highest rehospitalization rates among 6054 NICU survivors of all gestational ages [7]. Another study found that rehospitalization rates within 2 weeks of nursery discharge were higher among late preterm infants who never were admitted to the NICU [8].

Several of these studies have found similar reasons for these rehospitalizations. Escobar and colleagues found that the two most common reasons for rehospitalization in the first 2 weeks are jaundice and feeding difficulties [9]. They emphasized the high rate of admission for dehydration in late preterm infants to underscore the need for better education of parents about feeding issues faced by these infants who may appear more mature than they are. Tomashek and colleagues described readmission diagnoses among term and late preterm infants who were discharged early, with jaundice in 27% and 49% and infection in 33% and 29% of term and late preterm infants respectively [6]. A recent review article summarizes other short-term outcomes of 35- to 36-week gestation infants such as mortality and respiratory distress, in addition to rehospitalizations [10].

Although short-term problems during the birth hospitalization and rehospitalization are beginning to be recognized for late preterm infants, there is limited information on how these infants present to medical care and what interventions take place before, and inclusive of, a hospitalization. In a recent issue of *Pediatric Clinics of North America* devoted to pediatric emergencies, newborn emergencies in the first 30 days of were reviewed [11]. Newborns were not subclassified by gestational age, however. To the authors' knowledge, there are no published data describing outpatient presentation of late preterm infants in the immediate postnatal period. This article reports the experience in the authors' emergency department (ED) with newborn visits, with particular emphasis on late preterm infants.

Newborn visits to the emergency department: a comparison of term and late preterm infants

Medical care for the neonate after nursery discharge occurs in two main settings: the primary care office and the ED. The authors reviewed their experience of visits to the ED by newborns in their first 31 days of life, over a 1-year period from July 1, 2005, to June 30, 2006. The authors' institution consists of two free-standing tertiary care pediatric hospitals in a large metropolitan area. The EDs saw 122,585 pediatric patients during this 1-year period, of which 3059 (2.5%) were newborns between 0 and 31 days of age. In 1011 infants, gestational age was not documented; this lack of documentation is concerning given that these patients were newborns presenting to the ED, and their gestational age could have affected their management. Additionally, the hospital electronic medical record has predefined gestational age groups in the birth history template that sometimes are used. The two age groups of note are 32 to 35 weeks and 36 to 42 weeks. Eight patients were noted as being in the 32- to 35-week age group, and 440 were in the 36- to 42-week age group. Some late preterm infants may have been included in these groups, and therefore their preterm status not recognized. Four patients left before being seen by a physician. Of the1596 patients who had a specific gestational age documented, 764 were documented as full-term while 516 had a gestational age noted as being 37, 38, 39, 40, 41, or 42 weeks, for a total of 1280 (80.2%) documented term births. Twenty five (1.6%) were preterm (under 34 weeks gestational age); 282 (17.7%) were late preterm (34 to 36 weeks gestational age), and 9 (0.6%) were post-term (at least 43 weeks gestational age). The relatively low number of preterm infants seen in the ED in the authors' data set is probably a function of their inclusion criteria for analysis (age 0 to 31 days) and the fact that many preterm infants would remain hospitalized in the nursery or NICU during this age range. The proportion of visits by late preterm infants to the authors' ED (17.7%) is double the reported 8.8% rate of late preterm births nationally [2]. This may be a reflection of the institution's status as a tertiary care pediatric ED or a result of higher frequency of medical concerns in this subset of newborns. To better understand the unique issues related to late preterm infants, the authors compared the 1280 term infants seen in the ED to 282 late preterm infants.

Age at presentation

The age of the infant at presentation was available for every patient. Fig. 1 shows visits by age of patient divided into 0 to 7 days, 8 to 14 days, 15 to 21 days, 22 to 28 days, and 29 days or more in term newborns compared with late preterm infants. Patients were divided evenly between the four age ranges except the age group 29 days or more, which included only 4 days (29 to 31 days of age). More term infants presented to the ED in the second week of life, whereas more late preterm infants presented in the fourth week of life (Fig. 1A). Fig. 1B depicts the age at presentation to the ED of late preterm infants; no noticeable patterns emerge, except that more late preterm infants presented in the 22- to 28-day age range (fourth week of life).

Presenting complaint

The chief complaint of the patient at the time of presentation was recorded by the triage nurse for every visit. This included problems voiced by the parents and tentative diagnoses made by referring physicians. The

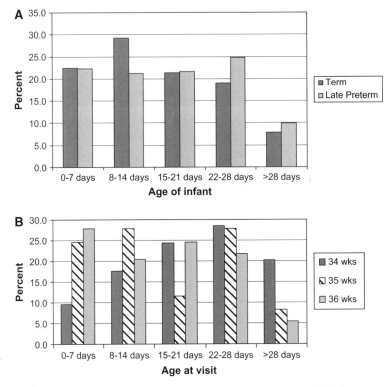

Fig. 1. (*A*) Age distribution of term (N = 1280) and late preterm (N = 282) infants at presentation to ED. (*B*) Age distribution of late preterm infants at presentation to ED. A significant number of infants presented at greater than or equal to 2 weeks of age, reflecting ongoing issues in this population.

top five complaints for term and late preterm infants accounted for most patient visits and were the same in each group: difficulty breathing/stopped breathing, fever, jaundice, vomiting, crying.

Acuity of presentation

Based on the presenting complaint and a quick assessment, patients arriving at the ED are assigned a triage category that denotes the acuity of their condition. This helps in prioritization of patients for immediate medical attention. Newborns in general are considered to be a higher priority than older patients with a similar presentation. Acuity is divided into four categories: critical, emergent, urgent, and nonurgent. Fig. 2 shows that most newborns presented in the emergent or urgent categories, in comparable ratios between term and late preterm infants. Although a higher proportion of late preterm infants presented in critical condition compared with term

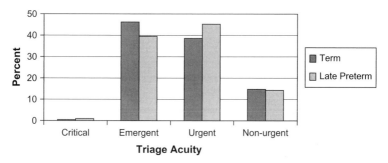

Fig. 2. Triage acuity at presentation to ED of term (N = 1280) and late preterm (N = 282) infants. Patients are classified into one of four categories based on the acuity of their initial presentation.

infants, the total number of newborns in critical condition was less than 1% (10 of 1562).

Gestational age at presentation

Term infants presented in the entire range from 37 weeks through 42 weeks, with many being noted simply as being "full term". Of the late preterm infants, 26.2% were 34 weeks gestational age, and 21.6% were 35 weeks. More than half, 52.1%, were 36 weeks (Fig. 3). This larger number of infants in the more mature late preterm category is surprising. Escobar and colleagues found that 34- to 36-week gestation infants who were never in the NICU were much more likely to be rehospitalized than other infant groups (including preterm infants) [8]. In view of that finding, one possible reason for the disproportionate number of infants of 36 weeks gestation presenting to the ED might be that these infants had short nursery stays, more like term infants, while those infants of 34 and 35 weeks gestation required longer stays in the nursery or NICU. So, despite an uneventful perinatal

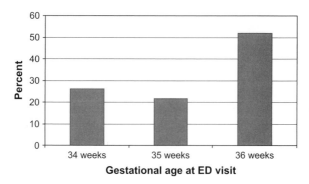

Fig. 3. Gestational age of late preterm infants at presentation to ED (N = 282). More than half of all late preterm infants were 36 weeks gestation.

course and discharge from the nursery, 36-week infants develop problems at home, prompting caregivers to seek medical attention. This trend underscores the need for critical evaluation of nursery discharge practices for late preterm infants.

Mode of delivery

The mode of delivery was documented as vaginal or normal for 715 term infants and 93 late preterm infants and as caesarean section for 275 term and 60 late preterm infants. For 290 term infants and 129 late preterm infants, the mode of delivery was not documented. Fig. 4 depicts the mode of delivery in term infants as compared with late preterm infants. Of note, as compared with 27.8% of term patients presenting to the ED delivered by caesarean section, 39.2% of late preterm infants had a caesarean section delivery. This higher rate of caesarean delivery in late preterm infants presenting to the ED may reflect a failure of smooth neonatal transition in these infants, or may be reflective of the recent increase in elective deliveries, and a concomitant rise in iatrogenic prematurity [12].

Range of diagnoses

The range of diagnoses noted at disposition from the ED in shown in Table 1. The authors grouped related diagnoses by system (eg, gastrointestinal [GI], respiratory, or neurologic) or common newborn conditions (eg, fever, apnea/apparent life-threatening event [ALTE], jaundice, feeding problems, or crying/fussiness). The six most commonly noted diagnoses accounted for most (over 75%) infants and were the same for term and late

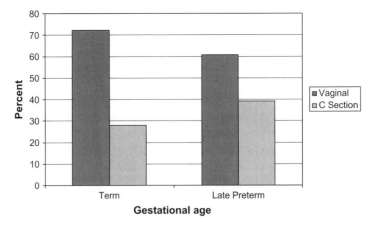

Fig. 4. Mode of delivery (vaginal or caesarean section) of term (N = 990) and late preterm (N = 153) infants presenting to the ED. Although most infants in both groups were delivered vaginally, late preterm infants were more likely to be delivered by caesarean section.

Table 1
Distribution of emergency department diagnoses in term and late preterm infants

Emergency department diagnosis	Term infants N (%)	Late preterm infants N (%)
Gastrointestinal	261 (20.5)	57 (20.4)
Respiratory	228 (17.9)	44 (15.8)
Fever	176 (13.8)	19 (6.8)
Jaundice	122 (9.6)	34 (12.2)
Infectious	84 (6.6)	23 (8.2)
Feeding problems	65 (5.1)	21 (7.5)
Apnea/ALTE	42 (3.3)	18 (6.5)
Dermatologic	42 (3.3)	5 (1.8)
Crying/fussiness	40 (3.1)	11 (3.9)
Normal examination	39 (3.1)	12 (4.3)
Ophthalmologic	34 (2.7)	5 (1.8)
Neurologic	30 (2.4)	1 (0.4)
Trauma	21 (1.6)	7 (2.5)
Abnormal labs	20 (1.6)	1 (0.4)
Dehydration	11 (0.9)	3 (1.1)
Cardiac	8 (0.6)	4 (1.4)
Hypothermia	3 (0.2)	7 (2.5)
Miscellaneous	51 (4.1)	6 (2.5)
Total	**1276**	**279**

preterm infants (GI, respiratory, fever, jaundice, infectious, feeding problems). Comparable to previous studies, the authors also found jaundice, infectious issues, feeding problems, and apnea/ALTE in a higher proportion
of late preterm infants, as compared with term infants [4,13,14]. Additionally, although not a very common presentation, more late preterm infants
were found to have hypothermia than term infants (2.5% versus 0.2%). Fever was a common presentation for both groups; however, it was seen much
less frequently in late preterm infants (term 13.8% versus late preterm 6.8%)
(Fig. 5). This finding supports the observation that the ability to mount a febrile response may be regulated developmentally.

Outcomes of the emergency department visit

Of the 1276 term infants and 279 late preterm infants evaluated in the
ED, 521 of 1276 (40.8%) term infants were hospitalized, compared with
103 of 279 (36.9%) late preterm infants (Fig. 6). Four term and three late
preterm infants left before being seen by a physician. There are several
points worthy of note concerning these admission rates. First, the authors'
institution is a tertiary care pediatric facility with an 11.4% overall rate of
admission from the ED, which may reflect a higher patient acuity in general.
Second, while these admission rates appear higher than those previously reported for late preterm infants, previous studies reported population-based
data [7,9,10]. Finally, these rates of hospitalization are comparable between
term and late preterm infants. At first glance, this appears contradictory to

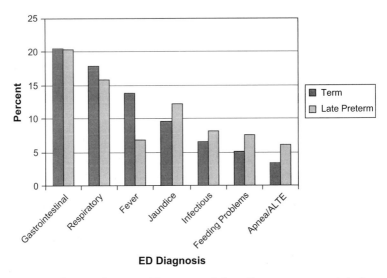

ED Diagnosis

Fig. 5. Top ED diagnoses in term and late preterm infants. Fever was common in both groups, but significantly less so in late preterm infants.

previously published higher rates of rehospitalization for late preterm infants [5,7,10,15,16]. Given, however, that late preterm infants presented to the authors' ED at twice the rate (17.7%) of late preterm births in the United States (8.8%), the absolute number of late preterm infant hospitalization is compatible with previously published readmission rates. Among admitted patients, the rate of disposition to the ICU or operating room in late preterm infants (12/103) was almost twice that of term infants (32/521) (11.7% versus 6.1%).

Late preterm infant: problems persist after discharge from nursery

Detailed medical record review was performed for all 279 late preterm infants. Various interventions, both diagnostic and therapeutic, were

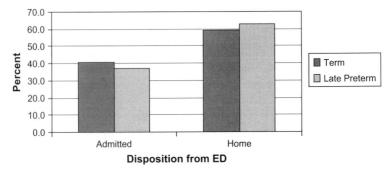

Disposition from ED

Fig. 6. Outcome of ED visit of term (N = 1276) and late preterm (N = 279) infants.

performed in the ED. One hundred thirty of 279 (46.6%) infants had laboratory evaluation (ie, complete blood count [CBC], electrolytes, bilirubin level, blood culture, or other tests). Urinalysis was performed in 60 (21.5%) infants, and lumbar puncture was performed in 44 (15.8%) infants. Radiologic imaging (chest radiograph, abdominal radiograph, CT, ultrasound and echocardiogram, fluoroscopy, or other images) was obtained in 82 (29.4%) infants. Some patients had more than one imaging study during a single visit.

Fifty four of 279 (19.4%) infants received a bolus of intravenous fluids, and 40 (14.3%) received antibiotics/antivirals. Five infants received critical care, including two who required intubation. Subspecialty consultation was requested for 27 (9.7%) infants, primarily for cardiac and surgical services.

Readmissions of late preterm infants from the emergency department

One hundred three of 279 (36.9%) late preterm infants seen in the ED in the first month of life required readmission to the hospital. These infants accounted for a total of 589 hospital days. The average length of stay was 5.7 days; most stayed for 3 days. There were various admitting diagnoses, of which the top six were apnea/ALTE (18), hyperbilirubinemia (17), neonatal fever/suspected sepsis (16), respiratory problems (13), feeding problems (7), and hypothermia (6). Almost all patients who were admitted required additional interventions during their hospitalization; only four were admitted for simple observation. These interventions included intravenous antibiotics and antivirals, imaging studies, intravenous fluids, additional laboratory evaluation, and subspecialty consultation.

The top six diagnoses accounted for most (about 75%) of late preterm patients admitted from the ED. The final diagnoses for these hospital admissions are noted in Table 2. Many infants admitted for apnea/ALTE and feeding problems were given a final diagnosis of gastroesophageal reflux disease (GERD). Three of the six infants with hypothermia had sepsis as the final diagnosis.

Table 2
Comparison of emergency department diagnosis to final diagnosis in hospitalized late preterm infants (top 75% diagnoses of 103 hospitalized patients)

Emergency department diagnosis	Final diagnosis
Apnea/ALTE (18)	GERD (11), bronchiolitis (3), sepsis (2), neurological (1), pertussis (1)
Hyperbilirubinemia (17)	Hyperbilirubinemia (17)
Fever (16)	Sepsis (2), UTI (1), meningitis (1), flu (1), rotavirus (1), URI (1), fever (9)
Respiratory (13)	Bronchiolitis (10), GERD (2), fever (1)
Feeding problems (7)	GERD (2), diarrhea (2), FTT (1), feeding problem (2)
Hypothermia (6)	Sepsis (3), hyperbilirubinemia (2), feeding problems (1)

Abbreviations: GERD, gastroesophageal reflux disease; URI, upper respiratory infection; UTI, urinary tract infection.

Twelve of the 103 late preterm infants who were hospitalized were admitted to the ICU, accounting for a total of 107 ICU days. One infant with staphylococcal pneumonia and empyema had a 36-day ICU stay.

Summary

This was a comprehensive review of the experience of late preterm infants as compared with term infants in a large pediatric ED, including rehospitalizations. The 17.7% rate of late preterm visits, as compared with the overall 8.8% rate of late preterm deliveries in the United States, might indicate increased parental concern or increased morbidity in this population. Although infants in both groups had similar complaints and diagnoses, the authors found a higher frequency of presentation for jaundice, infectious issues, feeding problems, and apnea/ALTE in late preterm infants. This is in concordance with similar findings in other studies within and outside the nursery. The authors found that over half of late preterm infants presenting to the ED were born at 36 weeks of gestation. This unexpected finding warrants further study of the early postnatal course and nursery discharge practices for these infants. The rate of caesarean section delivery in late preterm infants in the authors' data warrants further study of decisions regarding timing and mode of delivery. Finally, although rehospitalization rates were comparable among term and late preterm infants presenting to the ED, late preterm infants were more likely to be seen in the ED, thus accounting for an overall higher hospitalization rate for this population.

There are several initiatives underway to increase general awareness of the risks and problems faced by late preterm infants within the nursery. These initiatives need to extend beyond the nursery to outpatient providers and parents. Emphasis should be placed on feeding issues, jaundice, GERD, and temperature regulation, in addition to the common concerns of respiratory problems. Early follow-up with a pediatrician after discharge from the birthing unit may be helpful. More studies on short-term outcomes of late preterm infants compared with term infants may help delineate their morbidity and define guidelines for their care after nursery discharge.

References

[1] Medoff-Cooper B, Bakewell-Sachs S, Buus-Frank ME, et al. The AWHONN Near-Term Infant Initiative: a conceptual framework for optimizing health for near-term infants. J Obstet Gynecol Neonatal Nurs 2005;34(6):666–71.
[2] Martin JA, Hamilton BE, Sutton PD, et al. Births final data for 2003, National Center for Health Statistics, Hyattsville, MD. National Vital Statistics Reports 2005;54(2):1–116.
[3] Jenkins AW. Near-term but still a preemie. AWHONN Lifelines 2005;9(4):295–7.
[4] Wang ML, Dorer DJ, Fleming MP, et al. Clinical outcomes of near-term infants. Pediatrics 2004;114(2):372–6.
[5] Shapiro-Mendoza CK, Tomashek KM, Kotelchuck M, et al. Risk factors for neonatal morbidity and mortality among healthy, late preterm newborns. Semin Perinatol 2006;30(2): 54–60.

[6] Tomashek KM, Shapiro-Mendoza CK, Weiss J, et al. Early discharge among late preterm and term newborns and risk of neonatal morbidity. Semin Perinatol 2006;30(2):61–8.

[7] Escobar GJ, Joffe S, Gardner MN, et al. Rehospitalization in the first two weeks after discharge from the neonatal intensive care unit. Pediatrics 1999;104(1):e2.

[8] Escobar GJ, Greene JD, Hulac P, et al. Rehospitalisation after birth hospitalisation: patterns among infants of all gestations. Arch Dis Child 2005;90(2):125–31.

[9] Escobar GJ, Gonzales VM, Armstrong MA, et al. Rehospitalization for neonatal dehydration: a nested case–control study. Arch Pediatr Adolesc Med 2002;156(2):155–61.

[10] Escobar GJ, Clark RH, Greene JD, et al. Short-term outcomes of infants born at 35 and 36 weeks gestation: we need to ask more questions. Semin Perinatol 2006;30(1):28–33.

[11] Brousseau T, Sharieff GQ. Newborn emergencies: the first 30 days of life. Pediatr Clin North Am 2006;53(1):69–84.

[12] Davidoff MJ, Dias T, Damus K, et al. Changes in the gestational age distribution among U.S. singleton births: impact on rates of late preterm birth, 1992 to 2002. Semin Perinatol 2006;30(1):8–15.

[13] Martens PJ, Derksen S, Gupta S. Predictors of hospital readmission of Manitoba newborns within six weeks postbirth discharge: a population-based study. Pediatrics 2004;114(3): 708–13.

[14] Sarici SU, Serdar MA, Korkmaz A, et al. Incidence, course, and prediction of hyperbilirubinemia in near-term and term newborns. Pediatrics 2004;113(4):775–80.

[15] Escobar GJ, McCormick MC, Zupancic JA, et al. Unstudied infants: outcomes of moderately premature infants in the neonatal intensive care unit. Arch Dis Child Fetal Neonatal Ed 2006;91(4):F238–44.

[16] Oddie SJ, Hammal D, Richmond S, et al. Early discharge and readmission to hospital in the first month of life in the northern region of the UK during 1998: a case cohort study. Arch Dis Child 2005;90(2):119–24.

ELSEVIER
SAUNDERS

CLINICS IN
PERINATOLOGY

Clin Perinatol 33 (2006) 947–964

Neurodevelopmental Outcome of the Late Preterm Infant

Ira Adams-Chapman, MD

Department of Pediatrics, Division of Neonatology, Emory University School of Medicine,
469 Jesse Hill Junior Drive, Atlanta, GA 30303, USA

In contrast to the large body of literature detailing the neurodevelopmental (ND) outcome of the extremely low birth weight infant, there is very limited data about the developmental outcome of the late preterm infant. The developing brain is vulnerable to injury during this very active and important stage of fetal brain development; therefore, it is important to carefully monitor the neurologic outcome of these infants.

Infants with a gestational age less than 37 weeks gestation are considered "preterm" by definition; however, the associated neonatal morbidity in the late preterm infant is very different from the more immature infant. As a group, late preterm infants have fewer medical complications compared to extremely low birth weight infants; however, there is growing concern that the late preterm may also be at significant risk for brain injury and adverse long term neurodevelopmental outcome. Multiple factors related to their developmental immaturity may mediate the risk for brain injury and subsequent abnormal neurologic sequelae, including the risk for development of intraventricular hemorrhage (IVH) and periventricular leukomalacia (PVL), hypoxic respiratory failure, hyperbilirubinemia, and infection. It is also important to recognize that the late preterm brain is only a fraction of the full-term brain weight and a significant proportion of brain growth, development, and networking occurs during the last six weeks of gestation. These tissues are vulnerable to injury during this critical time period of development. Injury may result in direct injury to developing tissues or disruption of critical pathways needed for neuronal and glial development.

E-mail address: ira_adams-chapman@oz.ped.emory.edu

0095-5108/06/$ - see front matter © 2006 Elsevier Inc. All rights reserved.
doi:10.1016/j.clp.2006.09.004   *perinatology.theclinics.com*

Brain growth and development in the late preterm infant

Human brain development is a dynamic process that continues until the end of gestation. There is a critical period of brain growth and development that occurs in late gestation that is vital for the development of various neural structures and pathways. In fact, approximately 50% of the increase in cortical volume occurs between 34 and 40 weeks gestation, indicating that this is a very rapid period of brain growth [1–3]. Improved understanding of brain development has also led to a clearer understanding of the maturation-dependent vulnerability of the developing brain. Each of these factors contributes to the overall risk of brain injury in the late preterm infant.

Cerebral cortical development

Subplate/subcortical neurons are detectable at 10 weeks gestation and peak in number between 22 and 35 weeks gestation [2,4]. They originate from the ventricular zone and are important in directing thalamocortical pathways through activity-dependent mechanisms. Animal models have shown that injury to these cells results in alteration of axonal development and underdevelopment of associated neural structures [2,5].

Even though neuronal proliferation and migration to the cerebral cortex is complete by 24 weeks gestation, the maturation of these tissues (including gyral and sulcal formation) is incomplete, even in the late preterm infant. At 20 weeks gestation, the brain weighs approximately 10% of the brain weight at term, and weight increases in a linear fashion throughout gestation (Fig. 1). At 34 weeks gestation, the brain only weighs 65% of the term brain weight. Similarly, quantitative MRI data have shown that total brain volume increases linearly with increasing gestation age (Fig. 2) [3]. The relative distribution of cellular components also changes with increasing gestational

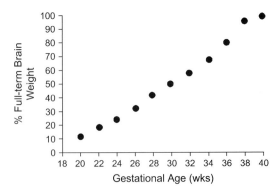

Fig. 1. Changes in fetal brain weight with increasing gestational age expressed as a percent of term brain weight. At 34 weeks gestational age, the overall brain weight is 65% of term weight. (*From* Kinney HC. The near term (late preterm) human brain and risk for periventricular leukomalacia: a review. Semin Perinatol 2006;30:82; with permission.)

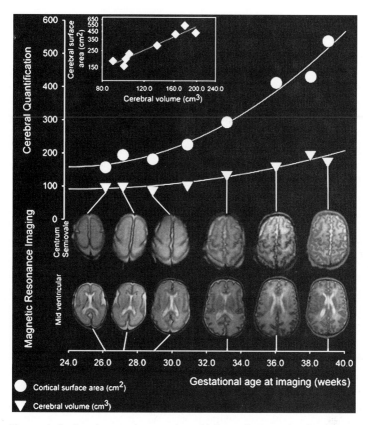

Fig. 2. Changes in brain volume and maturation with increasing gestational age. (*From* Kapellou O, Counsell SJ, Kennea N, et al. Abnormal cortical development after premature birth shown by altered allometric scaling of brain growth. PLOS Med 2006;3:e265; with permission.)

age. In early gestation, unmyelinated white matter is the predominant neural tissue. By midgestation, unmyelinated white matter and gray matter are found in similar amounts. After 30 weeks gestation, myelinated white matter is present and increases fivefold by the end of gestation. Gray matter volumes increase throughout gestation at a rate of 1.4% or 22 mL/wk and also have a similar rapid increase between 36 and 40 weeks because of neuronal differentiation and gyral formation [3]. Therefore, in the late preterm infant, the time period between 34 and 40 weeks gestation is critical, since the relative percentage of both gray matter and myelinated white matter to total brain volume increase exponentially.

White matter development

The preterm infant has various differential periods of vulnerability for white matter injury. The most immature infants have the greatest risk, and the most resilience is noted in the myelinated brain of early infancy [2,6]. Delineating the timing and sequence of myelination has led to a more precise understanding of the pathogenesis of white matter injury in the developing brain.

The immature oligodendrocyte is particularly vulnerable to injury and appears to play a key role in the pathogenesis of PVL. These cells originate in the ventricular zone and migrate to the developing white matter, where they proliferate, then differentiate into myelin-producing cells. Back and colleagues performed detailed immunofluorescent histochemical studies to track the development of the oligodendrocyte in the human brain and defined three stages of development based on staining patterns for antibodies to NG2 proteoglycan, O4, O1, and major basic protein (MBP) [7]. Early in gestation, between 18 to 27 weeks, late oligodendrocyte progenitor cells are the predominant cell lineage. Between 28 and 41 weeks, there is an increase in the immature oligodendrocyte. Myelin sheaths first are detected at approximately 30 weeks gestation, but active wrapping of axons does not occur until 3 to 5 months postnatal age and continues throughout the first year of life (Fig. 3) [2,6,7].

Historically, white matter injury was considered to be secondary to injury to the mature myelin-containing white matter tracks. However, recent evidence shows that the late oligodendrocyte progenitor cells are actually the dominant cell type during the window between 23 to 32 weeks gestation when the white matter is most likely to occur. This period in brain development actually precedes the onset of active myelin formation. These findings suggest that the late oligodendrocyte progenitors are the most likely target cells for injury in the pathogenesis of PVL. In addition, the incidence of PVL decreases after 32 weeks gestation, which also coincides with the onset of myelin production. The increase in myelinated white matter in the more mature brain appears to confer some protection from white matter injury. Huppi and colleagues reported supporting data from diffusion tensor MRI imaging showing decreasing water diffusion with increasing gestation

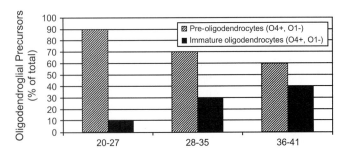

Fig. 3. Timing of appearance of the oligodendrocytes progenitors in the human cerebral white matter. (*From* Kinney HC. The near term (late preterm) human brain and risk for periventricular leukomalacia: a review. Semin Perinatol 2006;30:85; with permission.)

through the more heavily myelinated fiber, particularly between 30 and 40 weeks gestation [3,7].

Even though most of the emphasis on pathogenesis of white matter injury focuses on the extremely preterm infant, axonal synaptogenesis, maturation, and elongation occur primarily in the last half of gestation and postnatally [2,8]. Myelin-producing cells are detectable by immunohistochemistry in late gestation. Microscopic myelin, however, does not appear until 1 to 2 months postnatal age, and myelin tubes are not present until 11 to 13 months post-conceptual age [7]. Growth-associated protein -43 (GAP-43) is a marker of axonal growth and is a major phosphoprotein of neuronal growth cones in the developing brain. This protein continues to be expressed in high levels in the late preterm infant and persists for an additional 24 weeks postnatally during the period of active myelination [2,5].

Cerebellum development

There are limited data about the relationship between cerebellar development and function on overall neurodevelopmental outcome in the preterm infant [9]. Preterm infants often display an array of abnormal neurologic findings that could be attributed to cerebellar injury, including difficulty with fine motor control, coordination, and motor sequencing [9,10–12]. In addition, recent studies indicate that the cerebellum is also important in no-motor functions, including cognition, language, and social function [13]. The cerebellum is similarly in a very active phase of growth and development during the last trimester of pregnancy. Limperopoulos and colleagues examined MRI scans of infants at various gestational ages to determine the incidence of cerebellar abnormalities and to calculate changes in cerebellar volume with increasing gestational age [9]. Cerebellar volumes increased an average of 1.57 mL/wk postconceptual age in infants who had normal MRI findings compared with an increase of 1.46 mL/wk postconceptual age in those who had abnormal MRI findings ($P < .001$, r = 0.90). Furthermore, the volume of the cerebellum constitutes a larger relative percentage of the total brain volume as gestation increases. At 28 weeks, the cerebellum is approximately 4.5% of the total brain volume, with a linear increase up to 7.1% of the total brain volume by 42 weeks gestation. The mean cerebellar volume in the late preterm infant is only 5.5% of the volume at the end of gestation, suggesting that approximately 25% of the cerebellar volume will develop after late preterm birth (Fig. 4). In addition, mean cerebellar volumes were significantly lower in infants who had abnormal MRI findings and correlated with intracranial and total brain volumes. Data from previous studies have shown that the preterm infant is more likely to have decreased brain volumes with increasing age, particularly when there has been brain injury. Therefore, even though there are not specific data on cerebellar development from these studies, one could speculate that the cerebellar volumes would likely be decreased in these infants also. These authors

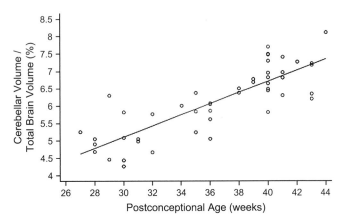

Fig. 4. Changes in cerebellar volume with increasing gestational age. (*From* Limperopoulos C, Soul JS, Gauvreau K, et al. Late gestation cerebellar growth is rapid and impeded by premature birth. Pediatrics 2005;115:688–95; with permission.)

documented impaired cerebellar growth in the preterm infant compared with those born at term, suggesting that cerebellar development is impeded by preterm delivery even in the child without MRI abnormalities. Cerebellar growth restriction is magnified further in those children who have associated CNS abnormalities [9].

Late gestation represents a period of proliferation and migration of the cerebellar granule cells. Injury to these cells will impact subsequent growth and development of cerebellar tissues. Similar to other regions in the CNS, cerebellar autoregulation is impaired in the preterm infant possibly related to border zone perfusion between the posterior inferior and inferior cerebellar arteries. Previous neuropathologic studies have shown an increased incidence of necrotic lesions in the cerebellum in preterm infants [14,15]. Preterm infants showed altered and impaired cerebellar growth even in the absence of structural abnormalities by MRI [14,16]. Others have described cerebellar atrophy in preterm infants with a history of PVL [16]. Functional connections between neural pathways linking cortical areas and the cerebellum may be disrupted by cerebellar injury. The immature cerebellum is dependent on input from trans-synaptic excitatory pathways from the cortex for normal growth and development of the cerebellum. Careful investigation for evidence of cerebellar injury in the preterm infant will be important in the evaluation of long term neurodevelopmental outcome. Since the cerebellum of the late preterm infant will exhibit a 25% increase in growth and development after delivery, it is clear that these late preterm infants are vulnerable to cerebellar injury and subsequent associated neurologic sequelae. Further research is indicated to determine to what extent cerebellar injury contributes to cognitive, motor, and behavioral difficulties in the late preterm population.

Brain injury and the late preterm infant

The major neuropathologic complications associated with poor long-term ND outcome are severe IVH and PVL. The relative risk for IVH and PVL decreases with increasing gestational age; however, late preterm infants are at risk for various other neonatal complications that may also be associated with an increased risk of brain injury and subsequent abnormal neurodevelopmental outcome. Additionally, recent data suggest that these infants may be at risk for early learning difficulties, suggesting injury to other cortical tissues [17].

Intraventricular hemorrhage and the late preterm infant

The incidence of IVH is related inversely to gestational age. As the developing CNS tissues mature, the risk for hemorrhage decreases exponentially. Typically, IVH in the preterm infant originates from the thin-walled endothelial cells within the subependymal germinal matrix. It is also important to recall that the germinal matrix is also the site of origin for cerebral and glial precursor cells; therefore injury to these tissues may contribute to abnormal and altered neuronal development. The germinal matrix undergoes continuous involution with increasing gestation and is almost completely involuted by 36 weeks gestation [8]. The surrounding tissues develop a more stable network as the fetus approaches term. Therefore, the late preterm infant is at significantly lower risk for intraventricular hemorrhage when compared with infants born less than 34 weeks gestation. In fact, in the absence of clinical symptoms, many neonatologists do not routinely perform cranial sonograms on preterm infants greater than 34 weeks gestation. Some speculate that the late preterm infant who develops an IVH may have sustained a more severe insult, given that the intrinsic risk should be decreased based on their maturity.

Periventricular leukomalacia and the late preterm infant

PVL affects approximately 3% to 4% of preterm infants weighing less than 1500 g; however, the incidence in the late preterm population is unknown. PVL is a known predictor of adverse neurologic outcome, including cerebral palsy and cognitive delays [6,8]. The late preterm infant is also at risk for white matter injury through multiple potential mechanisms, including: developmental vulnerability of the oligodendrocyte, glutamate-induced injury, cytokine and free radial-mediated injury, and a developmental lack of antioxidant enzymes to help regulate oxidative stress [2,6,18,19]. The circumstances leading to preterm delivery may also impact the risk for brain injury. Neonatal infection and chorioamnionitis have both been associated with white matter injury and adverse neurodevelopmental outcome and are seen not infrequently in the late preterm infant [6,8,25]. White matter injury may disrupt the development of other CNS tissues and fibers remote from the original site of injury.

Serial imaging of the preterm infant provides a surrogate for evaluating normal development of the brain at various gestational ages. In addition to gross evaluation of the brain, apparent diffusion coefficient (ADC) and relative anisotropy (RA) are measures to help define water diffusion and integrity of CNS structures. The ADC is the spatially averaged magnitude of water diffusion [20]. Relative anisotropy is a measure of preferred directionality of diffusion, and it increases in the presence of high ordered structures, such as myelinated axons [20]. Huppi and colleagues performed MRI studies after birth and then repeated the studies with diffusion tensor imaging at age-adjusted term gestation [21]. There was no difference in the ADC between infants with and without white matter injury; however, there was decreased diffusion in the densely packed tissues of the internal capsule in both groups. In contrast, infants who had evidence of white matter injury on the original MRI had significantly lower RA values at the original site of injury and the internal capsule, which is consistent with disruption of neural elements. They also noted a particular decrease in fibers in the posterior limb of the internal capsule that receives descending corticospinal tracks that travel from the central white matter. In infants with white matter injury, diffusion vector maps show altered size, density, orientation, and organization in both the central white matter and descending fibers. These findings are supported further by diffusion vector maps that show altered size, density, orientation, and organization of fiber tracts, both from the central white matter and descending fibers in infants with white matter injury. These findings suggest that white matter injury resulted in alteration of microstructural development of the central white matter and its descending fibers [21]. Neil and colleagues also reported that the ADC decreases with increasing gestational age in the gray and white matter in infants without evidence of white matter injury [22,23]. More importantly, they found that the increase in relative anisotropy occurs almost entirely at term, rather than a linear increase with increasing age, which is consistent with the biochemical data suggesting that the majority of myelination occurs during the last 6 weeks of gestation [20,23]. Infants who had white matter injury did not show the characteristic decrease in ADC or RA with increasing age, unlike normal infants [20]. Other studies have shown that preterm infants who sustain perinatal white matter injury have reduced volumes of gray matter and myelinated white matter at term gestation [24].

A major neuropathologic sequela of PVL is injury to the adjacent neural subplate, because this region has a critical role in cortical organization and neuronal networking. Disruption of these pathways may be responsible for the difficulty affected children often have with higher cognitive functioning and processing.

Kernicterus and associated neurodevelopmental outcome in the late preterm infant

Over recent years, it has become evident that guidelines for managing hyperbilirubinemia in term infants cannot be extrapolated safely to the late preterm population. Late preterm infants have a disproportionate risk of developing significant hyperbilirubinemia and an increased risk for long-term sequelae compared with term infants [26–31]. This most likely is secondary to a combination of factors, including immaturity of conjugation and enzymatic pathways, immature feeding patterns, and the age-dependent susceptibility of developing neurons and astrocytes to bilirubin-induced injury. With judicious management and care, most clinicians consider kernicterus to be a preventable disease; however, it continues to contribute to risk for adverse long-term ND outcome in the late preterm infant.

Neuropathology

Kernicterus is the term used to describe the neuropathologic changes associated with bilirubin-induced brain injury. Gross and microscopic examination of an affected brain shows yellow staining in multiple areas, including the basal ganglia (particularly the globus pallidus and subthalamic nucleus) and brainstem, oculomotor and vestibular nuclei [32]. Clinical manifestations correlate to these areas of brain injury as outlined in Box 1.

Acute bilirubin encephalopathy is defined by the presence of decreased feeding, lethargy, variable but abnormal tone, high-pitched cry, opisthotonus, fever, irritability, seizures, and death [8,32]. Affected infants also may have an abnormal auditory brainstem response (ABR) and acute abnormalities on MRI in the globus pallidus and subthalamic nucleus [32]. Chronic bilirubin encephalopathy is characterized by at least two or more of the following features:

- Movement disorder, including athetosis and dystonia with spasticity and hypotonia
- Hearing impairment
- Oculomotor abnormalities, including paralysis of upward gaze, lateral gaze and strabismus
- Dental enamel hypoplasia of the deciduous teeth [33]

Some studies have shown that the symptoms associated with acute toxicity may be reversible [31,32].

Elevated levels of unconjugated bilirubin are toxic to astrocytes and neurons, resulting in increased cell death, increased release of extracellular glutamate, and increased release of proinflammatory cytokines tumor necrosis factor α (TNF-α) and interleukin (IL)-1β and suppression of IL-6 [34–38]. This age-dependent susceptibility to bilirubin-induced neurotoxicity is enhanced in the presence of inflammation/infection [39]. These findings may,

---

Box 1. Clinical sequelae associated with kernicterus

Basal Ganglia
Abnormality of movement
Dystonia
Athetosis
Spasticity

Auditory Nuclei
Deafness
Hearing Impairment
Auditory Neuropathy

Brainstem Nuclei
Strabismus
Paralysis of Upward Gaze
Paralysis of Lateral Gaze
Apnea/regulation of breathing
Dental enamel hypoplasia of deciduous teeth

Data from Volpe JJ. Neurology of the Newborn. 4th edition. Philadelphia: W.B. Saunders; 2001.

---

in part, explain the apparent increased susceptibility of preterm infants to bilirubin toxicity with and without infection.

The blood–brain barrier slows the equilibrium of bilirubin between plasma and the brain. The duration and time of exposure to free bilirubin may be a critical determinant to the risk of toxicity. Wennberg proposed that this exposure time factor is critical and complicates interpretation of most ND outcome studies, which tend to examine only peak bilirubin levels [38].

Incidence of kernicterus in late preterm infants

The incidence of kernicterus in the late preterm population in unknown; however, it is clear that compared with term infants, late preterm infants are at increased risk for bilirubin neurotoxicity and kernicterus [26,28]. Some authors have reported a two- to fivefold increased risk of developing significant hyperbilirubinemia in late preterm infants compared with their term infant counterparts [26,28,31]. In a recent review by Sarici and colleagues, total serum bilirubin (TSB) levels were checked at 6 hours and then daily for 4 to 7 days. Interestingly, TSB values were not significantly different until days 5 to 7, when the near-term infant was more likely to have a higher level [28]. Careful attention should be paid to the later peak in bilirubin levels in the late preterm population, because this also will impact the needed duration of follow-up in this subgroup of patients. Hour-specific and gestational age-specific nomograms have been developed to help project the trajectory of rising bilirubin levels and predict which infants are likely to have bilirubin levels that rise to an unsafe range [27,28,39]. Other associated risk factors for development of severe hyperbilirubinemia also have been defined, and they should be considered in the predischarge assessment. The late preterm infant may have immature feeding patterns and poor suck–swallow coordination. This results in an increased risk for inadequate feeding, resulting in increased risk for hyperbilirubinemia and dehydration. In fact, data from the Pilot Kernicterus Registry reports that 30% of patients with kernicterus also had clinical evidence of dehydration as reflected by excessive weight loss and hypernatremia [26]. Feeding-related issues and hyperbilirubinemia are the most common causes for readmission within the first week of life, highlighting the importance of documenting an adequate feeding history, particularly in the late preterm infant [40]. Infants with sepsis may have an even lower threshold for kernicterus, which is consistent with animal and tissue culture data [38].

The 1994 AAP practice guidelines recommending a "kinder and gentler" approach to bilirubin management have been revised secondary to reports of an increased incidence of kernicterus, particularly in the late preterm infant. The new guidelines combine recommendations for bilirubin management and special emphasis on the predischarge assessment and postdischarge followup. There are specific recommendations for the evaluation and management of hyperbilirubinemia in the late preterm infant including a risk-based nomogram that is adjusted for prematurity. Furthermore, other associated risk factors such as genetics, albumin binding, postnatal age, integrity of the blood–brain barrier, and evidence of infection must be considered in the overall risk assessment of bilirubin levels.

Current AAP guidelines recommend initiation of phototherapy based on postconceptual age and TSB levels. Exchange transfusion is recommended if the infant has clinical evidence of acute bilirubin encephalopathy, or if the level is ever greater than 25 mg/dL; however exchange transfusion may be warranted at lower levels [27]. Data from the Kernicterus Registry, however, suggest that this threshold may be too high for the late preterm infant. In this cohort of infants, late preterm infants with total serum bilirubin levels greater than 25 mg/dL at the time of readmission were more likely to have severe neurologic sequelae compared with term infants (82.7% versus 70.8%, $P < .01$) [26]. Eight percent of term infants had no or mild sequelae compared with 3.45% of late preterm infants. In addition, evidence of neurotoxicity was noted at an earlier postnatal age in late preterm infants compared with term infants.

The resurgence in the incidence of kernicterus has allowed clinicians an opportunity to reevaluate parameters for safe discharge of the late preterm infant. Hospitals are encouraged to develop clinical pathways for routine care of all newborn infants which includes an assessment of feeding adequacy, documentation of hydration status, and routine pre-discharge bilirubin screening. Careful attention to any evidence of jaundice and inter-pretation of bilirubin levels based on a risk adjustment for known contrib-utors are critical components of the discharge process, particularly for the late preterm infant who is more likely to have difficulty in each of these areas. This additional information will help the clinican evaluate readiness for discharge and also more appropriately advise parents about optimal tim-ing of medical followup postdischarge.

Neurodevelopmental outcome associated with kernicterus in the late preterm infant

Though the literature is not exhaustive, some data are available regarding the long-term neurodevelopmental outcome of late preterm infants with moderate-to-severe hyperbilirubinemia. In addition to the major neurologic sequelae associated with kernicterus, many clinicians fear that these children are at higher risk for mild cognitive and motor impairment and behavior problems.

Several small studies suggested that infants with moderately elevated levels of hyperbilirubinemia were at risk for abnormal neurologic outcome. Soorani-Lunsing and colleagues reported an increased incidence of minor neurological findings at 3 to 12 months of age in a small cohort of infants with bilirubin levels no more than 26 mg/dL [41]. Similarly, Harris reported the ND outcome of six infants with TSB greater than 25 mg/dL with acute signs of encephalopathy from a single center [42]. Three out of four infants had abnormal initial MRI findings with increased signal in the basal ganglia. Two children had abnormal ABR during the acute event; however, only one infant had hearing impairment at follow-up. There was resolution of the abnormal neurologic findings in all but one infant. One infant in this small cohort had cerebral palsy and severe developmental delay [42].

In contrast, two major studies with longer ND follow-up showed no sig-nificant differences in developmental performance among infants with mod-erately elevated bilirubin levels, suggesting that the early abnormal findings resolve over time and with aggressive intervention [31,43].

Newman and colleagues recently performed a case–control study com-paring the neurologic outcome of 140 term and near-term infants with mod-erately elevated bilirubin levels from a community-based hospital with unaffected control infants at 2 or more years of age [31]. Most affected in-fants had peak bilirubin levels between 25 and 29 mg/dL (n = 130), and 10 infants had levels of at least 30 mg/dL. Consistent with previous findings, infants in the hyperbilirubinemia group were more likely to be less than 38 weeks gestation and were more likely to have been exclusively breast fed. The peak bilirubin levels in this cohort occurred between 3 and 7 days of life. Trained examiners administered the Wechsler Preschool and Primary Scale of Intelligence-Revised and the Beery-Buktenica Developmental Test of Visual-Motor Integration, 4th edition at 5 years of age. Parents who refused formal testing were asked to complete the Child Behavior Checklist questionnaire and the Parent Evaluation of Developmental Status questionnaire. These investigators found no significant differences in developmental testing scores between the two study groups (Table 1). Interestingly, neither the severity or duration of hyperbilirubinemia or gestational age had a significant effect on ND outcome in the hyperbilirubinemia subgroup. The authors also noted that infants with positive direct antibody testing and evidence of hemolysis and a bilirubin level of at least 25 mg/dL, and they were more likely to have lower IQ scores. This information must be evaluated with caution, however, because of the small number of infants in this subgroup. The Collaborative Perinatal Project reported outcomes at 7 years of age among 52 infants with TSB levels of at least 25 mg/dL compared to

Table 1

Results of testing with the Wechsler Preschool and Primary Scale of Intelligence–Revised (WPPSI-R) Test and the Beery–Buktenica Developmental Test of Visual-Motor Integration, 4th edition (VMI-4)

Test	Control group	Hyperbilirubinemia group	Adjusted difference (95% CI)[a]	P value
WPPSI-R[b]				
Verbal IQ				0.18
No. of subjects	162	81		
Mean score	101.1	103.5	2.5 (−1.1 to 6.1)	
Performance IQ				0.29
No. of subjects	165	81		
Mean score	106.0	107.0	0.5 (−2.9 to 4.0)	
Full scale IQ				0.42
No. of subjects	162	81		
Mean score	104.0	105.9	1.4 (−2.1 to 5.0)	
VMI-4[c]				
Visual-motor integration				0.74
No. of subjects	165	81		
Mean socre	102.1	103.3	0.6 (−2.8 to 3.9)	
Visual perception				0.60
No. of subjects	164	80		
Mean score	105.9	107.5	1.2 (−3.5 to 6.0)	
Motor coordination				0.54
No. of subjects	165	81		
Mean score	100.4	101.3	−1.3 (−5.6 to 2.9)	

[a] Adjusted differences were calculated with the use of multiple linear regression analysis. The models varied, but most models included paternal race or ethnic group and level of education. CI denotes confidence interval.

[b] Scores on the WPPSI-R test are distributed with a mean of 100 and an SD of 15. Scores in this study ranged from 46 to 149.

[c] Scores on the VMI-4 are distributed with a mean of 100 and an SD of 15. Scores in this study ranged from 45 to 150.

Data from Newman TB, Liljestrand P, Jeremy RJ, et al. Outcomes among newborns with total serum bilirubin levels of 25 mg per deciliter or more. N Eng J Med 2006;354:1896.

normal term control infants [43]. Investigators found no difference in developmental quotients between the two groups; however infants with levels greater than 20 mg/dL were more likely to have suspicious or abnormal findings on neurological examination. Fig. 5 summarizes the ND outcome of infants with moderate to severe hyperbilirubinemia from the major published studies. These findings highlight the low specificity of TSB in identifying those infants at risk for developing neurologic sequelae.

Hearing impairment

The brainstem auditory nuclei appear most vulnerable to bilirubin-induced injury. Permanent neurosensory hearing loss may be the only clinical manifestation of kernicterus in some infants. Alterations in ABR results have been reported at serum bilirubin levels less than 20 mg/dL. As the levels increase, the tracing changes from increased interwave intervals to decreased amplitude and eventual loss of wave III and IV. Changes in wave I may be seen in more severely affected infants. ABR changes may reverse or improve after phototherapy or exchange transfusion; however, this may take several months to normalize [44]. Premature and late preterm infants may be particularly vulnerable to bilirubin-induced damage to hearing [32].

Chisin and colleagues described a unique pattern of hearing loss in children associated with hyperbilirubinemia in 1979, which had the same findings as those in the more recently described syndrome of auditory neuropathy/auditory dyssynchrony (AN/AD) [45,46]. This syndrome is characterized by absent or abnormal ABR response, normal otoacoustic

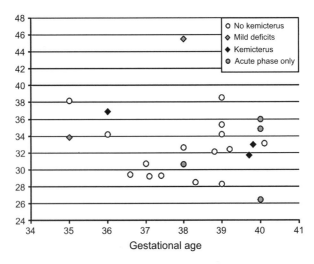

Fig. 5. Outcome of newborns readmitted with severe hyperbilirubinemia. (*From* Wennberg RP, Ahlfors CE, Bhutani VK, et al. Toward understanding kernicterus: a challenge to improve the management of jaundiced newborns. Pediatrics 2006;117:479; with permission.)

Table 2
School-age outcomes of healthy near term infants (34 to 37 weeks) versus healthy term infants(38 to 42 weeks)

Outcome	Age (years)	% Near term (n=22552)	% Full term (n=164,628)	Relative risk (95% CI) adjusted
Development delay/disability	0–3	4.8	3.2	1.46 (1.42–1.50)
PreK at 3[a]	3	4.8	4.0	1.18 (1.14–1.21)
PreK at4[a]	4	7.7	6.6	1.15 (1.13–1.18)
Not ready to start school	4	4.7	4.1	1.09 (1.05–1.12)
Special education	5	13.6	11.8	1.13 (1.11–1.15)
Retention	5	7.6	6.2	1.11 (1.08–1.14)
Suspension	5	1.4	1.2	0.97 (0.91–1.04)

[a] Referral to Flordia's Part B program, Prekindergarten for Children with Disabilities.
Data from Morse SB, Tang Y, Roth J. Abstract 4355. Pediatr Res 2006;1(Suppl):158.

emissions, normal cochlear microphonic response, and variable degrees of hearing impairment. The children have difficulty with language acquisition in the absence of significant hearing loss and often present with language delays, behavior problems, and learning disability [47–49]. Approximately 50% of patients diagnosed with AN/AD have a history of prematurity or hyperbilirubinemia (Fig. 2).

School-age neurodevelopmental outcome of late preterm infants

As the population of near-term infants continues to increase, clinicians are more carefully evaluating their short- and long-term morbidity, including neurodevelopmental outcome. In general, there is a paucity of published data on the ND outcome in this population. Morse and colleagues recently reported data from preschool readiness testing in Florida [17]. They evaluated results from standardized evaluations of over 22,000 near-term infants compared with 164,628 term infants. Late preterm infants were more likely to have a diagnosis of developmental delay within the first 3 years of life. These infants are more likely to be referred for special needs preschool resources. They are also more likely to have problems with school readiness (Table 2). This is a very important clinical observation due to the major economic impact that it will have on the educational system in order to provide additional educational services for this growing population of late preterm children.

Summary

Improved understanding of human brain development has elucidated a clearer understanding of the maturation-dependent vulnerability of the late preterm brain. A significant proportion of development in the cortical gray matter, white matter, and cerebellum occurs during the last 6 weeks of gestation. It is critically important to define the causes of brain injury to guide development of neuroprotective strategies for the late preterm infant. Data recently presently by McCormick and colleagues indicates the heavier low birth weight infants (birth weight 2001 to 2499 g) who received early intervention had sustained benefit in educational performance in early adulthood in contrast to the smaller low birth weight infants [50]. This suggests that the late preterm infant with neurologic injury may derive greater benefit from therapeutic interventions. This further highlights the importance of understanding the inherent risk to this subgroup of patients and designing appropriate interventions for prevention and treatment. The rapidly increasing number of infants born between 34 and 37 weeks gestation highlights the magnitude of the economic impact on community resources and the educational system if these infants are indeed found to have increased risk for brain injury and adverse neurodevelopmental outcome.

References

[1] Guihard-Costa AM, Larroche JC. Differential growth between the fetal brain and its infratentorial part. Early Hum Dev 1990;23:27–40.
[2] Kinney HC. The near-term (late preterm) human brain and risk for periventricular leukomalacia: a review. Semin Perinatol 2006;30:81–8.
[3] Huppi PS, Warfield S, Kikinis R, et al. Quantitative magnetic resonance imaging of brain development in premature and mature newborns. Ann Neurol 1998;43:224–35.
[4] Samuelsen GB, Larsen KB, Bogdanovic N, et al. The changing number of cells in the human fetal forebrain and its subdivisions: a sterological analysis. Cereb Cortex 2003;13:115–22.
[5] Haynes RL, Borenstein NS, Desilva TM, et al. Axonal development in the cerebral white matter of the human fetus and infant. J Comp Neurol 2005;484:156–67.
[6] Rezaie P, Dean A. Periventricular leukomalacia, inflammation and white matter lesions within the developing nervous system. Neuropathology 2002;22:106–32.
[7] Back SA, Luo NL, Borenstein NS, et al. Late oligodendrocyte progenitors coincide with the developmental window of vulnerability for human perinatal white matter injury. J Neurosci 2001;15:1302–12.
[8] Volpe JJ. Neurology of the newborn. 4th edition. Philadelphia: WB Saunders; 2001.
[9] Limperopoulos C, Soul JS, Gauvreau K, et al. Late gestation cerebellar growth is rapid and impeded by premature birth. Pediatrics 2005;111:688–95.
[10] Goyen TA, Lui K, Woods R. Visual–motor, visual–perceptual, and fine motor outcomes in very low birth weight children at 5 years. Dev Med Child Neurol 1998;40:76–81.
[11] Allin M, Matsumoto H, Santhouse AM, et al. Cognitive and motor function and the size of the cerebellum in adolescents born very prematurely. Brain 2001;124:60–6.
[12] Aylward GP. Cognitive and neuropsychological outcomes: more than IQ scores. Ment Retard Dev Disabil Res Rev 2002;8:234–40.
[13] Hadders-Algra M, Huisjes JH, Touwen BC. Perinatal risk factors and minor neurological dysfunction: significance for behavior and school achievement at nine years. Dev Med Child Neurol 1988;30:482–91.
[14] Grunnet ML, Shilds WD. Cerebellar hemorrhage in the premature infant. J Pediatr 1976;88:605–8.
[15] Armstrong DL, Hay M, Terrian DM. Modulation of cerebellar granule cell activity by iontophoretic application of serotonergic agents. Brain Res Bull 1987;19:699–704.

[16] Argyropoulou MI, Xydis V, Drougia A, et al. MRI measurements of the pons and cerebellum in children born preterm; associations with the severity of periventricular leukomalacia and perinatal risk factors. Neuroradiology 2003;45:730–4.

[17] Morse SB, Tang Y, Roth J. Abstract 4355. Pediatric Research Supplement 2006;158.

[18] Folkerth RD, Haynes RL, Borenstein NS, et al. Developmental lag in superoxide dismutases relative to other antioxidant enzymes in premyelinated human telencephalic white matter. J Neuropathol Exp Neurol 2004;63:990–9.

[19] Haynes RL, Borenstein N, Desilva TM, Folkerth RD, Liu LG, Volpe JJ. Developmental lag of superoxide dismutases relative to another antioxidant enzymes in premyelinated human telenccephalic white matter. J Neuropathol Exp Neurol 2004;14:265–74.

[20] Miller SP, Vigneron DB, Henry RG, et al. Serial quantitative diffusion tensor MRI of the premature brain: Development in newborns with and without injury. J Magn Reson Imaging 2002;16:621–32.

[21] Huppi PS, Murphy B, Maier SE, et al. Microstructural brain Development after perinatal cerebral white matter injury assessed by diffusion tensor magnetic resonance imaging. Pediatrics 2001;107:455–60.

[22] Neil J, Miller J, Mukherjee P, et al. Diffusion tensor imaging of normal and injured developing human brain—a technical review. NMR Biomed 2002;15:543–52.

[23] Neil JJ, Shiran SI, McKinstry RC, et al. Normal brain in human newborns: apparent diffusion coefficient and diffusion anisotropy measured by using diffusion tensor MR imaging. Radiology 1998;209:57–66.

[24] Inder TE, Huppi PS, Warfield S, et al. Periventricular white matter injury in the premature infant is followed by reduced cerebral cortical gray matter volume at term. Ann Neurol 1999; 46:755–60.

[25] Adams-Chapman I, Stoll BJ. Neonatal infection and long term neurodevelopmental outcome in the preterm. Curr Opin Infect Dis 2006;19:290–7.

[26] Bhutani VK, Johnson L. Kernicterus in late preterm infants cared for as term healthy infants. Semin Perinatol 2006;30:89–97.

[27] Maisels MJ, Baltz RD, Bhutani VK, et al. Management of hyperbilirubinemia in the newborn infant 35 or more weeks of gestation. Pediatrics 2004;114:297–316.

[28] Sarici SU, Serdar MA, Korkmaz A, et al. Incidence, course and prediction of hyperbilirubinemia in near-term and term newborns. Pediatrics 2004;113:775–80.

[29] Newman TB, Xiong B, Gonzales VM, et al. Prediction and prevention of extreme neonatal hyperbilirubinemia in a mature health maintenance organization. Arch Pediatr Adolesc Med 2000;154:1140–7.

[30] Newman TB, Liljestrand P, Escobar GJ. Infants with bilirubin levels of 30 mg/dL or more in a large managed care organization. Pediatrics 2003;111:1303–11.

[31] Newman TB, Liljestrand P, Jeremy RJ, et al. Outcomes among newborns with total serum bilirubin levels of 25 mg per deciliter or more. N Engl J Med 2006;354:1889–900.

[32] Shapiro SM. Definition of the clinical spectrum of kernicterus and bilirubin-induced neurologic dysfunction (BIND). J Perinatol 2005;25:54–9.

[33] Perlstein M. Neurologic sequelae of erythroblastosis fetalis. Am J Dis Child 1950;79: 605–6.

[34] Fernandes A, Silva RFM, Falcao AS, et al. Cytokine production, glutamate release and cell death in rat cultures astrocytes with unconjugated bilirubin and LPS. J Neuroimmunol 2004; 153:64–75.

[35] Wennberg RP, Hance AJ. Experimental bilirubin encephalopathy: importance of total bilirubin, protein binding and blood-brain-barrier. Pediatr Res 1986;20:789–92.

[36] Wennberg RP. Animal models of bilirubin encephalopathy. Adv Vet Sci Comp Med 1993; 37:87–113.

[37] Wennberg RP, Ahlfors CE, Bhutani VK, et al. Toward Understanding Kernicterus: A challenge to improve the management of jaundiced newborns. Pediatrics 2006;117: 474–85.

[38] Falcao AS, Fernandes A, Brito MA, et al. Bilirubin-induced inflammatory response, gluta-mate release, and cell death in rat cortical astrocytes are enhanced in younger cells. Neuro-biol Dis 2005;20:199–206.

[39] Bhutani VK, Johnson L, Sivieri EM. Predictive ability of a predischarge hour-specific serum bilirubin for subsequent significant hyperbilirubinemia in healthy term and near term new-borns. Pediatrics 1999;103:6–14.

[40] Brown AK, Damus K, Kim MH, et al. Factors relating to readmission of term and near-term neonates in the first two weeks of life. Early Discharge Survey Group of the Health Profes-sional Advisory Board of the Greater New York Chapter of the March of Dimes. J Perinat Med 1999;27:263–75.

[41] Soorani-Lunsing I, Woltil HA, Hadders-Algra M. Are moderate degrees of hyperbilirubine-mia in healthy term neonates really safe for the brain? Pediatr Res 2001;50:701–5.

[42] Harris MC, Bernbaum JC, Polin JR, et al. Developmental follow-up of breastfed term and near term infants with marked hyperbilirubinemia. Pediatrics 2001;107:1075–80.

[43] Newman TB, Klebanoff M. 33,272 Infants, 7-year follow-up: total serum bilirubin, transfu-sion reexamined. Pediatrics 2002;110:1032.

[44] Gupta AK, Mann SB. Is auditory brainstem response a bilirubin toxicity marker? Am J Oto-laryngol 1998;19:232–6.

[45] Chisin R, Perlman M, Sohmer H. Cochlear and brain stem responses in hearing loss follow-ing neonatal hyperbilirubinemia. Ann Otol Rhinol Laryngol 1979;88:352 [Check page numbers.].

[46] Starr A, Picton TW, Sininger Y, et al. Auditory neuropathy. Brain 1996;119:741–53.

[47] Berlin CI, Hood L, Morlet T, et al. Auditory neuropathy/dys-synchrony: diagnosis and man-agement. Ment Retard Dev Disabili Res Rev 2003;9:225–31.

[48] Rance G, Beer DE, Cone-Wesson B, et al. Clinical findings for group of infants and young children with auditory neuropathy. Ear Hear 1999;20:238–52.

[49] Sininger Y. Overview of auditory neuropathy. Audiology Online. Available at: http://www.audiologyonline.com.

[50] McCormick MC, Brooks-Gunn J, Buka SL, et al. Early intervention in low birth weigh pre-mature infants: results at 18 years of age for the Infant Health and Development Program. Pediatrics 2006;117:771–80.

ELSEVIER
SAUNDERS

Clin Perinatol 33 (2006) 965–972

CLINICS IN
PERINATOLOGY

Index

Note: Page numbers of article titles are in **boldface** type.

0095-5108/06/$ - see front matter © 2006 Elsevier Inc. All rights reserved.
doi:10.1016/S0095-5108(06)00101-1